Perioperative Pharmacotherapy

Guest Editor

ALAN D. KAYE, MD, PhD

ANESTHESIOLOGY CLINICS

www.anesthesiology.theclinics.com

Consulting Editor

LEE A. FLEISHER, MD, FACC

December 2010 • Volume 28 • Number 4

SAUNDERS an imprint of ELSEVIER, Inc.

W.B. SAUNDERS COMPANY
A Division of Elsevier Inc.

1600 John F. Kennedy Boulevard, Suite 1800 • Philadelphia, PA 19103-2899

http://www.theclinics.com

ANESTHESIOLOGY CLINICS Volume 28, Number 4
December 2010 ISSN 1932-2275, ISBN-13: 978-1-4557-0585-6

Editor: Rachel Glover
Developmental Editor: Jessica Demetriou

Anesthesiology Clinics (ISSN 1932-2275) is published quarterly by Elsevier Inc., 360 Park Avenue South, New York, NY 10010-1710. Months of issue are March, June, September, and December. Periodicals postage paid at New York, NY and at additional mailing offices. Subscription prices are $141.00 per year (US student/resident), $287.00 per year (US individuals), $351.00 per year (Canadian individuals), $459.00 per year (US institutions), $569.00 per year (Canadian institutions), $198.00 per year (Canadian and foreign student/resident), $398.00 per year (foreign individuals), and $569.00 per year (foreign institutions). To receive student and resident rate, orders must be accompanied by name of affiliated institution, date of term, and the *signature* of program/residency coordinator on institutions letterhead. Orders will be billed at individual rate until proof of status is received. Foreign air speed delivery is included in all *Clinics'* subscription prices. All prices are subject to change without notice. POSTMASTER: Send address changes to *Anesthesiology Clinics,* Elsevier Health Sciences Division, Subscription Customer Service, 3251 Riverport Lane, Maryland Heights, MO 63043. Customer Service (orders, claims, online, change of address): Elsevier Health Sciences Division, Subscription Customer Service, 3251 Riverport Lane, Maryland Heights, MO 63043. Tel:1-800-654-2452 (U.S. and Canada); 314-447-8871 (outside U.S. and Canada). Fax: 314-447-8029. E-mail: journalscustomerservice-usa@elsevier.com (for print support); journalsonlinesupport-usa@elsevier.com (for online support).

Reprints. For copies of 100 or more of articles in this publication, please contact the Commercial Reprints Department, Elsevier Inc., 360 Park Avenue South, New York, NY 10010-1710. Tel.: 212-633-3812; Fax: 212-462-1935; E-mail: reprints@elsevier.com.

Anesthesiology Clinics, is also published in Spanish by McGraw-Hill Inter-americana Editores S. A., P.O. Box 5-237, 06500 Mexico D. F., Mexico.

Anesthesiology Clinics, is covered in *MEDLINE/PubMed (Index Medicus), Current Contents/Clinical Medicine, Excerpta Medica, ISI/BIOMED*, and *Chemical Abstracts*.

Printed and bound by CPI Group (UK) Ltd, Croydon, CR0 4YY

Transferred to Digital Print 2011

Contributors

CONSULTING EDITOR

LEE A. FLEISHER, MD, FACC
Robert D. Dripps Professor and Chair of Anesthesiology and Critical Care, University of Pennsylvania School of Medicine, Philadelphia, Pennsylvania

GUEST EDITOR

ALAN D. KAYE, MD, PhD
Professor and Chairman, Department of Anesthesiology, Director, Pain Services, Professor, Department of Pharmacology, Louisiana State University School of Medicine, New Orleans, Louisiana

AUTHORS

AREZOU SADIGHI AKHA, MD, MS
UCLA/TORI Site Monitor, Clinical Research Unit, Jonsson Comprehensive Cancer Center, University of California, Los Angeles, California

MUHAMMAD ANWAR, MD
Department of Anesthesiology, Yale University, New Haven, Connecticut

ETHAN O. BRYSON, MD
Department of Anesthesia, Mount Sinai Medical Center, New York, New York

DOMINIC S. CAROLLO, MS, MD
Department of Anesthesiology, Ochsner Medical Center, New Orleans, Louisiana

DANIEL CHIEN, BS
Research Associate, Department of Anesthesiology, Mount Sinai School of Medicine, New York, New York

MAJ AARON M. FIELDS, MD
Staff Anesthesiologist, Wilford Hall Medical Center, Lackland Air Force Base; Associate Program Director, San Antonio Uniformed Services Health Education Consortium, Brooke Army Medical Center, Division of Anesthesia Critical Care, Fort Sam Houston, Texas

STUART A. FORMAN, MD, PhD
Associate Professor of Anesthesia, Department of Anesthesia, Critical Care and Pain Medicine, Massachusetts General Hospital, Boston, Massachusetts

CHARLES J. FOX, MD
Associate Professor of Anesthesiology, Tulane University Medical Center, New Orleans, Louisiana

JULIE A. GAYLE, MD
Assistant Professor of Clinical Anesthesiology, Department of Anesthesiology, Louisiana State University Health Sciences Center, New Orleans, Louisiana

CLIFFORD GEVIRTZ, MD, MPH
Associate Professor, Department of Anesthesiology, Louisiana State University Health Sciences Center, New Orleans, Louisiana

JONATHAN S. JAHR, MD
Professor of Clinical Anesthesiology, Department of Anesthesiology, David Geffen School of Medicine at UCLA, Ronald Reagan UCLA Medical Center, Los Angeles, California

PHILIP J. KADOWITZ, PhD
Department of Pharmacology, Tulane University Medical Center, New Orleans, Louisiana

PHILLIP L. KALARICKAL, MD, MPH
Assistant Professor of Anesthesiology, Tulane University Medical Center, New Orleans, Louisiana

ADAM M. KAYE, PharmD, FASCP, FCPhA
Associate Clinical Professor, Department of Pharmacy Practice, Thomas J. Long School of Pharmacy and Health Sciences, University of the Pacific, Stockton, California

ALAN D. KAYE, MD, PhD
Professor and Chairman, Department of Anesthesiology, Director, Pain Services, Professor, Department of Pharmacology, Louisiana State University School of Medicine, New Orleans, Louisiana

KIANUSCH KIAI, MD, MS
Clinical Associate Professor of Anesthesiology, David Geffen School of Medicine at UCLA, Ronald Reagan UCLA Medical Center, Los Angeles, California

VIVIAN K. LEE, MD
Resident, Department of Anesthesiology, David Geffen School of Medicine at UCLA, Ronald Reagan UCLA Medical Center, Los Angeles, California

ALVIN LI
College of Letters and Science, University of California, Los Angeles, California

SCOTT LIPSON, MD
Department of Anesthesia, Mount Sinai Medical Center, New York, New York

HENRY LIU, MD
Associate Professor of Anesthesiology, Director of Cardiac Anesthesia, Tulane University Medical Center, New Orleans, Louisiana

RONALD D. MILLER, MD, MS
Professor, Department of Anesthesia and Perioperative Care, University of California, San Francisco, California

CPT DAUN JOHNSON MILLIGAN, MD
Anesthesia Staff and Anesthesia Critical Care Fellow, San Antonio Uniformed Services Health Education Consortium, Brooke Army Medical Center, Division of Anesthesia Critical Care, Fort Sam Houston, Texas

VENOD NARINE, BS
Research Associate, Department of Anesthesiology, Mount Sinai School of Medicine, New York, New York

BOBBY D. NOSSAMAN, MD
Adjunct Associate Professor of Pharmacology, Department of Pharmacology, Tulane University Medical Center; Staff, Anesthesiology, Department of Anesthesiology, Ochsner Medical Center, New Orleans, Louisiana

VAUGHN E. NOSSAMAN, MS/MS
Department of Pharmacology, Tulane University Medical Center, New Orleans, Louisiana

PAMELA P. PALMER, MD, PhD
Chief Medical Officer, AcelRx Pharmaceuticals, Inc, Redwood City; Clinical Professor, Department of Anesthesia and Perioperative Care, University of California, San Francisco, California

JASON L. PARK, MD
Department of Anesthesiology, Ochsner Medical Center, New Orleans, Louisiana

USHA RAMADHYANI, MD
Department of Anesthesiology, Ochsner Medical Center, New Orleans, Louisiana

JOSEPH ROSA III, MD
Clinical Professor of Anesthesiology, David Geffen School of Medicine at UCLA, Ronald Reagan UCLA Medical Center, Los Angeles, California

COREY SCHER, MD
Professor, Department of Anesthesiology, Montefiore Medical Center, Bronx, New York

RINOO SHAH, MD
Department of Anesthesiology, Guthrie Clinic-Big Flats, Horseheads, New York

JEFFREY Y. TSAI, MS
Research Associate, Louisiana State University Health Sciences Center, New Orleans, Louisiana

NALINI VADIVELU, MD
Department of Anesthesiology, Yale University, New Haven, Connecticut

RUTH S. WATERMAN, MD
Department of Anesthesiology, Tulane University Medical Center, New Orleans, Louisiana

SHIHAI ZHANG, MD, PhD
Professor of Anesthesiology, Director of Cardiac Anesthesiology, Union Hospital of Tongji Medical College, Huazhong University of Science and Technology, Wuhan, Hubei, China

Contents

Pamela P. Palmer and Ronald D. Miller

Moderate-to-severe acute postoperative pain is commonly controlled with opioids administered via programmable intravenous (IV) patient-controlled analgesia (PCA) infusion pumps. Intravenously administered opioids provide effective relief of postoperative pain, and IV PCA enables patients to control their level of analgesia, which has advantages over nurse-administered approaches, including more satisfied patients and improved pain relief. Unfortunately, commonly used opioid analgesics can cause significant adverse effects. Furthermore, IV PCA has drawbacks, such as device programming errors, system errors, medication errors, limitations in patient mobility, and potential for IV tubing kinks, clogging, and transmission of infection. The IV route of administration is also characterized by a rapid, high peak in analgesic drug concentration followed by rapidly decreasing concentrations. Consequently, respiratory depression, excessive sedation, and inadequate pain control can occur. Furthermore, the technical assembly of an infusion pump is often complex and time-consuming. PCA modalities that incorporate superior opioid analgesics, such as sufentanil, and novel noninvasive routes of administration offer great promise for enhancing the patient and caregiver experience with the use of postoperative PCA.

Nalini Vadivelu and Muhammad Anwar

Several decades ago, the analgesic properties of buprenorphine were discovered. Its approval for the use as an agent for the treatment of opioid abuse has led to increasing numbers of patients presenting for surgery on buprenorphine. This article describes the challenges, advantages, and disadvantages of the use of buprenorphine as an analgesic for postoperative pain in patients with and without preoperative maintenance therapy.

Ethan O. Bryson, Scott Lipson, and Clifford Gevirtz

Opioid abuse is a devastating, costly, and growing problem in the United States, and one for which treatment can be complicated by barriers such as access to care and legal issues. Only 12% to 15% of the opioid-dependent population is enrolled in methadone maintenance programs.

A significant breakthrough occurred with passage of the Drug Addiction Treatment Act of 2000 (DATA 2000). For the first time in approximately 80 years, physicians could legally prescribe opioid medications for the treatment of opioid addiction. The opiate, so designated, was buprenorphine (Subutex).

Acetaminophen has unique analgesic and antipyretic properties. It is globally recommended as a first-line agent for the treatment of fever and pain due to its few contraindications. Acetaminophen lacks the significant gastrointestinal and cardiovascular side effects associated with nonsteroidal anti-inflammatory drugs and narcotics. An intravenous formulation of acetaminophen is available in Europe and is currently undergoing extensive clinical development for use in the United States. This use may have important implications for management of postoperative pain and fever. This review summarizes recent clinical trial experiences with intravenous acetaminophen for the treatment of postoperative pain and fever in adult and pediatric subjects.

Recovery from ambulatory surgical procedures can be limited by postoperative pain. Inadequate analgesia may delay or prevent patient discharge and can result in readmission. More frequently, postoperative pain produces discomfort and interrupts sleep, contributing to postoperative fatigue. The development of effective analgesic regimens for the management of postoperative pain is a priority especially in patients with impaired cardiorespiratory, hepatic, or renal function. Tramadol and tapentadol hydrochloride are novel in that their analgesic actions occur at multiple sites. Both agents are reported to be mu-opioid receptor agonists and monoamine-reuptake inhibitors. In contrast to pure opioid agonists, both drugs are believed to have lower risks of respiratory depression, tolerance, and dependence. The Food and Drug Administration has approved both drugs for the treatment of moderate-to-severe acute pain in adults. This article provides an evidence-based account of the role of tramadol and tapentadol in modern clinical practice.

With a growing number of new anticoagulant/antiplatelet agents being developed, it is likely that an increasing number of patients taking these drugs will present for surgery and other procedures. A familiarity with mechanisms of action and drug interactions helps to maintain optimal patient safety in the perioperative period. Furthermore, it is crucial for anesthesiologists to remain current on recommendations regarding discontinuation or need to continue the newer anticoagulants/antiplatelet drugs in patients presenting for surgery and/or regional anesthesia. Further studies are needed for monitoring of many of these newer agents and to identify antidotes.

Recombinant Factor VIIa in Trauma Patients Without Coagulation Disorders

Corey Scher, Venod Narine, and Daniel Chien

Recombinant activated factor VIIa (rFVIIa) has many clinical applications for patients with congenital bleeding disorders and in a variety of clinical settings. Additional studies in the future are ongoing and should provide the clinical anesthesiologist an additional option during certain bleeding states. Specific recommendations as to timing of administration and frequent monitoring of ionized calcium status are suggested at this time. Optimization of fibrinogen levels, platelet levels, pH, and body temperature will enhance efficacy of rFVIIa.

Sugammadex: Cyclodextrins, Development of Selective Binding Agents, Pharmacology, Clinical Development, and Future Directions

Arezou Sadighi Akha, Joseph Rosa III, Jonathan S. Jahr, Alvin Li, and Kianusch Kiai

Neuromuscular blocking agents are widely used in perioperative medicine to aid in endotracheal intubation, facilitate surgery, and in critical care/ emergency medicine settings. Muscle relaxants have profound clinical uses in current surgical and intensive care and emergency medical therapy. This article reviews cyclodextrins, development of selective binding agents, clinical development, and future directions of sugammadex.

Dexmedetomidine: Clinical Application as an Adjunct for Intravenous Regional Anesthesia

Usha Ramadhyani, Jason L. Park, Dominic S. Carollo, Ruth S. Waterman, and Bobby D. Nossaman

The selective α-2 adrenoceptor agonist, dexmedetomidine, has been shown to be a useful, safe adjunct in perioperative medicine. Intravenous regional anesthesia is one of the simplest forms of regional anesthesia and has a high degree of success. However, intravenous regional anesthesia is limited by the development of tourniquet pain and its inability to provide postoperative analgesia. To improve block quality, prolong postdeflation analgesia, and decrease tourniquet pain, various chemical additives have been combined with local anesthetics, although with limited success. The antinociceptive effects of α-2 adrenoceptor agonists have been shown in animals and in humans. However, less is known about the clinical effects of dexmedetomidine when coadministered with local anesthetics in patients undergoing intravenous regional anesthesia. This review examines what is currently known to improve our understanding of the properties and application of dexmedetomidine when used as an adjunct in intravenous regional anesthesia.

THE CLINICS ARE NOW AVAILABLE ONLINE!

Access your subscription at:
www.theclinics.com

Foreword:

Perioperative Pharmacotherapy

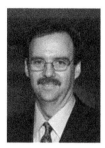

Lee A. Fleisher, MD
Consulting Editor

Anesthesiologists have always been considered the clinical pharmacologists of medicine, utilizing drugs to induce and maintain anesthesia and analgesia while also maintaining homeostasis. For many years, new and novel agents were introduced which allowed us to advance the care of our patients and surgery on more complex patients. More recently, there have been fewer such advances despite newer techniques available to create such agents. In this issue of *Anesthesiology Clinics*, a series of articles has been written to demonstrate that there remains areas in which drug discovery and development is continuing, which will allow us to continue to advance our science.

I am fortunate to have Alan David Kaye, MD, PhD, serve as Guest Editor for this issue. Dr Kaye is currently Professor and Chair of Anesthesiology at LSU School of Medicine. In addition to receiving his MD from the University of Arizona, he received a PhD in Pharmacology from Tulane University and completed an Anesthesiology Residency and Interventional Pain Fellowship. He has been an active investigator and involved in editorial boards and editing textbooks. He has assembled a diverse group of authors and topics to enlighten us on current and upcoming advances in pharmacology.

Lee A. Fleisher, MD
University of Pennsylvania School of Medicine
3400 Spruce Street, Dulles 680
Philadelphia, PA 19104, USA

E-mail address:
fleishel@uphs.upenn.edu

Anesthesiology Clin 28 (2010) xiii
doi:10.1016/j.anclin.2010.09.002
1932-2275/10/$ — see front matter © 2010 Elsevier Inc. All rights reserved.

anesthesiology.theclinics.com

Preface:

Drugs—How They Improve Our Lives and Our Patients' Lives

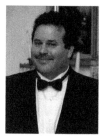

Alan D. Kaye, MD, PhD
Guest Editor

In many academic articles that I have read and written, drugs are described in very abstract and theoretical ways. These drugs might possess novel mechanisms or improved duration of activity. These agents might be less toxic or possess reduced side effects. Clearly, drugs dramatically affect our life spans, as well as our quality of life. For many years as a PhD researcher with a pulmonary vascular laboratory, I looked at them narrowly and impersonally. As the years have gone by, I have a much greater appreciation for their wonders.

I lead a relatively healthy life, and my first critical experience came during my wife's first pregnancy. At 20 weeks, my son Aaron was about to be delivered too soon; my wife's uterus 100% effaced, and his mortality was hanging in the balance. An infusion of terbutaline, the Beta 2 selective smooth muscle relaxant, resulted in uterine relaxation and a perfectly healthy child. He is now a top athlete and student filling out his college applications. Another critical experience occurred during my sixth year as Chairman of Anesthesia at Texas Tech Health Sciences Center in Lubbock. It was 2005; my strength and energy suddenly vanished. Life, vigor, and productivity returned with a thyroid supplement for my newly diagnosed hypothyroidism.

It was not long ago that our life spans were much shorter. Tens of thousands of people died due to plague, an organism easily treated with sulfonamides. Dysentery was the single greatest cause of death of Confederate and Union soldiers during our epic Civil War. Some of our greatest figures in history had shortened lives related to what we would consider treatable states. George Washington probably died of acute bacterial epiglottis. The poet Lord Byron died prematurely from an epileptic seizure. Harry Houdini probably died from acute appendicitis. Arthur Ashe died, in part, from transmission of the human immune deficiency virus.

Anesthesiology Clin 28 (2010) xv–xvii
doi:10.1016/j.anclin.2010.08.012
1932-2275/10/$ – see front matter © 2010 Elsevier Inc. All rights reserved.

anesthesiology.theclinics.com

Principally during the last fifty years, we have increased our understanding of disease states, and the technology to detect these states has also grown with leaps and bounds. Drug development has resulted in an increasing longevity and quality of life. Last week I was called to a code, the patient appearing lifeless and without hope. After administration of atropine, epinephrine, sodium bicarbonate, and calcium, he was rescued and stabilized. These drug-mediated miracles are commonplace and routine in our practices.

In the last decade, we have seen complete cataloging of the human genome and an increase in drug targets from five hundred to over one thousand. No longer is it a guaranteed death sentence to have human immune deficiency virus, many types of cancers, or sepsis. There is now new hope in drug targeting for vascular atherosclerosis, cardiomyopathy, many cancers, and Alzheimer's disease. We find ourselves constantly at a new beginning with drugs, including in our fields of anesthesia and pain medicine. The first angiotensin receptor antagonists that were the principal topic of my thesis are now generic antihypertensive agents. Structural activity relationships and complex three-dimensional analyses of therapeutic targets have produced further advances. Freudenberg received a patent for a cyclodextrin structure in 1953, while, in 2010, we appreciate the role of a cyclodextrin structured agent, sugammadex, in neuromuscular drug reversal. Forty years ago, we first identified an opiate receptor. In recent years, we have made substantial increases in understanding of endogenous opiates and subgroup opioid receptors throughout the body. With these understandings, our future will see better targeting agents for acute and chronic pain states. It is an exciting time filled with hope in modern medicine and in our field. Anesthesia has never been safer thanks, in part, to drug development.

In this section on the *Anesthesia Clinics*, there are many exciting pharmacology reviews giving us a glimpse into future practice. There are five focused reviews on drugs designed and utilized in pain management and drug addiction: buprenorphine, acetaminophen, an oral sufentanil preparation, and tapentadol. These reviews are timely because so many new drugs have come to market to modulate and to better target pain and inflammation. Likewise, there has been an explosion in the use of a number of anticoagulants that modulate the coagulation cascade. The two reviews in this edition of the journal provide a clear understanding of how many of these newer agents work, discussion of the new recombinant activated factor VII (Novo7), and guidelines for these drugs in clinical anesthesia and pain practice.

Evolving understanding and clinical use of dexmetomidine, in the operating room, intensive care unit, and peripheral sites, have reshaped the way we sedate a large population of our patients. This review describes highly clinically relevant perioperative agents.

There are also reviews on pharmacological options in the management of patients with hypertension, cardiac disease, and new cardiac anesthesia agents in the operating room and intensive care unit. There is a special review on the role of statins in cardiac anesthesia, an exciting and relevant topic. Cardiovascular drug development is a topic that our own laboratory worked on for over twenty years and many of our animal findings have been translatable to humans in attempting to develop treatment protocols for these complex disease states. Also reviewed is a drug we studied over a decade ago, levosimendan, a calcium sensitizer utilized for acutely decompensated congestive heart failure and shown to reduce cardiac troponin release after cardiac surgery.

Last, we examine the future of induction and inhalation agents and structure-based modifications. This review demonstrates that our practice will continuously change as basic scientists modify existing clinically relevant compounds and develop newer generations into the future. Further, this topic is provocative and should be appealing to our readers.

History affords us lessons and clues to be better prepared for our present and future. We must remain critical about expectations regarding quality and standardization of our drugs in order to maintain appropriate bioavailability and therapeutic outcomes. We must be leaders as many people within our hospitals suddenly are finding it their business to influence our practices and decision-making. It is a golden age for drugs and we should continue to improve the quality of life on this planet. Let us all be up to the challenge.

Alan D. Kaye, MD, PhD
Departments of Anesthesiology and Pharmacology
Louisiana State University School of Medicine
1542 Tulane Avenue, Room 656
New Orleans, LA 70112, USA

E-mail address:
alankaye44@hotmail.com

Current and Developing Methods of Patient-Controlled Analgesia

Pamela P. Palmer, MD, PhD[a,b],*, Ronald D. Miller, MD, MS[b]

KEYWORDS

- Analgesia • Morphine • Opioid • Patient-controlled
- Postoperative • Sufentanil

In the past decade, numerous advances have been made in perioperative regional anesthesia techniques, which enhance the control of moderate-to-severe postoperative pain. These include long-acting epidural opioids, patient-controlled epidural analgesia, ultrasound-guided peripheral nerve infusions, catheter-delivered infusions directly into the surgical incision, and other techniques. Despite these great strides in pain management technology, intravenous (IV) patient-controlled analgesia (PCA) using opioids is the most commonly used mode of postoperative analgesia.

IV PCA has several advantages over nurse-administered approaches, such as patients being able to control their own analgesia by titrating opioid doses in small increments and patients needing to be alert enough to administer the next dose providing inherent safety.[1–8] Furthermore, compared with many regional anesthesia techniques, implementation of IV PCA is not dependent on the skill of an anesthesiologist (needed for regional catheter placement techniques).[1,5,8] However, complications of IV PCA use include dosing and ordering errors,[9] IV PCA machine programming and system errors,[9] mobility restrictions of IV administration,[1] potential for analgesic gaps due to issues with IV tubing,[10] potential for infection due to the need for venous access,[11] and opioid-related adverse events.[12] The problems with and characteristics of opioid use in IV PCA for postoperative pain management are discussed, and new PCA modalities are described. These new approaches may be equally efficacious but could be easier to use, less invasive, and less prone to error.

Financial disclosures and/or conflicts of interest: Medical writing assistance was provided by Nancy Bella, PharmD, of MedErgy and was funded by AcelRx. Dr Palmer is an employee and stockholder of AcelRx. Dr Miller is on the Clinical Advisory Board of Masimo.

[a] AcelRx Pharmaceuticals, Inc, 575 Chesapeake Drive, Redwood City, CA 94063, USA
[b] Department of Anesthesia and Perioperative Care, University of California, Box 0648, 521 Parnassus Avenue, Clinic Sci C317, San Francisco, CA 94143-0648, USA
* Corresponding author. AcelRx Pharmaceuticals, Inc, 575 Chesapeake Drive, Redwood City, CA 94063.
E-mail address: ppalmer@acelrx.com

Anesthesiology Clin 28 (2010) 587–599
doi:10.1016/j.anclin.2010.08.010   **anesthesiology.theclinics.com**
1932-2275/10/$ – see front matter © 2010 Elsevier Inc. All rights reserved.

USE OF IV PCA FOR POSTOPERATIVE ANALGESIA
Advantages of IV PCA

Opioids are valuable and powerful analgesics for the management of moderate-to-severe postoperative pain. The most commonly used opioids for IV PCA are morphine, hydromorphone, and fentanyl.[13] Typical IV PCA settings for effectively managing postoperative pain in most patients are summarized in **Table 1**.[5] Meperidine is no longer a viable option for IV PCA because of accumulation of its toxic metabolite, normeperidine, particularly in patients with renal impairment[14]; therefore, the Institute for Safe Medication Practices (ISMP)[9] recommends avoidance of meperidine for pain control and the American Pain Society (APS)[15] does not recommend using meperidine for the treatment of acute pain.

The concept behind PCA is to provide small, on-demand opioid doses that allow patients to safely titrate to their own therapeutic plasma level of opioid. The demand dose of opioid has a significant impact on the success of PCA; the typical demand dose of morphine, hydromorphone, and fentanyl used for IV PCA (see **Table 1**) is generally that which provides the optimal balance of analgesia and safety.[16]

Although less frequently used in opioid-naive patients, a constant basal rate of opioid analgesic may be administered in addition to the on-demand dose, but this approach is often problematic. Basal infusions increase the risk of respiratory depression without providing increased analgesia.[17–19] In a 2004 analysis, the incidence of respiratory depression with IV PCA alone (ranging from 0.19% to 0.29%) was less than that with IV PCA with basal infusion (ranging from 1.09% to 3.8%).[17] The increased incidence of respiratory depression with basal infusions may result from the loss of the safety associated with patient feedback during IV PCA pain management.[18] Because of these safety concerns, the APS cautions against using basal infusions except in opioid-tolerant patients.[20]

Disadvantages of IV PCA

IV PCA errors
Medication errors have been frequently reported with IV PCA. The infusion pump used to deliver IV PCA is a separately approved device that must be programmed to deliver the specific opioid ordered. Various devices exist, and different device manufacturers use different programming steps, which introduces the potential for programming errors. The ISMP[9] reports that programming errors are the most frequently reported practice-related problem with IV PCA. Programming errors can lead to oversedation, respiratory depression, death, or inadequate pain control.[8] Pumps that default to low drug-concentration settings are particularly dangerous. Specifically, if too low an analgesic concentration is entered by mistake, the pump increases the volume of infusion to compensate, resulting in an overdose.[21,22]

Table 1			
Settings for common opioids used in IV PCA			
Drug	**Demand Dose**	**Lockout Interval (min)**	**Basal Infusion Rate**[a]
Morphine	1–2 mg	5–10	≤0.5 mg/h
Hydromorphone	0.25–0.5 mg	5–10	≤0.4 mg/h
Fentanyl	10–50 µg	5–10	≤50 µg/h

[a] Basal infusions are not recommended; use only if necessary in opioid-tolerant patients.
Data from Momeni M, Crucitti M, De KM. Patient-controlled analgesia in the management of postoperative pain. Drugs 2006;66:2321–37.

To reduce errors in prescribing IV PCA, preprinted medication order sheets are often used. Smart PCAs, devices that contain computerized drug libraries and accommodate the entry of specific protocols for drug administration via bar code, may also help to avoid dosing errors by working within predefined dose limits. To avoid medication safety problems, smart PCA pumps are programmed to stop working or to alert the clinician to doses outside the limits.[1,23] A study of critically ill patients demonstrated that medication errors and preventable drug-related adverse events were detected by using smart infusion pumps.[24]

Significant errors still occur even with smart PCAs. Approximately 56,000 adverse events, including several injuries and deaths from smart PCAs, were reported to the US Food and Drug Administration (FDA) over a 5-year period (2005–2009), prompting 70 Class II infusion pump recalls (the recalled device could cause temporary or reversible adverse effects) and 14 Class I infusion pump recalls (the recalled device could cause serious injury or death).[25] The frequent incidence of adverse events associated with infusion pumps has led the FDA to launch an Infusion Pump Initiative, which establishes stricter requirements for infusion pump manufacturers, assist with improving infusion pump devices, and increase user awareness of potential dangers with PCA pumps.[25] Examples of such errors include software defects; user interface issues, such as unclear instructions (which may lead to misprogramming of medication doses or infusion rates); and mechanical or electrical failures.[25]

In addition to IV PCA errors endangering the patient, the costs attributable to these errors are considerable. In one recent analysis of US data, medication-related errors had an average cost of $733 per error.[26] Using the error rate of 406.8 errors per 10,000 patients with more than 13 million patients who require PCA each year, the annual cost of IV PCA medication-related errors in the United States is about $388 million.[26] For IV PCA device-related errors, the estimated annual cost was $12 million.[26] This estimate does not include potential legal costs associated with adverse events, including deaths from IV PCA device-related errors. In addition to financial costs, IV PCA requires considerable nursing care, including time for pump setup and patient instruction on the use of the IV PCA device.[27,28] Nurses can spend approximately 150 to 250 minutes per patient in the setup and use of IV PCA pumps for postoperative pain relief.[29,30]

IV route of administration

Several complications with the IV route of administration make its use problematic for postoperative pain control. The IV route leaves the patient vulnerable to gaps in analgesia that may result from kinked tubing, infiltrated catheters, and dislodged catheters.[10] In pooled analysis of data from 2 open-label, randomized trials, 658 patients who received morphine IV PCA postoperatively had an incidence of analgesic gaps of 12%, many resulting from infiltrated and dislodged catheters.[10] The IV route leaves patients susceptible to infections, with a 7% to 9% incidence of phlebitis and a 0.2% to 0.4% incidence of bacteremia caused by IV peripheral venous catheters.[11] Furthermore, IV administration is characterized by rapid, high maximum plasma concentrations (C_{max}), which are followed fairly rapidly by trough plasma concentrations, leading to frequent redosing. A retrospective study of more than 1000 patients receiving IV PCA morphine for postoperative pain found that the mean use of morphine in the first 24-hour period of PCA was 65.2 mg.[31] Based on these data and using a standard 1-mg demand dose, calculation of an interdosing interval suggests that patients would have to press the PCA button every 22 minutes to maintain analgesia. Also, tethering the patient via the IV tubing to the PCA infusion pump and IV pole limits the patient's mobility and range of ambulation, which may interfere with recovery of function or lead to postoperative complications.[1] This feature is especially cumbersome when the patient is no longer restricted to receiving IV fluids, and the IV pole is tethered to the patient only for PCA opioid administration, making trips to the bathroom, ability to shower, and walking on the ward more difficult.[1] Patients are also at risk of excessive sedation, respiratory depression, and other serious opioid-related adverse events if IV pump device malfunctions occur because opioid delivery is IV, and overdosing may be undetected by the staff or patient until such adverse events occur.[32]

CHARACTERISTICS OF SPECIFIC OPIOIDS USED FOR PCA

Numerous issues exist with the typical opioids used with IV PCA, including adverse events,[12] respiratory and hemodynamic effects,[33] influence of age on opioid requirements,[31,34,35] and accumulation of active metabolites. These adverse events include nausea and vomiting, pruritus, urinary retention, and sedation. A 2005 meta-analysis summarized the mean incidences of these adverse events: mild sedation, 56.5%; nausea, 32.0%; vomiting, 20.7%; pruritus, 13.8%; urinary retention, 13.4%; and excessive sedation, 5.3%.[36] **Table 2** summarizes the incidence of adverse events recorded in a retrospective analysis of IV PCA with 3 of the most commonly used opioids—morphine, hydromorphone, and fentanyl—in 254 patients who had undergone hip or knee surgery in 3 similar hospitals.[13] A 2004 analysis of publications involving the management of postoperative pain found that the mean rate of respiratory adverse events with IV PCA ranged from 1.2% (hypoventilation) to 11.5% (oxygen desaturation).[33]

Morphine has been the prototypical opioid for decades and still is the most commonly used opioid to manage postoperative pain. Yet, morphine is a poor choice of postoperative opioid. From preclinical studies of the different therapeutic indices of various opioids (**Table 3**) to the issue of active metabolites and the adverse-event profile of morphine, there can be room for improvement in using newer opioid analgesics for postoperative PCA.[37] The strengths and weaknesses of the most commonly used postoperative opioid analgesics are as follows.

Table 2
Incidence of adverse events with opioids commonly used for IV PCA

Adverse Event (%)	Morphine	Hydromorphone	Fentanyl
Nausea/vomiting	31	33	18
Pruritus	16	10	3
Urinary retention	16	10	3
Sedation	8	9	1
Respiratory depression	8	7	4
Headache	7	2	3
Confusion	5	1	0
Agitation	2	0	1
Hallucination	0	1	0

Data from Hutchison RW, Chon EH, Tucker WF Jr, et al. A comparison of a fentanyl, morphine, and hydromorphone patient-controlled intravenous delivery for acute postoperative analgesia: a multicenter study of opioid-induced adverse reactions. Hosp Pharm 2006;41:659–63.

Table 3		
Efficacy and therapeutic indices of morphine, fentanyl, and sufentanil		
Opioid	ED_{50} (mg/kg)	Therapeutic Index[a]
Morphine	3.2	71
Fentanyl	0.01	277
Sufentanil	0.007	26,716

Abbreviations: ED_{50}, median effective dose; LD_{50}, median lethal dose.
[a] Ratio of $LD_{50}:ED_{50}$.
Data from Mather LE. Opioids: a pharmacologist's delight! Clin Exp Pharmacol Physiol 1995;22:833–6.

Morphine

Although morphine is the most commonly used opioid for IV PCA, accumulation of its active metabolites, morphine-3-glucuronide (M3G) and morphine-6-glucuronide (M6G), represents a risk for a prolonged duration of action and untoward effects.[5,38,39] Morphine is metabolized primarily by the kidney; therefore, M3G can accumulate more rapidly in renally impaired and elderly patients and may cause side effects.[36,38,40] M6G is more potent than morphine but builds up more slowly than M3G and may not be a problem during short-term use.[41] IV PCA morphine has a frequent rate of adverse events, including nausea, vomiting, pruritus, urinary retention, sedation, and respiratory depression (see **Table 2**).[13] The low therapeutic index for IV PCA morphine demonstrated in preclinical models indicates that morphine is not an ideal option for postoperative pain relief for all patients.

Hydromorphone

Many patients with renal impairment or morphine allergies are treated instead with hydromorphone.[42] Hydromorphone is metabolized primarily by the liver and is approximately 5 times more potent than morphine. The clinical effects of hydromorphone are dose-related, and its adverse-event profile is similar to that of morphine.[5,13,42–44] Hydromorphone can cause excessive sedation and somnolence. A systematic review of adverse events associated with the postoperative use of 6 major opioids (buprenorphine, fentanyl, hydromorphone, meperidine, morphine, and sufentanil) found that after meperidine (67.9%), the opioid with the most frequent incidence of central nervous system side effects (mainly sedation) was hydromorphone (42.7%).[12] Also, the hydromorphone-3-glucuronide metabolite may cause excitation in large doses. In addition, because of the similarity of name of morphine and hydromorphone and the significant differences in their potencies, the use of hydromorphone has caused confusion, resulting in harmful errors in the programming of IV PCA.[9]

Fentanyl

Fentanyl has no active metabolites and displays a wider therapeutic index than morphine in preclinical models (approximately 300 LD_{50}/ED_{50}[median lethal/effective dose]; **Table 3**).[37] Fentanyl is 80 to 100 times as potent as morphine[42] and may have less respiratory depression than morphine. In a secondary analysis of a retrospective cohort study of 8955 patients who received one of 3 opioids for postoperative pain (morphine, fentanyl, or meperidine), 0.6% of patients who received fentanyl experienced respiratory depression compared with 2.8% of patients who received morphine.[45] However, fentanyl may be associated with more IV PCA programming errors, because it is dosed in micrograms and not milligrams. In addition, fentanyl is very lipophilic; therefore, its pharmacokinetic profile is characterized by a rapid, high C_{max} followed by a short alpha-redistribution half-life, resulting in a rapid onset but short duration of action.[5,42] Consequently, patients may need to redose frequently or use a higher on-demand dose, or they may require a basal rate, which is not recommended because of the increased risk of respiratory depression. On-demand doses of 20 µg or less with fentanyl IV PCA result in low patient satisfaction and a high rate of unsuccessful patient dosing attempts.[46,47] The infusion durations of more than 4 hours are another concern, resulting in a dramatic increase in the context-sensitive half-time of the drug (time required to reach 50% of C_{max} after infusion is stopped) because of its high volume of distribution and long elimination half-life (longer than morphine).[5,48,49] This may result in an undesirable prolonged drug effect with extended use.

Sufentanil

Sufentanil is a fentanyl analogue and, like fentanyl, has no active metabolites. It is 5 to 10 times more potent than fentanyl but has the highest therapeutic index (approximately 25,000) of any post-operatively used opioid in preclinical models. This high therapeutic index may be clinically relevant, because of a less frequent incidence of respiratory depression with sufentanil compared with morphine, alfentanil, and fentanyl.[5,50–55] A randomized, double-blind trial in 30 healthy volunteers showed that sufentanil provided more effective analgesia and caused less respiratory depression compared with fentanyl.[52] In a separate randomized study in 30 patients who had undergone abdominal surgery, sufentanil had fewer decreased oxygen saturation values (3.4%) compared with morphine (23.3%) and alfentanil (18.9%).[50]

Sufentanil is highly lipophilic (twice as lipophilic as fentanyl), so it has an even more rapid alpha-redistribution and shorter duration of action when administered IV. Therefore, sufentanil has not been widely used in IV PCA. However, unlike fentanyl, its context-sensitive half-time does not increase appreciably as a function of infusion duration.[48,49] Furthermore, sufentanil, unlike fentanyl, does not display a delayed paradoxic increase in plasma concentration during the elimination phase. A randomized, double-blind pharmacokinetic study in 41 patients who had undergone coronary artery bypass graft surgery found that 9 patients who had received a single bolus dose of fentanyl exhibited secondary plasma concentration peaks occurring from 4 to 15 hours after injection, with increases in plasma concentrations ranging from 29% to 79%.[56] In contrast, only one patient who received sufentanil had a secondary peak with an increase of 43% at 7 hours after injection.[56] These secondary plasma concentration peaks explain the well-known delayed postoperative respiratory depression observed with fentanyl.[57,58] Therefore, based on its high therapeutic index and reliable pharmacokinetic profile, sufentanil may be an optimal opioid for postoperative PCA if the short duration of action of the IV route could be remedied.

ADVANCES IN SYSTEMIC OPIOID PCA THERAPY

New modalities are being developed for systemic PCA that are less invasive and have simplified dosing regimens compared with IV PCA. These include transdermal, sublingual, inhalation, intranasal (IN), and oral PCA systems. Some of these systems are pre-programmed, which eliminates the potential for programming and medication errors and decreases the time required for preparation. All these options reduce the risk of

IV line complications and allow for greater ease of patient mobility compared with IV PCA.

Transdermal PCA

The fentanyl iontophoretic transdermal system (IONSYS; Ortho-McNeil, Raritan, NJ, USA) is a preprogrammed noninvasive method of PCA.[1,5,10,59] With this system, which attaches via adhesive to the patient's upper outer arm or chest, fentanyl is transferred iontophoretically across the skin when the patient pushes the button on the unit.[60] The system has a 10-minute lockout interval and each actuation by the patient results in a 10-minute duration of transdermal drug delivery.[60] The dose of fentanyl delivered over time, however, is not consistent. The delivered dose of fentanyl averages 16 µg on initial application of the patch to the skin, a dose previously found to be inadequate for many patients,[46,47] with the intended dose of 40 µg per actuation not occurring until 10 hours after patch application.[60] In a Phase III, open-label, active comparator trial, which allowed 3 hours of IV breakthrough opioid rescue after study initiation, the fentanyl iontophoretic transdermal system was shown to be therapeutically equivalent to IV PCA morphine based on patient global assessments of the method of pain control.[61] Other endpoints that did not differ significantly from IV PCA morphine included frequency of early discontinuations due to inadequate analgesia and pain intensity scores at 24 hours after dosing.[61] Although Phase III studies were successful, key concerns with the use of IONSYS were the need to provide supplemental analgesia for about 40% (range of 34%–45%) of patients during the first 3 hours of treatment in placebo-controlled studies (and the active comparator study against IV PCA) and the incidence of application site reactions.[60,61] In the 3 placebo-controlled trials, an adverse event of erythema at the patch site was recorded for 14% of patients.[60] Also, 60% of patients reported some redness at the application site, although mostly mild, 24 hours after removal of the system.[60] This system was withdrawn from the market by the marketing authorization holder in September 2008, because of a manufacturing defect found in some units. Corrosion of one of the components within the circuit board could cause self-activation of the system and, therefore, put patients at risk of an overdose. The root cause of the defect is under analysis, and the return of the system to the market is uncertain. Currently, the marketing authorization is suspended.[62]

Sublingual PCA

The Sufentanil NanoTab PCA System (AcelRx Pharmaceuticals, Redwood City, CA, USA) is designed for sublingual administration of sufentanil. The system comes in the form of a NanoTab (a 3-mm diameter oral transmucosal dosage form intended to minimize the salivary response) placed sublingually, with a preprogrammed, handheld device with lockout features and radio-frequency identification (RFID) to allow single-user identification. Although IV sufentanil has a short plasma half-time because of rapid redistribution, when oral transmucosal absorption of sufentanil was evaluated in Phase I pharmacokinetic studies in healthy volunteers, results indicated that the pharmacokinetic profile of sublingual sufentanil was highly suitable for use as a titratable postoperative analgesic.[63] Sufentanil NanoTabs have a fairly high bioavailability and a low variability in time to maximal plasma concentrations.[63] The sublingual Nano-Tab allows sufentanil to maintain a longer plasma half-time and a blunted, safer C_{max} compared with IV administration.[63] Repeat-dosing studies demonstrated the potential for safe and reliable redosing with a 20-minute lockout period.[63] Successful Phase II clinical trials for pain relief in postoperative settings of major orthopedic and abdominal surgery have been completed.[64–66] In these Phase II studies, the Sufentanil

NanoTab PCA System is demonstrated to deliver effective postoperative analgesia with a low side-effect profile. Phase III clinical trials of this device are planned.

Inhalation PCA

Several products using the inhaled route of opioid delivery for postoperative PCA have been evaluated. An inhaled morphine system (AERx Pain Management System; Aradigm Corporation, Hayward, CA, USA) that had many of the safety features typical of PCA (ie, lockout period, multiple patient-initiated dosing) demonstrated comparable efficacy and safety to standard IV PCA morphine in a Phase II study.[67] Inhaled fentanyl (AeroLEF; YM Biosciences, Mississauga, ON, Canada) delivered using a breath-activated nebulizer has also demonstrated efficacy in Phase II studies in patients with postoperative pain after orthopedic surgery.[68,69] Phase III studies have not yet been initiated for either product.

Intranasal PCA

Administration of opioids via the IN route uses formulations of dry powder or solutions made up in water or saline. The nasal mucosa provides rapid absorption and distribution of drugs, because it is highly perfused.[1,70] IN morphine (Rylomine; Javelin Pharmaceuticals, Inc, Cambridge, MA, USA) was shown to be effective for postoperative moderate-to-severe orthopedic pain in Phase II studies[71] and is currently in Phase III development; however, the single unit-dose nasal spray device does not have many of the safety features associated with PCA, including multiple on-demand dosing or a timed lockout. Other opioids have been delivered via the IN route using nasal spray devices, but, similar to IN morphine, these studies lacked devices that contain the typical PCA safety features. A comparison of IN PCA fentanyl with IV PCA fentanyl in patients who underwent orthopedic, abdominal, or thyroid surgery showed that both methods were similarly effective at providing pain relief and were similarly accepted by patients.[72] Sufentanil has also been successfully used via the IN route postoperatively in pediatric and adult patients.[73,74] However, the IN method causes nasal irritation, nasal congestion, upper respiratory infection, sinus congestion, rhinitis, pharyngitis, or epistaxis, particularly after long-term usage.[75]

Oral PCA

The Medication on Demand (MOD) Oral PCA Device (Avancen, Mount Pleasant, SC, USA) is a unit locked onto an IV pole within the patient's reach. An RFID wristband is programmed into the device and placed on the patient's wrist. At the end of the lockout interval, a green ready light indicates the availability of the next dose. After patients record their level of pain on the device's pain scale (0–10) and swipes the wristband over the front of the device, the tray is able to be turned to the open position, and the patient can remove a pill. An evaluation of a version of this device to deliver oral hydromorphone, oxycodone, morphine, and acetaminophen to hospital inpatients with cancer showed that 95% patients found that it provided better pain control than nurse-delivered oral doses. Also, more than 90% of nurses reported that it saved them time, and over 80% of nurses found it to be reliable, easy to program, and easy for acquiring data on medication dispensed.[76] Although this oral PCA device is a nice alternative to nurse-delivered oral tablets, its utility for treating moderate-to-severe postoperative pain would be limited, especially in the "nil by mouth" patient.

SUMMARY

IV PCA remains a mainstay of postoperative pain management, but inherent draw-backs with this method and the commonly used opioids indicates the need for easier-to-use, patient-controlled modalities that are less prone to error and have fewer side effects. Methods of PCA administration via routes other than IV have been developed recently and are showing promise in clinical trials. These novel routes of delivery may improve the pharmacokinetic profile of certain opioids that were not optimally delivered via IV, such as sufentanil, and may have the added benefit of dedicated delivery devices that do not require programming. Given that errors with IV PCA are a risk to patient safety and increase costs considerably, further development of these alternative PCA methods should be pursued to minimize such errors while providing effective and tolerable management of postoperative pain.

ACKNOWLEDGMENTS

The authors would like to acknowledge Nancy Bella, PharmD, of MedErgy for providing medical writing assistance that was funded by AcelRx. The authors retained full editorial control over the content of the article, and Dr Miller received no financial compensation for authoring the article.

REFERENCES

1. Viscusi ER. Patient-controlled drug delivery for acute postoperative pain management: a review of current and emerging technologies. Reg Anesth Pain Med 2008;33:146–58.
2. Kaloul I, Guay J, Cote C, et al. The posterior lumbar plexus (psoas compartment) block and the three-in-one femoral nerve block provide similar postoperative analgesia after total knee replacement. Can J Anaesth 2004;51:45–51.
3. White PF, Kehlet H. Improving postoperative pain management: what are the unresolved issues? Anesthesiology 2010;112:220–5.
4. Sumida S, Lesley MR, Hanna MN, et al. Meta-analysis of the effect of extended-release epidural morphine versus intravenous patient-controlled analgesia on respiratory depression. J Opioid Manag 2009;5:301–5.
5. Momeni M, Crucitti M, De KM. Patient-controlled analgesia in the management of postoperative pain. Drugs 2006;66:2321–37.
6. Hudcova J, McNicol E, Quah C, et al. Patient controlled opioid analgesia versus conventional opioid analgesia for postoperative pain. Cochrane Database Syst Rev 2006;4:CD003348.
7. Ballantyne JC, Carr DB, Chalmers TC, et al. Postoperative patient-controlled analgesia: meta-analyses of initial randomized control trials. J Clin Anesth 1993;5: 182–93.
8. Macintyre PE. Safety and efficacy of patient-controlled analgesia. Br J Anaesth 2001;87:36–46.
9. Institute for Safe Medication Practices. Medication safety alert. High alert medication feature: reducing patient harm from opiates. Available at: http://www.ismp.org/Newsletters/acutecare/articles/20070222.asp. Accessed May 20, 2010.
10. Panchal SJ, Damaraju CV, Nelson WW, et al. System-related events and analgesic gaps during postoperative pain management with the fentanyl ionto-phoretic transdermal system and morphine intravenous patient-controlled analgesia. Anesth Analg 2007;105:1437–41.

11. Webster J, Osborne S, Rickard C, et al. Clinically-indicated replacement versus routine replacement of peripheral venous catheters. Cochrane Database Syst Rev 2010;3:CD007798.
12. Wheeler M, Oderda GM, Ashburn MA, et al. Adverse events associated with postoperative opioid analgesia: a systematic review. J Pain 2002;3:159–80.
13. Hutchison RW, Chon EH, Tucker WF Jr, et al. A comparison of a fentanyl, morphine, and hydromorphone patient-controlled intravenous delivery for acute postoperative analgesia: a multicenter study of opioid-induced adverse reactions. Hosp Pharm 2006;41:659–63.
14. Simopoulos TT, Smith HS, Peeters-Asdourian C, et al. Use of meperidine in patient-controlled analgesia and the development of a normeperidine toxic reaction. Arch Surg 2002;137:84–8.
15. American Pain Society. Principles of analgesic use in the treatment of acute pain and cancer pain. 6th edition. Glenview (IL): American Pain Society; 2008.
16. Owen H, Plummer JL, Armstrong I, et al. Variables of patient-controlled analgesia. 1. Bolus size. Anaesthesia 1989;44:7–10.
17. Hagle ME, Lehr VT, Brubakken K, et al. Respiratory depression in adult patients with intravenous patient-controlled analgesia. Orthop Nurs 2004;23:18–27.
18. Schug SA, Torrie JJ. Safety assessment of postoperative pain management by an acute pain service. Pain 1993;55:387–91.
19. Sidebotham D, Dijkhuizen MR, Schug SA. The safety and utilization of patient-controlled analgesia. J Pain Symptom Manage 1997;14:202–9.
20. American Pain Society. Principles of analgesic use in the treatment of acute pain and cancer pain. 5th edition. Glenview (IL): American Pain Society; 2003. p.1–73.
21. Abbott PCA. Plus II patient-controlled analgesic pumps prone to misprogramming resulting in narcotic overinfusions. Health Devices 1997;26:389–91.
22. Vicente KJ, Kada-Bekhaled K, Hillel G, et al. Programming errors contribute to death from patient-controlled analgesia: case report and estimate of probability. Can J Anesth 2003;50:328–32.
23. Keohane CA, Hayes J, Saniuk C, et al. Intravenous medication safety and smart infusion systems: lessons learned and future opportunities. J Infus Nurs 2005;28: 321–8.
24. Rothschild JM, Keohane CA, Cook EF, et al. A controlled trial of smart infusion pumps to improve medication safety in critically ill patients. Crit Care Med 2005;33:533–40.
25. Center for Devices and Radiological Health, US Food and Drug Administration. Infusion Pump Improvement Initiative. April 2010.
26. Meissner B, Nelson W, Hicks R, et al. The rate and costs attributable to intravenous patient-controlled analgesia errors. Hosp Pharm 2009;44:312–24.
27. Choiniere M, Rittenhouse BE, Perreault S, et al. Efficacy and costs of patient-controlled analgesia versus regularly administered intramuscular opioid therapy. Anesthesiology 1998;89:1377–88.
28. Hutchison RW, Anastassopoulos K, Vallow S, et al. Intravenous patient-controlled analgesia pump and reservoir logistics: results from a multicenter questionnaire. Hosp Pharm 2007;42:1036–44.
29. Bonnet F, Eberhart L, Wennberg E, et al. Fentanyl HCl iontophoretic transdermal system versus morphine IV-PCA for postoperative pain management: survey of healthcare provider opinion. Curr Med Res Opin 2009;25:293–301.
30. Evans C, Schein J, Nelson W, et al. Improving patient and nurse outcomes: a comparison of nurse tasks and time associated with two patient-controlled analgesia modalities using delphi panels. Pain Manag Nurs 2007;8:86–95.

31. Macintyre PE, Jarvis DA. Age is the best predictor of postoperative morphine requirements. Pain 1996;64:357–64.

32. Miaskowski C. Patient-controlled modalities for acute postoperative pain management. J Perianesth Nurs 2005;20:255–67.

33. Cashman JN, Dolin SJ. Respiratory and haemodynamic effects of acute postoperative pain management: evidence from published data. Br J Anaesth 2004;93:212–23.

34. Leung JM, Sands LP, Paul S, et al. Does postoperative delirium limit the use of patient-controlled analgesia in older surgical patients? Anesthesiology 2009;111:625–31.

35. Macintyre PE. Intravenous patient-controlled analgesia: one size does not fit all. Anesthesiol Clin North America 2005;23:109–23.

36. Dolin SJ, Cashman JN. Tolerability of acute postoperative pain management: nausea, vomiting, sedation, pruritis, and urinary retention. Evidence from published data. Br J Anaesth 2005;95:584–91.

37. Mather LE. Opioids: a pharmacologist's delight! Clin Exp Pharmacol Physiol 1995;22:833–6.

38. Ratka A, Wittwer E, Baker L, et al. Pharmacokinetics of morphine, morphine-3-glucuronide, and morphine-6-glucuronide in healthy older men and women. Am J Pain Manag 2004;14:45–55.

39. Sear JW, Hand CW, Moore RA, et al. Studies on morphine disposition: influence of general anaesthesia on plasma concentrations of morphine and its metabolites. Br J Anaesth 1989;62:22–7.

40. Sear JW, Hand CW, Moore RA, et al. Studies on morphine disposition: influence of renal failure on the kinetics of morphine and its metabolites. Br J Anaesth 1989;62:28–32.

41. Baker L, Hyrien O, Ratka A. Contributions of morphine-3-glucuronide and morphine-6-glucuronide to differences in morphine analgesia in humans. Am J Pain Manag 2003;13:16–28.

42. Grass JA. Patient-controlled analgesia. Anesth Analg 2005;101:S44–61.

43. Quigley C. Hydromorphone for acute and chronic pain. Cochrane Database Syst Rev 2002;1:CD003447.

44. Hong D, Flood P, Diaz G. The side effects of morphine and hydromorphone patient-controlled analgesia. Anesth Analg 2008;107:1384–9.

45. Cepeda MS, Farrar JT, Baumgarten M, et al. Side effects of opioids during short-term administration: effect of age, gender, and race. Clin Pharmacol Ther 2003;74:102–12.

46. Camu F, Van Aken H, Bovill JG. Postoperative analgesic effects of three demand-dose sizes of fentanyl administered by patient-controlled analgesia. Anesth Analg 1998;87:890–5.

47. Prakash S, Fatima T, Pawar M. Patient-controlled analgesia with fentanyl for burn dressing changes. Anesth Analg 2004;99:552–5.

48. Egan TD, Lemmens HJ, Fiset P, et al. The pharmacokinetics of the new short-acting opioid remifentanil (GI87084B) in healthy adult male volunteers. Anesthesiology 1993;79:881–92.

49. Hughes MA, Glass PS, Jacobs JR. Context-sensitive half-time in multicompartment pharmacokinetic models for intravenous anesthetic drugs. Anesthesiology 1992;76:334–41.

50. Ved SA, Dubois M, Carron H, et al. Sufentanil and alfentanil pattern of consumption during patient-controlled analgesia: a comparison with morphine. Clin J Pain 1989;5(Suppl 1):S63–70.

51. Clark NJ, Meuleman T, Liu WS, et al. Comparison of sufentanil-N_2O and fentanyl-N_2O in patients without cardiac disease undergoing general surgery. Anesthesiology 1987;66:130–5.

52. Bailey PL, Streisand JB, East KA, et al. Differences in magnitude and duration of opioid-induced respiratory depression and analgesia with fentanyl and sufentanil. Anesth Analg 1990;70:8–15.

53. De Castro J. Practical applications and limitations of analgesic anesthesia: a review. Acta Anaesthesiol Belg 1976;27:107–28.

54. Monk JP, Beresford R, WardSufentanil A. A review of its pharmacological properties and therapeutic use. Drugs 1988;36:286–313.

55. Savoia G, Loreto M, Gravino E. Sufentanil: an overview of its use for acute pain management. Minerva Anestesiol 2001;67:206–16.

56. Brusset A, Levron JC, Olivier P, et al. Comparative pharmacokinetic study of fentanyl and sufentanil after single high-bolus doses. Clin Drug Invest 1999;18:377–89.

57. Stoeckel H, Schuttler J, Magnussen H, et al. Plasma fentanyl concentrations and the occurrence of respiratory depression in volunteers. Br J Anaesth 1982;54:1087–95.

58. Becker LD, Paulson BA, Miller RD, et al. Biphasic respiratory depression after fentanyldroperidol or fentanyl alone used to supplement nitrous oxide anesthesia. Anesthesiology 1976;44:291–6.

59. Power I. Fentanyl HCl iontophoretic transdermal system (ITS): clinical application of iontophoretic technology in the management of acute postoperative pain. Br J Anaesth 2007;98:4–11.

60. IONSYS™ (fentanyl iontophoretic trandermal system) [package insert]. Raritan, NJ: Ortho-McNeil, Inc; 2006. Available at: http://www.accessdata.fda.gov/drugsatfda_docs/label/2006/021338lbl.pdf. Accessed June 20, 2010.

61. Viscusi ER, Reynolds L, Chung F, et al. Patient-controlled transdermal fentanyl hydrochloride vs intravenous morphine pump for postoperative pain: a randomized controlled trial. JAMA 2004;291:1333–41.

62. European Medicines Agency. Evaluation of medicines for human use. Questions and answers on the recommendation to suspend the marketing authorisation of Ionsys. Available at: http://www.ema.europa.eu/humandocs/PDFs/EPAR/ionsys/Ionsys_Q&A_60985608en.pdf. Accessed May 21, 2010.

63. Palmer PP, Hamel LG, Skowronski RJ. Single- and repeat-dose pharmacokinetics of sublingual sufentanil NanoTab in healthy volunteers [abstract A1222]. Presented at: the Annual Meeting of the American Society of Anesthesiologists. New Orleans (LA), October 17–21, 2009.

64. Griffin DW, Skowronski RJ, Dasu BN, et al. A phase 2 open-label functionality, safety, and efficacy study of the sufentanil NanoTab™ PCA System in patients following elective unilateral knee replacement surgery. Poster presented at: the 35th Annual Spring Meeting and Workshops of the American Society of Regional Anesthesia and Pain Medicine. Toronto, Ontario, Canada, April 22–25, 2010.

65. Minkowitz HS, Skowronski RJ, Palmer PP. A phase 2 multicenter, randomized, placebo-controlled study to evaluate the clinical efficacy, safety, and tolerability of sublingual sufentanil NanoTab™ in patients following elective unilateral knee replacement surgery. Poster presented at: the 35th Annual Spring Meeting and Workshops of the American Society of Regional Anesthesia and Pain Medicine. Toronto, Ontario (Canada), April 22–25, 2010.

66. Singla NK, Skowronski RJ, Palmer PP. A phase 2 multicenter, randomized, placebo-controlled study to evaluate the clinical efficacy, safety, and tolerability

of sublingual sufentanil NanoTab™ in patients following major abdominal surgery. Poster presented at: the 35th Annual Spring Meeting and Workshops of the American Society of Regional Anesthesia and Pain Medicine. Toronto, Ontario (Canada), April 22–25, 2010.

67. Thipphawong JB, Babul N, Morishige RJ, et al. Analgesic efficacy of inhaled morphine in patients after bunionectomy surgery. Anesthesiology 2003;99: 693–700.

68. Brull R, Chan V, University Health Network TWTO. A randomized controlled trial demonstrates the efficacy, safety and tolerability of Aerosolized Free and Liposome-Encapsulated Fentanyl (AeroLEF) via pulmonary administration. Poster presented at the American Pain Society (APS) Annual Meeting. Tampa (FL), May 8–10, 2008.

69. Clark A, Rossiter-Rooney M, Valle-Leutri F, et al. Aerosolized Liposome-Encapsulated Fentanyl (AeroLEF™) via pulmonary administration allows patients with moderate to severe post-surgical acute pain to self-titrate to effective analgesia. Presented at the American Pain Society 2008 Annual Meeting. Tampa (FL), May 8–10, 2008.

70. Vadivelu N, Mitra S, Narayan D. Recent advances in postoperative pain management. Yale J Biol Med 2010;83:11–25.

71. Stoker DG, Reber KR, Waltzman LS, et al. Analgesic efficacy and safety of morphine-chitosan nasal solution in patients with moderate to severe pain following orthopedic surgery. Pain Med 2008;9:3–12.

72. Toussaint S, Maidl J, Schwagmeier R, et al. Patient-controlled intranasal analgesia: effective alternative to intravenous PCA for postoperative pain relief. Can J Anesth 2000;47:299–302.

73. Heshmati F, Noroozinia H, Abbasivash R, et al. Intranasal sufentanil for postoperative pain control in lower abdominal pediatric surgery. Ir J Pharmacol Ther 2006;5:131–3.

74. Mathieu N, Cnudde N, Engelman E, et al. Intranasal sufentanil is effective for postoperative analgesia in adults. Can J Anaesth 2006;53:60–6.

75. Dale O, Hjortkjaer R, Kharasch ED. Nasal administration of opioids for pain management in adults. Acta Anaesthesiol Scand 2002;46:759–70.

76. Rosati J, Gallagher M, Shook B, et al. Evaluation of an oral patient-controlled analgesia device for pain management in oncology inpatients. J Support Oncol 2007;5:443–8.

Buprenorphine in Postoperative Pain Management

Nalini Vadivelu, MD*, Muhammad Anwar, MD

KEYWORDS

- Buprenorphine • Analgesic • Mu receptors
- Postoperative pain control

Interest in the use of buprenorphine as an analgesic has increased in recent years. Its unique agonist-antagonist properties makes it a useful analgesic with a potential lower abuse liability in humans. Buprenorphine has been used as an analgesic in the postoperative period for the treatment of moderate-to-severe pain. Buprenorphine has also been found to have antihyperalgesic properties, which might make it an agent to consider for prevention and reduction of central sensitization. In addition, its high affinity for the mu receptor along with its slow dissociation from the receptors has led to new challenges when controlling postoperative pain in patients on buprenorphine maintenance therapy. This article highlights the challenges present in the postoperative period of using buprenorphine as an analgesic in patients with and without preoperative maintenance therapy.

PHARMACOLOGY AND PHARMACOKINETICS OF BUPRENORPHINE

Buprenorphine, a derivative of thebaine, is a semisynthetic opioid analgesic. It binds to mu, kappa, and delta opioid receptor subtypes and has a slow dissociation from these receptors. Its actions on both mu and kappa receptors make it useful as an analgesic and for the maintenance therapy in patients with a history of drug abuse. It is a centrally acting partial mu agonist and a kappa and delta antagonist.[1] Buprenorphine can occupy the mu receptor almost maximally; therefore, it decreases the availability of the mu receptor making it useful in decreasing withdrawal symptoms.[2] Buprenorphine binds to the mu receptor with high affinity but with a lower intrinsic binding capacity when compared with a full mu agonist.[1]

Buprenorphine has a rapid onset secondary to its high lipophilicity, which is greater than the lipophilicity of morphine. Buprenorphine penetrates the blood brain barrier more easily than morphine. The onset also depends on the route; for example, the onset of action of buprenorphine is 5 to 15 minutes for the intravenous or

Department of Anesthesiology, Yale University, 333 Cedar Street, New Haven, CT 06520, USA
* Corresponding author.
E-mail address: nalinivg@gmail.com

Anesthesiology Clin 28 (2010) 601–609
doi:10.1016/j.anclin.2010.08.015
1932-2275/10/$ – see front matter © 2010 Elsevier Inc. All rights reserved.

intramuscular routes and 15 to 45 minutes for the sublingual route. The duration of action of buprenorphine is 6 to 8 hours.[3] Jasinski and colleagues[4] have suggested that the long duration of action of buprenorphine is due to its slow dissociation from mu receptors. Constipation rates in patients on buprenorphine are also low.[5] Buprenorphine can be used in the presence of renal failure. Similar clearance of buprenorphine was found in patients with normal and impaired renal function.[6]

Buprenorphine is a potent analgesic. Sittl[7] suggests that buprenorphine has an antinociceptive potency about 75 to 100 times greater than that of morphine. Buprenorphine has a dose-dependent effect on analgesia with no respiratory depression.[8] Dahan and colleagues[9] demonstrated that buprenorphine has a ceiling effect on respiratory depression, but not on analgesia. Dahan and colleagues,[9] in a study on 20 volunteers, showed that there was a ceiling effect on respiratory depression by not on analgesia. This was demonstrated over a dose range of 0.05 to 0.6 mg buprenorphine in humans. Buprenorphine shows analgesic effects, but no respiratory depression, at doses up to 10 mg. Therefore, buprenorphine may have a differential effect on respiration and analgesia.

In 1994, Walsh and colleagues[10] demonstrated that there is no ceiling for analgesia in patients receiving sublingual buprenorphine from 1 to 32 mg. Buprenorphine has been showed to have strong antihyperalgesic effects that can exceed its analgesic effects.[11]

METABOLISM OF BUPRENORPHINE

Cytochrome P450 mediates the metabolism of buprenorphine in the liver.[12,13] Buprenorphine is metabolized in the liver and the gut to norbuprenorphine. Buprenorphine and its metabolite, norbuprenorphine, undergo glucuronidation. Norbuprenorphine is an N-dealkylated metabolite that is reported to have one-fourth the potency of buprenorphine.[14] Norbuprenorphine can produce respiratory depression 10 times greater than buprenorphine; however, the respiratory depression caused by norbuprenorphine can be reversed by naloxone.[15] Buprenorphine appears to be excreted by the biliary route and gut and urine. It is thought that about 15 percent of the original dose of buprenorphine is excreted in the urine.[16] Levels of buprenorphine metabolites appear to be increased in renal failure patients with similar buprenorphine levels as compared with controls.[6] It must be remembered that buprenorphine cannot be dialyzed—most likely owing to its slow dissociation and high affinity to the mu receptor.[15,17]

SIDE EFFECTS

Buprenorphine is a lipophilic drug with a high affinity for mu receptors and slow dissociation rate, as well as decreased absorption into the cerebrospinal fluid. The high lipophilicity can affect the degree of side effects seen with buprenorphine as compared with morphine. Nausea, vomiting, euphoria, sedation, delayed gastric emptying, and pupillary constriction can all be seen with buprenorphine—but to a lesser degree than with morphine.[10]

CLINICAL APPLICATION OF BUPRENORPHINE AS ANALGESIA

Buprenorphine for the control of postoperative pain has been used in several routes, leading to new treatment options worldwide. Johnson and colleagues[3] showed that effective management of postoperative pain can be achieved in patients who are not dependent on uploads. Buprenorphine was introduced in the United States in 1981 as an analgesic via the parenteral route with the trade name of Buprenex.

Use of buprenorphine as an analgesic in Europe, however, had started much earlier—in the parenteral form at the dose of 0.3 mg/mL and in the sublingual form at the dose of 0.2 to 0.4 mg. Studies have shown parenteral buprenorphine to be a potent analgesic with a dose of 0.3 mg of buprenorphine to be equivalent to 10 mg of morphine sulfate in patients who are not dependent on opioids. Buprenorphine has since been used for pain control via the intrathecal, sublingual, intramuscular, epidural, and transdermal routes as evidenced by several clinical trials.

EPIDURAL BUPRENORPHINE

Buprenorphine has been used successfully via the epidural route without significant respiratory depression[18] and with good analgesia.[19] Epidural buprenorphine is most likely absorbed rapidly from the epidural space into the systemic circulation and acts centrally in the supraspinal regions to produce analgesia similar to intravenous buprenorphine.[20] Adequate epidural analgesia with buprenorphine for postoperative pain relief has been achieved for coronary artery bypass surgery,[21] gynecologic surgery,[22] genitourinary surgery in children,[23] upper and lower abdominal surgeries,[24] and for the treatment of rib fractures.[25] The epidural dose of buprenorphine ranges from 4 to 8 μg per hour, which is as effective as epidural morphine at a dose of 80 μg per hour for most surgeries. Lower abdominal surgeries might require a higher dose of 15 μg per hour of epidural buprenorphine.[26]

Buprenorphine is a semisynthetic lipophilic opioid that is less water-soluble than morphine; thus, the effectiveness of the epidural can depend on the site of injection of the drug. Takata and colleagues[27] found that hepatectomy patients had good pain relief with long duration when buprenorphine was injected into the thoracic epidural space, but not when injected into the lumbar epidural space. This was in contrast to epidural morphine, which produced excellent and long lasting pain relief when injected at the lumbar or the thoracic levels.

INTRATHECAL BUPRENORPHINE

Buprenorphine has been shown to provide more prolonged pain control in cesarean-section–delivery patients compared with controls who did not take buprenorphine. Celleno and Capogna[28] compared the effects of intrathecal hyperbaric bupivacaine with two groups taking 0.03 and 0.045 mg of intrathecal buprenorphine in addition to the hyperbaric bupivacaine and found that there was a longer pain-free interval in patients receiving buprenorphine. They also found that, within the patient groups receiving buprenorphine, a longer effect was seen in patients receiving the higher dose of buprenorphine.

INTRAVENOUS BUPRENORPHINE FOR ANALGESIA

Intravenous buprenorphine has been shown to provide analgesia as adequate as intravenous morphine. Abrahamsson and colleagues[29] showed that buprenorphine provides analgesia for up to 13 hours in dose ranges from 5 to 15 μg/kg.

SUBLINGUAL BUPRENORPHINE FOR ANALGESIA

Sublingual buprenorphine is a well-known agent for maintenance therapy for patients with opioid abuse. However, there have been studies demonstrating the effectiveness of sublingual buprenorphine for providing pain relief in the postoperative period. Witjes and colleagues[30] showed that sublingual buprenorphine provided adequate pain relief as the sole agent in about 80% of patients in the postoperative period after cholecystectomy.

SUBCUTANEOUS BUPRENORPHINE

Buprenorphine can be given subcutaneously for pain relief in the early postoperative period at a dose of 30 µg per hour.[31] This route is especially useful for patients with poor intravenous access.

Intramuscular buprenorphine is also especially useful in the presence of poor intravenous access. The duration of pain relief is approximately 6 hours, with a peak effect at about 1 hour, and onset at about 15 minutes. It can be used for patients requiring round-the-clock opioid therapy in the presence of acute or chronic pain.

INTRAARTICULAR ROUTE OF BUPRENORPHINE

Buprenorphine has shown to significantly reduce the amount of analgesia required after knee arthroscopy when injected intraarticularly. A study by Varrassi and colleagues[32] showed that intraarticular bupivacaine and intraarticular buprenorphine produced comparable pain control after knee arthroscopy.

BUPRENORPHINE IN REGIONAL ANESTHESIA

Buprenorphine could have peripherally mediated opioid analgesia and be a useful adjunct in regional anesthesia. Candido and colleagues[33] showed that addition of buprenorphine to local anesthetic in axillary brachial plexus blocks prolonged postoperative analgesia.

TRANSDERMAL BUPRENORPHINE

The high lipid solubility of buprenorphine makes it a suitable agent to be used via the transdermal route. This route uses hydrogels for the delivery of buprenorphine with the application of iontophoresis.[34] Transdermal buprenorphine has been used for the treatment of chronic pain.[35–37] Transdermal buprenorphine is being used in Europe for the treatment of acute pain, cancer pain, and neuropathic pain.[7,38] The patch is available at 35, 52.5, and 70 µg per hour for 3 days. The onset of action of transdermal buprenorphine is 12 to 24 hours and the duration of action of each patch transdermal buprenorphine is 3 days.[39]

PAIN CONTROL OF PATIENTS ON PREOPERATIVE BUPRENORPHINE

Opioid-dependent patients are often treated with buprenorphine. Worldwide, opioid dependence has been on the increase in the last decade and many of these patients present for surgery and for postoperative pain control. In 1996, buprenorphine was available in France as a substitution treatment for heroin addicts. In the United States, the Food and Drug Administration approved buprenorphine to be marketed only in the form of sublingual tablets (Subutex) or with naloxone (Subuxone) to treat opioid dependence. The rescheduling of buprenorphine from a schedule V to a schedule III narcotic was published in the Federal Register in October, 2002. Methadone, also used for the treatment of opioid abuse, is a schedule II drug. Schedule II drugs have more abuse potential than schedule III drugs.

Postoperative pain control of patients on preoperative buprenorphine can be a challenge[40] and can complicate postoperative pain management.[41] The possibility that the tight binding with the mu receptor could lead to partial opioid blockade with resultant reduction in postoperative analgesia when treated with opioids has been raised as a point of concern. There is also concern for relapse in patients taking buprenorphine for opioid dependence, which may also complicate pain management in the postoperative period. This should be taken into consideration while caring for opioid-dependent patients on buprenorphine in the postoperative period. *The National Drug Abuse Treatment Clinical Trials Network Prescription Opioid Addiction Treatment Study*, presented at the American Psychiatric Association annual meeting in 2010[42], showed that tapering with buprenorphine over 9 months led to almost universal relapse in persons dependent on prescription opioids.

Reviews of literature include several studies on and management strategies for preoperative pain in patients who are on buprenorphine as maintenance therapy for drug abuse.[41–44]

Alford and colleagues[44] have recommended that patients be converted to full opioid agonist preoperatively. Roberts and Meyer-Witting[43] suggest that buprenorphine be continued throughout the perioperative period and full agonist opioid be used for pain control when monitoring for respiratory depression and pain control. They also suggest that buprenorphine be discontinued up to 72 hours before the surgery and converted to a full agonist such as methadone to eliminate the existence of any partial blockade.

Ballantyne and La Forge[45] recommend that buprenorphine be discontinued for about a week before surgery.

Several studies in contrast to this concept suggest that full opioid agonists are effective in buprenorphine-treated patients. Budd and Collett[16] concluded that full opioid agonists are effective in acute and chronic pain syndromes in the presence of buprenorphine use and that buprenorphine does not produce persistent blockade of the mu receptor. There are other reports that demonstrate the effective use of full opioid agonists such as morphine in patients treated with buprenorphine and that buprenorphine use can be continued into the postoperative period. Mitra and Sinatra[46] recommend that patients on maintenance therapy take their morning dose of buprenorphine or methadone on the day of surgery to decrease the risk of opioid withdrawal during surgery.

Mehta and Langford[47] recommend the use of short-acting full opioid agonists for postoperative pain control in patients using transdermal buprenorphine. Morphine has shown to be an effective breakthrough medication in patients on transdermal buprenorphine. A study by Mercadante and colleagues[48] of 29 cancer patients demonstrated the effectiveness of morphine for pain control as a breakthrough medication in patients receiving transdermal buprenorphine.

A study by Jones and colleagues[49] done on obstetric patients also demonstrated the successful use of opioid agonists in the presence of buprenorphine maintenance.[49]

Finally, buprenorphine has been used effectively to control postoperative pain in buprenorphine-maintained patients.[40] Budd and Collett[16] suggest that sublingual buprenorphine could be used effectively as a breakthrough agent to control pain in patients on buprenorphine in the postoperative period.

ADVANTAGES

Buprenorphine can be safely used in the presence of renal failure.[50] The long duration of action[3] and safety of buprenorphine via the transdermal route makes it a useful agent for use in elderly patients.[51] Buprenorphine appears to have antihyperalgesic effects that can be useful for chronic-pain patients undergoing surgery in the postoperative period. Koppert and colleagues[52] studied the antihyperalgesic and analgesic effects of buprenorphine in humans via sublingual and the intravenous route with the magnitude of pain and secondary hyperalgesia assessed by transcutaneous stimulation. They found that the antihyperalgesic effects were stronger than the analgesic effects of buprenorphine using both the intravenous and the sublingual route. They also found that the antihyperalgesic effects were stronger and of longer duration as compared with the pure mu receptor agonist studied in the same model. Buprenorphine may have potential in the prevention and reduction of central sensitization in difficult chronic pain states during the postoperative period.

DISADVANTAGES

Drugs such as opioids, sedatives, hypnotics, anesthetic agents, antidepressants, and psychostimulants, which can induce or inhibit cytochrome P450 and can potentiate the central effects of buprenorphine. Buprenorphine should be used with extreme caution when used with benzodiazepines. Lai and Teo[53,54] showed that 19 of the 21 buprenorphine-related deaths in Singapore occurred with concurrent use with buprenorphine. Benzodiazepines with buprenorphine can exert a synergistic effect on the central nervous system and cause sedation and respiratory depression.[55]

SUMMARY

Several decades ago, the analgesic properties of buprenorphine were discovered. Buprenorphine has been administered via different routes—including epidural, intrathecal, intramuscular, sublingual, transdermal, and intraarticular—for the control of pain in the postoperative period. Newer routes, such as sublingual and transdermal, have increased the possibility of its developing into a useful analgesic for the treatment of postoperative pain. In addition, it could be an useful adjunct to local anesthetic for pain control in peripheral nerve blocks for the control of postoperative pain.[33]

Its approval for the use as an agent for the treatment of opioid abuse has led to increasing numbers of patients presenting for surgery on buprenorphine. Pain control in the postoperative period with patients on preoperative buprenorphine can be complicated and is a challenge. Concern for decreased analgesia in the postoperative period exists. Different management strategies have been put forward with an attempt to tackle this issue. Alford and colleagues[44] recommend the discontinuation of buprenorphine and conversion to pure opioid agonist before surgery while several others have shown effective pain control with pure opioid agonists such as morphine in the presence of buprenorphine in the postoperative period. Budd and Collett[16] suggest that, in addition to being controlled with opioid agonist, postoperative pain control in patients with preoperative buprenorphine may be controlled with sublingual buprenorphine. More research and outcome studies are necessary to confirm its usefulness for the control of postoperative pain in patients with acute pain or a preoperative history of chronic pain, in the treatment of patients with preoperative buprenorphine, and in the prevention and reduction of central sensitization postoperatively.

REFERENCES

1. Negus SS, Mello NK, Linsenmayer DC, et al. Kappa opioid antagonist effects of the novel kappa antagonist 5'-guanidinonaltrindole (GNTI) in an assay of schedule-controlled behavior in rhesus monkeys. Psychopharmacology (Berl) 2002;163(3–4):412–9.
2. Greenwald M, Johanson C, Moody D, et al. Effects of buprenorphine maintenance dose on mu-opioid receptor availability, plasma concentrations, and

antagonist blockade in heroin-dependent volunteers. Neuropsychopharmacology 2003;28(11):2000-9.

3. Johnson RE, Fudala PJ, Payne R. Buprenorphine: considerations for pain management. J Pain Symptom Manage 2005;29(3):297-326.

4. Jasinski DR, Pevnick JS, Griffith JD. Human pharmacology and abuse potential of the analgesic buprenorphine: a potential agent for treating narcotic addiction. Arch Gen Psychiatry 1978;35(4):501-16.

5. Griessinger N, Sittl R, Likar R. Transdermal buprenorphine in clinical practice–a post-marketing surveillance study in 13,179 patients. Curr Med Res Opin 2005;21(8):1147-56.

6. Hand C, Sear J, Uppington J, et al. Buprenorphine disposition in patients with renal impairment: single and continuous dosing, with special reference to metabolites. Br J Anaesth 1990;64(3):276-82.

7. Sittl R. Transdermal buprenorphine in cancer pain and palliative care. Palliat Med 2006;20(Suppl 1):s25-30.

8. Dahan A, Yassen A, Bijl H, et al. Comparison of the respiratory effects of intravenous buprenorphine and fentanyl in humans and rats. Br J Anaesth 2005;94(6):825-34.

9. Dahan A, Yassen A, Romberg R, et al. Buprenorphine induces ceiling in respiratory depression but not in analgesia. Br J Anaesth 2006;96(5):627-32.

10. Walsh SL, Preston KL, Stitzer ML, et al. Clinical pharmacology of buprenorphine: ceiling effects at high doses. Clin Pharmacol Ther 1994;55(5):569-80.

11. Simonnet G, Rivat C. Opioid-induced hyperalgesia: abnormal or normal pain? Neuroreport 2003;14(1):1-7.

12. Kobayashi K, Yamamoto T, Chiba K, et al. Human buprenorphine N-dealkylation is catalyzed by cytochrome P450 3A4. Drug Metab Dispos 1998;26(8):818-21.

13. Heel RC, Brogden RN, Speight TM, et al. Buprenorphine: a review of its pharmacological properties and therapeutic efficacy. Drugs 1979;17(2):81-110.

14. Ohtani M, Kotaki H, Nishitateno K, et al. Kinetics of respiratory depression in rats induced by buprenorphine and its metabolite, norbuprenorphine. J Pharmacol Exp Ther 1997;281(1):428-33.

15. Gal TJ. Naloxone reversal of buprenorphine-induced respiratory depression. Clin Pharmacol Ther 1989;45(1):66-71.

16. Budd K, Collett BJ. Old dog–new (ma)trix. Br J Anaesth 2003;90(6):722-4.

17. Knape J. Early respiratory depression resistant to naloxone following epidural buprenorphine. Anesthesiology 1986;64(3):382-4.

18. Scherer R, Schmutzler M, Giebler R, et al. Complications related to thoracic epidural analgesia: a prospective study in 1071 surgical patients. Acta Anaesthesiol Scand 1993;37(4):370-4.

19. Inagaki Y, Mashimo T, Yoshiya I. Mode and site of analgesic action of epidural buprenorphine in humans. Anesth Analg 1996;83(3):530-6.

20. Giebler R, Scherer R, Peters J. Incidence of neurologic complications related to thoracic epidural catheterization. Anesthesiology 1997;86(1):55-63.

21. Mehta Y, Juneja R, Madhok H, et al. Lumbar versus thoracic epidural buprenorphine for postoperative analgesia following coronary artery bypass graft surgery. Acta Anaesthesiol Scand 1999;43(4):388-93.

22. Miwa Y, Yonemura E, Fukushima K. Epidural administered buprenorphine in the perioperative period. Can J Anaesth 1996;43(9):907-13.

23. Kamal R, Khan F. Caudal analgesia with buprenorphine for postoperative pain relief in children. Paediatr Anaesth 1995;5(2):101-6.

24. Kaetsu H, Takeshi M, Chigusa S, et al. [Analgesic effects of epidurally adminis-tered fentanyl for postoperative pain relief—comparison with buprenorphine]. Masui 1992;41(12):1870–4 [in Japanese].

25. Govindarajan R, Bakalova T, Michael R, et al. Epidural buprenorphine in management of pain in multiple rib fractures. Acta Anaesthesiol Scand 2002;46(6):660–5.

26. Hirabayashi Y, Mitsuhata H, Shimizu R, et al. [Continuous epidural buprenorphine for postoperative pain relief in patients after lower abdominal surgery]. Masui 1993;42(11):1618–22 [in Japanese].

27. Takata T, Yukioka H, Fujimori M. [Epidural morphine and buprenorphine for post-operative pain relief after hepatectomy]. Masui 1990;39(1):13–8 [in Japanese].

28. Celleno D, Capogna G. Spinal buprenorphine for postoperative analgesia after caesarean section. Acta Anaesthesiol Scand 1989;33(3):236–8.

29. Abrahamsson J, Niemand D, Olsson A, et al. [Buprenorphine (Temgesic) as a pero-perative analgesic. A multicenter study]. Anaesthesist 1983;32(2):75–9 [in German].

30. Witjes W, Crul B, Vollaard E, et al. Application of sublingual buprenorphine in combination with naproxen or paracetamol for post-operative pain relief in chole-cystectomy patients in a double-blind study. Acta Anaesthesiol Scand 1992; 36(4):323–7.

31. Matsumoto S, Mitsuhata H, Akiyama H, et al. [The effect of subcutaneous admin-istration of buprenorphine with patient controlled analgesia system for post-oper-ative pain relief]. Masui 1994;43(11):1709–13 [in Japanese].

32. Varrassi G, Marinangeli F, Ciccozzi A, et al. Intra-articular buprenorphine after knee arthroscopy. A randomised, prospective, double-blind study. Acta Anaes-thesiol Scand 1999;43(1):51–5.

33. Candido K, Winnie A, Ghaleb A, et al. Buprenorphine added to the local anes-thetic for axillary brachial plexus block prolongs postoperative analgesia. Reg Anesth Pain Med 2002;27(2):162–7.

34. Fang J, Hwang T, Huang Y, et al. Transdermal iontophoresis of sodium noniva-mide acetate. V. Combined effect of physical enhancement methods. Int J Pharm 2002;235(1–2):95–105.

35. Budd K. Buprenorphine and the transdermal system: the ideal match in pain management. Int J Clin Pract Suppl 2003;133:9–14 [discussion: 23–4].

36. Simpson K. Individual choice of opioids and formulations: strategies to achieve the optimum for the patient. Clin Rheumatol 2002;21(Suppl 1):S5–8.

37. Likar R, Griessinger N, Sadjak A, et al. [Transdermal buprenorphine for treatment of chronic tumor and non-tumor pain]. Wien Med Wochenschr 2003;153(13–14): 317–22 [in German].

38. Kress H. Clinical update on the pharmacology, efficacy and safety of transdermal buprenorphine. Eur J Pain 2009;13(3):219–30.

39. Sorge J, Sittl R. Transdermal buprenorphine in the treatment of chronic pain: results of a phase III, multicenter, randomized, double-blind, placebo-controlled study. Clin Ther 2004;26(11):1808–20.

40. Book S, Myrick H, Malcolm R, et al. Buprenorphine for postoperative pain following general surgery in a buprenorphine-maintained patient. Am J Psychi-atry 2007;164(6):979.

41. Marcucci C, Fudin J, Thomas P, et al. A new pattern of buprenorphine misuse may complicate perioperative pain control. Anesth Analg 2009;108(6):1996–7.

42. The national drug abuse treatment clinical trials network prescription opioid addiction treatment study presented at the American Psychiatric Association annual meeting 2010.

43. Roberts D, Meyer-Witting M. High-dose buprenorphine: perioperative precautions and management strategies. Anaesth Intensive Care 2005;33(1):17–25.
44. Alford D, Compton P, Samet J. Acute pain management for patients receiving maintenance methadone or buprenorphine therapy. Ann Intern Med 2006; 144(2):127–34.
45. Ballantyne J, LaForge K. Opioid dependence and addiction during opioid treatment of chronic pain. Pain 2007;129(3):235–55.
46. Mitra S, Sinatra R. Perioperative management of acute pain in the opioid-dependent patient. Anesthesiology 2004;101(1):212–27.
47. Mehta V, Langford R. Acute pain management for opioid dependent patients. Anaesthesia 2006;61(3):269–76.
48. Mercadante S, Villari P, Ferrera P, et al. Safety and effectiveness of intravenous morphine for episodic breakthrough pain in patients receiving transdermal buprenorphine. J Pain Symptom Manage 2006;32(2):175–9.
49. Jones H, Johnson R, Milio L. Post-cesarean pain management of patients maintained on methadone or buprenorphine. Am J Addict 2006;15(3):258–9.
50. Balázs E, Ruszwurm A, Székely M, et al. [Old age and kidneys]. Orv Hetil 2008; 149(17):789–94 [in Hungarian].
51. Vadivelu N, Hines R. Management of chronic pain in the elderly: focus on transdermal buprenorphine. Clin Interv Aging 2008;3(3):421–30.
52. Koppert W, Ihmsen H, Körber N, et al. Different profiles of buprenorphine-induced analgesia and antihyperalgesia in a human pain model. Pain 2005; 118(1–2):15–22.
53. Lai S, Yao Y, Lo D. A survey of buprenorphine related deaths in Singapore. Forensic Sci Int 2006;162(1–3):80–6.
54. Lai SH, Teo CE. Buprenorphine-associated deaths in Singapore. Ann Acad Med Singapore 2006;35(7):508–11.
55. Ibrahim R, Wilson J, Thorsby M, et al. Effect of buprenorphine on CYP3A activity in rat and human liver microsomes. Life Sci 2000;66(14):1293–8.

Anesthesia for Patients on Buprenorphine

Ethan O. Bryson, MD[a], Scott Lipson, MD[a],
Clifford Gevirtz, MD, MPH[b,*]

KEYWORDS

• Opioids • Buprenorphine • Naloxine • Methadone • Addiction

Opioid abuse is a devastating, costly, and growing problem in the United States, and one for which treatment can be complicated by barriers such as access to care and legal issues.

Only 12% to 15% of the opioid-dependent population is enrolled in methadone maintenance programs.[1] A significant breakthrough occurred with passage of the Drug Addiction Treatment Act of 2000 (DATA 2000). For the first time in approximately 80 years, physicians could legally prescribe opioid medications for the treatment of opioid addiction. The opiate, so designated, was buprenorphine (Subutex) (**Fig. 1**).

Two years later, the U.S. Food and Drug Administration (FDA) approved buprenorphine/naloxone (Suboxone), a sublingual preparation of buprenorphine and naloxone, intended for the treatment of opioid-dependent individuals.[2] Unlike other opioid-abuse treatments, these formulations can be prescribed legally and managed by specially certified clinicians in an office-based setting, as opposed to the ongoing monitoring and observation required for methadone-maintenance programs.

At the current stage of medication development for opioid addiction, buprenorphine is nearly ideal, because it can be adjusted rapidly with minimal risk for inducing severe consequences. Buprenorphine also has a low abuse potential when combined with naloxone. In this combination product, attempts to use the drug through snorting, injecting, or cooking the tablet releases the antagonist drug naloxone, which in turn produces the withdrawal syndrome in opioid-dependent patients.

Both the increased access to treatment and the improved safety profile make buprenorphine/naloxone an attractive and significant treatment option. Anesthesiologists must be familiar with this medication, because it poses unique challenges in acute pain management for the growing population of patients maintained on buprenorphine/naloxone who present to the perioperative environment.

[a] Department of Anesthesia, Mount Sinai Medical Center, 1 Gustave Levy Plaza, New York, NY 10029, USA
[b] Department of Anesthesiology Louisiana State University Health Sciences Center, 433 Bolivar Street, New Orleans, LA 70112, USA
* Corresponding author.
E-mail address: cliffgevirtzmd@yahoo.com

Anesthesiology Clin 28 (2010) 611–617
doi:10.1016/j.anclin.2010.08.005
1932-2275/10/$ – see front matter © 2010 Elsevier Inc. All rights reserved.

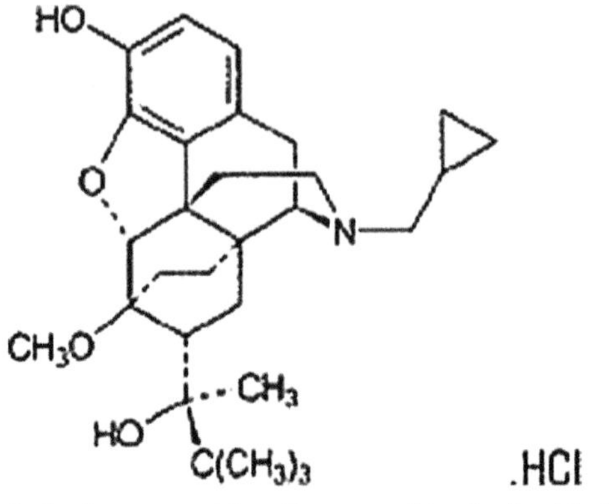

Fig. 1. Structural formula for buprenorphine. Buprenorphine hydrochloride is a white powder, weakly acidic with limited solubility in water (17 mg/mL). Chemically, buprenorphine is 17-(cyclo-propylmethyl)–α–(1,1-dimethylethyl)–4,5–epoxy-18,19-dihydro-3-hydroxy-6-methoxy-α-methyl-6,14-ethenomorphinan-7-methanol, hydrochloride [5α,7αS|]-. Buprenorphine hydrochloride has the molecular formula C29H41NO4 HCl and the molecular weight is 504.10.

OPIOID RECEPTORS

Initial studies identified three types of opioid receptors: mu, kappa, and sigma.[3] This classification has since been expanded to include the newly identified delta and epsilon receptors, three different subtypes of mu receptors, three different subtypes of kappa receptors, and two distinct forms of the delta receptor.

Different opioid receptors seem to be responsible for the different effects caused by the agents that bind to them. Endogenous opioids seem to have little selectivity for specific opioid receptors, whereas synthetic opioids may be designed to be highly selective for a specific receptor.[4] Most clinically used opioids (eg, morphine, oxycodone, fentanyl) are selective for the mu opioid receptors.

The expanded safety profile of buprenorphine has made it the first opioid treatment option that can be managed and prescribed by any certified medical doctor in an office-based setting. This management allows patients to live a more regular life while getting treatment for their addiction.

Characteristics of Buprenorphine/Naloxone

The use of buprenorphine is increasing. Of the estimated 1.2 million patients dependent on opioids in 2005,[5] only approximately 100,000 had been placed on buprenorphine treatment.[6] According to the manufacturer, by 2008 the estimate for use worldwide had risen to 400,000 patients.[7] Currently, buprenorphine is sold under the trade name of Suboxone, which is a formulation of buprenorphine and naloxone, in a 4:1 ratio. Subutex is a formulation that contains only buprenorphine and is used as the first induction onto the partial agonist drug during detoxification from illicit medications.

In the combination form, naloxone is added to the buprenorphine formulation in an attempt to prevent diversion and subsequent misuse through the parenteral or intranasal routes. The naloxone is not absorbed in clinically relevant amounts by the patient if taken sublingually as intended, thus leaving the opioid agonist effects of buprenorphine to predominate. Interestingly, naloxone does not necessarily prevent diversion; in fact, the buprenorphine/naloxone product has some value on the street for mitigating the effects of withdrawal associated with opioid abuse when preferred opioids are not available. When taken parenterally by patients physically dependent on full agonist opioids, the opioid antagonism of naloxone may cause withdrawal effects.

Suboxone is currently a Schedule III drug under the Convention on Psychotropic Substances Controlled Substances Act. Just before approval by the FDA, Suboxone was rescheduled from Schedule V, the schedule with the lowest restriction and penalties for misuse, to Schedule III, to reflect its potential for diversion and abuse.

Under this classification, any doctor who becomes specially certified to prescribe buprenorphine/naloxone may treat opioid addiction in the office. The certification process is simple and requires practitioners only to participate in one 8-hour continuing medical educational program and send a formal notice to the Department of Health and Human Services that they intends to prescribe these medications for detoxification purposes. A separate registration is not required if the medication is prescribed for intraoperative or pain management purposes only. Similarly, the intravenous form is specifically labeled "not for detoxification."

Buprenorphine, a semisynthetic opioid, acts as a partial mu opioid agonist and as an antagonist at the k opioid receptors. Although buprenorphine has a very high potency, 25-fold to 50-fold higher than morphine at low doses, its full opioid agonist affects are lower. Therefore, it has an improved safety profile compared with methadone.[8]

The affinity of buprenorphine for mu and kappa receptors is high, 1000-fold higher then morphine, and dissociation from the receptors is extremely slow. Compared with fentanyl, which has a dissociation half time of 7 minutes, the dissociation half-time for buprenorphine from the mu receptor is 166 minutes. These traits of buprenorphine limit the opioid "high" associated with pure mu agonists such as methadone. At higher doses, the agonist effects of the drug plateau, providing a ceiling effect, allowing a larger therapeutic window.

Starting doses of 4 to 8 mg are used to treat moderate to severe pain. The usual maximum recommended dose is 24 mg/d, and is needed only in patients previously taking large doses of opiates (eg, >120 mg/d of methadone or 200 mg/d of morphine). It is important to understand that the pharmacodynamics of the drug require a slower titration for pain relief (ie, add 4 mg every 20 minutes) rather than proceeding straight to the maximum dose.

Use during pregnancy

Because of the lack of comprehensive data on the safety of buprenorphine during pregnancy, pregnant women who conceive while on buprenorphine treatment should be advised to transfer to methadone maintenance. However, some pregnant women may decline this transfer. Clinical situations may arise where it seems "less unsafe" for a pregnant woman to continue buprenorphine during pregnancy than to relapse to dependent heroin use. Therefore, in pregnant women who use heroin, the balance of risks must be considered. The dangers of maintaining dependent opioid use, particularly illicit heroin use, during pregnancy may well be significantly greater than the risks of buprenorphine maintenance for these women and their babies. The substantial body of knowledge regarding the safety of methadone treatment during pregnancy must also be weighed in the calculus of decision-making.

An advantage for the neonate was discerned by Johnson and colleagues,[9] who conducted a meta-analysis of the incidence of withdrawal symptoms from buprenorphine in neonates. Although an estimated 55% to 94% of infants born to opioid-dependent mothers in the United States show signs of opioid withdrawal, buprenorphine has been reported to produce little or no autonomic signs or symptoms of opioid withdrawal after abrupt termination in adults. The authors reviewed 21 published reports representing approximately 15 evaluable cohorts of infants exposed to buprenorphine in utero. Of approximately 309 infants exposed, a neonatal abstinence syndrome (NAS) was reported in 62% infants, with 48% requiring treatment; apparently more than 40% of these cases are confounded by illicit drug use. The NAS associated with buprenorphine generally appears within 12 to 48 hours, peaks at 72 to 96 hours, and lasts for 120 to 168 hours. These results seem similar to or less than those observed after in utero exposure to methadone. From a review of the literature, buprenorphine seems to be safe and effective in both mother and infant, with an NAS that may differ from methadone both qualitatively and quantitatively.

Pediatric use

Michel and Zernikow[10] reviewed the pediatric data on buprenorphine, especially with respect to the long-term application in children experiencing chronic pain and to pediatric pharmacokinetic and pharmacodynamic data after repeated sublingual or long-term transdermal administration. After single-dose buprenorphine, children seem to exhibit a larger clearance related to body weight and a longer duration of action compared with adults.

If combined with other opioids or sedatives or if the metabolite norbuprenorphine (norBUP) cumulates, the risk of respiratory depression is difficult to estimate. Clear-cut evidence that there is a ceiling of buprenorphine-induced respiratory depression is lacking with regard to children. Because of its various application routes, long duration of action, and metabolism largely independent of renal function, buprenorphine is of special clinical interest in pediatrics, especially for postoperative pain and cancer pain control. There is no reason to expect that effects in children are fundamentally different from those in adults.

However, Geib and colleagues[11] reported a series of five toddlers with respiratory and mental status depression after unintentional buprenorphine exposure. Despite buprenorphine's partial agonist activity and ceiling effect on respiratory depression, all children required hospital admission and either opioid-antagonist therapy or mechanical ventilation. Results of routine urine toxicology screening for opioids were negative in all cases. Confirmatory testing was sent for one child and returned with a positive result. The increasing use of buprenorphine as a home-based therapy for opioid addiction in the United States raises public health concerns for the pediatric population.

Use in renal failure

Hand and colleagues[12] studied buprenorphine clearance in patients with normal and impaired renal function and found that it was similar (934 and 1102 mL min-1, respectively), as were dose-corrected plasma concentrations of buprenorphine. In patients with renal failure, plasma concentrations of norBUP increased by a median of 5 times, and buprenorphine 3-gluconate concentrations by a median of 15 times. However, because both of these metabolites are not clinically active, the doses used in renal failure do not need to be modified.

Use in liver disease

Berson and colleagues[13] reported on four cases of former heroin addicts infected with hepatitis C virus who had been placed on substitution therapy with buprenorphine. These patients exhibited a marked increase in serum alanine amino transferase after injecting buprenorphine intravenously, and three of them also became jaundiced. Interruption of buprenorphine injections was associated with prompt recovery, even though two of these patients continued buprenorphine sublingually. A fifth patient with the hepatitis C and human immunodeficiency viruses, developed jaundice and asterixis with panlobular liver necrosis and microvesicular steatosis after using sublingual buprenorphine and small doses of paracetamol and aspirin.

These investigators concluded that although buprenorphine hepatitis is most uncommon even after intravenous misuse, addicts placed on buprenorphine substitution should be repeatedly warned not to use it intravenously. Higher drug concentrations could trigger hepatitis in a few intravenous users, possibly those whose mitochondrial function is already impaired by viral infections and other factors.

This issue was further examined by Petry and colleagues,[14] who assessed changes in liver enzyme levels among opioid-dependent patients treated with buprenorphine. They evaluated liver enzyme levels among 120 individuals before treatment and after a minimum of 40 days of buprenorphine treatment (2, 4, or 8 mg/70 kg/d). Among patients with a history of hepatitis, aspartate aminotransferase (AST) and alanine aminotransferase levels significantly increased ($P<.05$) with buprenorphine treatment. The investigators determined that the odds of observing an increase in AST depend on the buprenorphine dose ($P<.05$; odds ratio, 1.23 per 1-mg increase in dose). These results suggest that liver enzyme levels should be monitored very carefully when patients with hepatitis are treated with buprenorphine. Anesthesiologists would be well advised to use agents that are not extensively metabolized by the liver and to use techniques that maintain hepatic blood flow.

SPECIAL CONSIDERATIONS FOR ACUTE AND CHRONIC PAIN CONTROL

Although limited published data are available involving patients on buprenorphine who present for procedures or surgery requiring anesthesia, case reports have offered suggestions for the management of perioperative pain.

The successful management of postcesarean section pain in two patients maintained on buprenorphine was achieved using intravenous morphine patient-controlled analgesia (PCA) and oral oxycodone at markedly elevated doses.[15] In both cases the patients were able to continue buprenorphine therapy throughout their hospital stay. Each was able to experience acceptable levels of pain control with a total dose of 180 mg/d of morphine. When switched to oral medications, one patient was able to achieve pain relief with 60 mg/d of oxycodone and 6 g of acetaminophen; however, the second patient required 600 mg of ibuprofen every 8 hours in addition to this regimen.

Supplemental doses of sublingual buprenorphine have successfully been used to control postoperative pain in a patient maintained on buprenorphine.[16] This patient received general anesthesia for the removal of breast implants and was instructed to take supplemental buprenorphine, 2 to 4 mg every 4 to 6 hours, in addition to her 24 mg/d maintenance dose, as needed for pain. She was able to experience adequate pain relief with supplemental buprenorphine, requiring a total dose of 72 mg on postoperative day 1, and tapering back to 24 mg/d by postoperative day 11.

Recommendations have been proposed for controlling acute pain in patients maintained on buprenorphine through using shorter-acting opioid analgesics in addition to the maintenance dose of buprenorphine, and titrating to effective pain control.[17] Through dividing the buprenorphine maintenance dose over the course of 24 hours and relying on the analgesic properties of buprenorphine, replacing the buprenorphine with methadone and then adding another opioid analgesic, or replacing the buprenorphine with another opioid analgesic altogether, adequate pain relief can be achieved in the acute setting.

In any case, patients maintained on buprenorphine typically require much higher doses of opioid agonists to experience adequate pain relief.

Options for Pain Control in Patients on Buprenorphine Maintenance

Some patients on buprenorphine may desire to avoid opioids, if at all possible, because of the risk of restarting opiate addiction. If a patient is on buprenorphine maintenance therapy, several options for intraoperative and postoperative pain control can be considered, including preemptive administration of celecoxib or pregabalin, preloading of the incision sites with local anesthetic before incision, placement of an epidural catheter for intraoperative and postoperative use, and postoperative ketorolac administration.

High-dose buprenorphine used for opioid substitution has a long half-life, which combines with its strong affinity for the mu opioid receptor and slow receptor dissociation to account for the long duration of action of the drug.[18]

Studies have shown that the opioid-blocking action of buprenorphine can persist for several days after discontinuation of the medication, which would make conventional pain therapy difficult or impossible. In one study of male subjects with a recent history of opioid addiction, sublingual buprenorphine at a dose of 8 mg/d for 1 week blocked the subjective and respiratory depressant effects of hydromorphone, 4 mg intramuscularly, for up to 5 days after discontinuation of the buprenorphine.[19]

Because buprenorphine is a partial agonist, patients maintained on this drug have a significantly increased tolerance for opioids and may require extremely high doses to achieve analgesia. This affinity of buprenorphine for mu receptors is so high that it reportedly has been used to reverse heroin overdose.[20] No controlled trials show the extent to which required doses of opioid agonists administered to patients maintained on buprenorphine are increased. One option for the treatment of acute pain is to increase the dose of buprenorphine itself to achieve pain relief, although there is a ceiling effect and if analgesia is not achieved other options must be considered. The use of nonopioid analgesics, local or regional techniques, or a combination of techniques may prove to be effective for patients taking buprenorphine or other partial agonists, or agonist/antagonists such as pentazocine, butorphanol, and nalbuphine.

SUMMARY

The FDA approved Suboxone in 2002 for detoxification and maintenance treatment of opioid dependence as an alternative to methadone. In combination with naloxone, it has been prescribed to an increasing number of patients. Results of a recent multicenter study indicate preference for buprenorphine/naloxone over buprenorphine alone (54% vs 31%, respectively), citing the preferable tablet size and taste and sublingual dissolution of the former compound.[21]

Furthermore, a budgetary impact analysis in Spain showed that additional costs were minimal (€9, or approximately $12).[13,22] Because buprenorphine is a partial opioid agonist with high affinity for mu receptors, patients maintained on this agent are prevented from experiencing the euphoria associated with opioid use, and require substantially higher doses of opioids to achieve the same level of pain control. When these patients present for procedures or surgery requiring anesthesia, standard opioid-based anesthetic techniques are not sufficient and alternate anesthetic agents must be used. The anesthesiologist must be aware of this need and be prepared to adjust analgesic dosages accordingly.

REFERENCES

1. Raisch DW, Fye CL, Boardman KD, et al. Opioid dependence treatment, including buprenorphine/naloxone. Ann Pharmacother 2002;36:312–21.
2. Ling W. Buprenorphine for opioid dependence. Expert Rev Neurother 2009;9(5): 609–16.
3. Pleuvry BJ. The endogenous opioid system. Anaesth Pharmacol Rev 1993;1: 114–23.

4. Coda BA. Opioids. In: Barash PG, editor. Clinical anesthesia. 5th edition. Phila-delphia: Lippincott; 2006. p. 353–83.
5. Inter-University Consortium for Political and Social Research. National Survey on Drug Use and Health, 2005. Available at: www.icpsr.umich.edu/cocoon/ICPSR/STUDY/04596.xml. Accessed September 21, 2010.
6. The Determinations Report: A Report on the Physician Waiver Program Estab-lished by the Drug Addiction Treatment Act of 2000 ("DATA"). Available at: http://buprenorphine.samhsa.gov/SAMHSA_Determinations_Report.pdf.   Ac-cessed September 21, 2010.
7. Suboxone facts for patients [patient brochure]. Richmond (VA): Reckitt Benckiser Pharmaceuticals Inc; 2008.
8. Orman JS, Keating GM. Buprenorphine/naloxone: a review of its use in the treat-ment of opioid dependence. Drugs 2009;69(5):577–607.
9. Johnson RE, Jones HE, Fischer G. Use of buprenorphine in pregnancy: patient management and effects on the neonate. Drug Alcohol Depend 2003; 70(Suppl 1):S87–101.
10. Michel E, Zernikow B. Buprenorphine in children. A clinical and pharmacological review. Schmerz 2006;20:40–50.
11. Geib AJ, Babu K, Burns M, et al. Adverse effects in children after unintentional buprenorphine exposure. Pediatrics 2006;118:1746–51.
12. Hand CW, Sear JW, Uppington J. Buprenorphine disposition in patients with renal impairment: single and continuous dosing, with special reference to metabolites. Br J Anaesth 1990;64:276–82.
13. Berson A, Gervais A, Cazals D, et al. Hepatitis after intravenous buprenorphine misuse in heroin addicts. J Hepatol 2001;34:346–50.
14. Petry NM, Bickel WK, Piasecki D, et al. Elevated liver enzyme levels in opioid-dependent patients with hepatitis treated with buprenorphine. Am J Addict 2000;9:265–9.
15. Jones HE, Johnson RE, Milio L. Post-cesarean pain management of patients maintained on methadone or buprenorphine. Am J Addict 2006;15(3):258–9.
16. Book SW, Myrick H, Malcolm R, et al. Buprenorphine for postoperative pain following general surgery in a buprenorphine-maintained patient. Am J Psychi-atry 2007;164:979.
17. Alford DP, Compton P, Samet JH. Acute pain management for patients receiving main-tenance methadone or buprenorphine therapy. Ann Intern Med 2006;144(2):127–34.
18. Robert DM, Meyer-Witting M. High-dose buprenorphine: perioperative precau-tions and management strategies. Anaesth Intensive Care 2005;33:17–25.
19. Schuh KJ, Walsh SL, Stitzerr ML. Onset, magnitude and duration of opioid blockade produced by buprenorphine and naltrexone in humans. Psychophar-macology 1999;145:162–74.
20. Welsh C, Sherman SG, Tobin KE. A case of heroin overdose reversed by sublin-gually administered buprenorphine/naloxone (Suboxone®). Addiction 2008;103: 1226–8.
21. Dalouede JP, Caer Y, Galland P, et al. Preference for buprenorphine/naloxone and buprenorphine among patients receiving buprenorphine maintenance therapy in France: a prospective, multicenter study. J Subst Abuse Treat 2010;38(1):83–9.
22. Martine-Raga J, Gonzalez Salz F, Pascual C, et al. Suboxone (buprenorphine/naloxone) as an agonist opioid treatment in Spain: a budgetary impact analysis. Eur Addict Res 2010;16(1):31–42.

Intravenous Acetaminophen

Jonathan S. Jahr, MD*, Vivian K. Lee, MD

KEYWORDS

- Intravenous acetaminophen • Acute pain • Fever • Analgesia
- Perioperative • Multimodal analgesia

Acetaminophen was first used clinically in 1887 but only much later—during the mid-1950s—was it widely marketed in the United States.[1] It has since gone on to become one of the mostly widely used and safest antipyretic and analgesic drugs available.[1–3] Acetaminophen has a high therapeutic index (approximately 10),[1] indicative of its efficacy-to-safety ratio and a long and respected legacy as a safe and effective choice for treating pain and fever in a wide range of patient types. This is particularly true in the hospital setting, where it may be successfully combined with other analgesics to manage postoperative pain.

Acetaminophen is a synthetic, nonopiate, centrally acting analgesic and antipyretic derived from *p*-aminophenol. It has not been shown to affect platelet function, increase surgical bleeding, or affect kidney function[4] and is, therefore, appropriate for use at any time during the perioperative period. The opioid-sparing qualities of acetaminophen have been recognized,[5] and these properties may lead to acetaminophen being incorporated effectively as an adjunct therapy. Unlike nonsteroidal anti-inflammatory drugs (NSAIDs), acetaminophen has no substantial peripheral anti-inflammatory activity.[6]

Despite more than a century of study, the mechanism of action of acetaminophen is not definitively known, although it is believed that part of its analgesic action may be associated with centrally acting cyclooxygenase (COX) inhibition with weak peripheral effects.[6–8] This central action could explain the antipyretic effect of acetaminophen, and the minimal peripheral effects could be responsible for the lack of gastric irritation and clotting abnormalities often associated with NSAIDs. Owing to its efficacy, safety, and lack of the side effects associated with other analgesics, acetaminophen has been considered a fundamental component of the multimodal analgesic approach to which NSAIDs and other drugs are added.[9] Moreover,

Financial disclosures: J.S. Jahr - Speaker's Bureau, Cadence Pharmaceuticals; Principal Investigator on UPSA/BMS Phase 3 study and BMS Phase 3 studies.
Department of Anesthesiology, David Geffen School of Medicine at UCLA, Ronald Reagan UCLA Medical Center, 757 Westwood Plaza, Suite 3304, Los Angeles, CA 90095-7403, USA
* Corresponding author.
E-mail address: jsjahr@mednet.ucla.edu

Anesthesiology Clin 28 (2010) 619–645
doi:10.1016/j.anclin.2010.08.006 **anesthesiology.theclinics.com**

acetaminophen has been formally recommended for first-line use as one of the possible components of multimodal analgesic regimens for postoperative pain management by the American Society of Anesthesiologists.[10]

In the postoperative period, effective acute pain control is essential for optimal recovery and patient satisfaction. Nonetheless, management of postoperative pain remains suboptimal—in one survey, approximately 80% of patients reported moderate to acute pain after surgery,[11] and other reports indicate that approximately 50% of patients experience uncontrolled pain.[12] Postsurgical pain is associated with more than patient discomfort; it is also the most common cause of unanticipated readmissions for same-day surgery.[12] The need to address postoperative pain complications is compounded by the increasing number of surgical procedures performed in the United States. In 2006 alone, 46 million inpatient procedures were reported.[13]

Adequate postoperative pain control provides advantages to patients beyond immediate clinical benefits, such as increased satisfaction and improved sleep. Recovery may be more rapid, resulting in less time in the postanesthesia care unit; shorter hospital stays; less need for rehabilitative services; lower risks of postoperative complications, such as the development of long-term or chronic pain conditions,[12] which may be associated with acute postoperative pain[14]; fewer neuroendocrine side effects of injury; and a lower risk of deep vein thrombosis and pulmonary effects.[15]

Acetaminophen is commonly available in oral and suppository formulations, which are not always appropriate for perioperative use. The recent clinical development of an intravenous (IV) formulation for use in the United States may have important implications for the perioperative management of pain, because IV delivery allows for administration of analgesics for pre-emptive management of pain. IV administration of analgesics is the preferred route in the immediate postoperative period, especially in situations where a patient is unable to take medications by mouth (eg, nothing by mouth status, severe nausea, odynophagia, or dysphagia), when a faster onset of analgesia is desired, or when it may be prudent to attenuate postoperative pain as early and effectively as possible, before the onset of acute pain.[16] IV acetaminophen supports this need for rapid analgesia, in part because patients dos not have to be fully recovered from general anesthesia before receiving the medication, permitting the initiation of effective analgesic therapy in the early phase of the postoperative period.[16–18]

Recent evidence-based developments in postoperative pain management have focused on balancing effective analgesia with patient safety by optimizing analgesic delivery and refining multimodal analgesia techniques. The conceptual framework of multimodal analgesia was introduced approximately 2 decades ago as a method for improving pain control and reducing the incidence of opioid-related adverse events.[19,20] One multimodal strategy for the management of postoperative pain is represented in a stepwise structure (**Fig. 1**).[21] The rationale for this strategy is based on the known additive or synergistic effects between different classes of analgesics, which allow a reduction in any one individual drug dose, thus potentially lowering the incidence of that medication's adverse effects. Several studies have described the clinically significant beneficial effects of multimodal analgesia on pain control and the recovery process.[19] The reduced incidence of adverse effects and improved pain control demonstrated with multimodal analgesia techniques may result in shorter hospitalization times, improved recovery and function, and decreased health care costs.[22]

IV acetaminophen has been approved for the treatment of acute pain and fever in approximately 80 countries outside of the United States since its approval in 2001,

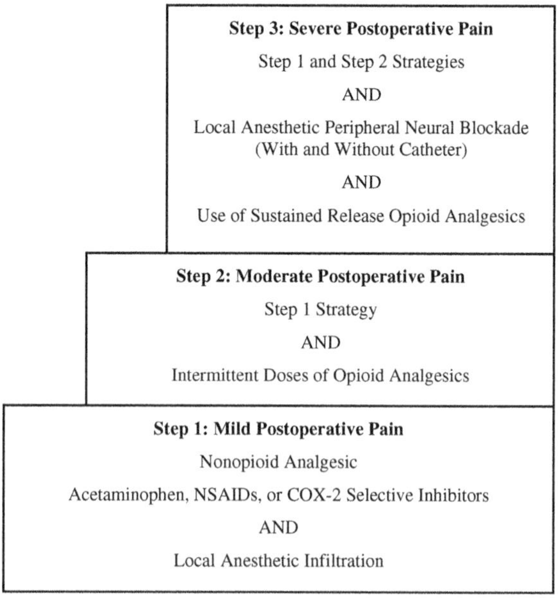

Fig. 1. The proposed ladder of therapy for multimodal postoperative pain management. Step 1 therapy represents mild pain. Step 2 and Step 3 therapies are added as the intensity of anticipated or actual degree of postoperative pain increases. (*Reprinted from* Crews JC. Multimodal pain management strategies for office-based and ambulatory procedures. JAMA 2002;288:629–32; with permission.)

as reported in mid-2009; more than 437 million doses had been distributed in Europe.[23] As development of IV acetaminophen continues in the United States, it is intriguing to explore how such a formulation may have an impact on the current state of postoperative analgesia. IV administration of acetaminophen may provide rapid and predictable analgesia that can be subsequently maintained by oral delivery.[24] IV administration may also result in a more rapid onset of analgesia with more predictable pharmacokinetics than the oral or rectal formulations.[1,3] Speed of onset compared with the oral route may at times be especially important.[3] The advantages afforded by IV acetaminophen may result in its assuming a key role in multimodal pain management, because it has been found safe to use along with other drugs and has few clinically significant drug interactions.[24,25]

PHARMACOKINETIC AND PHARMACODYNAMIC PROPERTIES

IV delivery of acetaminophen results in rapid and high plasma concentrations and a clinical analgesic effect that occurs within 5 minutes of administration.[26] IV acetaminophen has been shown to achieve higher maximum concentration (C_{max}) and earlier time to maximum concentration (T_{max}) than bioequivalent oral or rectal formulations with less intrasubject variability.[1,3,27–29] The standard dose used in US adult clinical trials was 1 g, infused over 15 minutes, every 4 to 6 hours to a daily maximum of 4 g. The mean C_{max} after a standard 15-minute infusion has been reported to be 29.9 mg/L,[30] which is approximately 70% higher than the mean C_{max} observed at an equivalent oral dose.[29] The higher C_{max} with IV acetaminophen does not seem to compromise the safety profile or the production of glutathione conjugates compared with oral acetaminophen, because the C_{max} at this dose remains far below the 150 mg/L concentration considered the threshold for potential hepatotoxicity.[31] The median time to reach T_{max} for IV acetaminophen, which occurs at the end of the 15-minute infusion,[30] is much faster than typically reported for oral or rectal formulations (>45 minutes).[1]

With respect to its analgesic and antipyretic effects, acetaminophen's pharmacodynamic effect seems to correlate well with cerebrospinal fluid (CSF) levels. Acetaminophen readily penetrates an intact blood-brain barrier, and acetaminophen concentrations in the CSF are linearly dose proportional, with plasma levels after IV doses of 500 mg to 2000 mg.[32] In children and adults, acetaminophen is detectable in the CSF within minutes after IV administration (studies evaluated both IV acetaminophen and IV propacetamol, the prodrug to acetaminophen, which required reconstitution before administration and resulted in frequent injection-site pain reactions, leading to its replacement by the ready-to-use and better tolerated IV acetaminophen).[33,34] The rapid CSF penetration and earlier and higher C_{max} observed with IV acetaminophen seem responsible for its more rapid onset of action and peak efficacy compared with oral or rectal acetaminophen.[35]

Acetaminophen metabolism is well characterized and is not dependent on route of administration. Acetaminophen is metabolized by the liver via three pathways: glucuronidation (approximately 85%), sulfation, and oxidation.[36] The oxidation pathway produces N-acetyl-p-benzoquinone imine (NAPQI), a highly reactive intermediate, primarily by cytochrome P450 isoenzyme, CYP2E1.[37] NAPQI conjugation with intracellular glutathione results in products excreted in the urine as thiol metabolites.[36,37] NAPQI may cause hepatotoxicity if glutathione stores are depleted, most commonly after a massive, acute acetaminophen overdose.

Regardless of route of delivery, the terminal elimination half-life of acetaminophen is approximately 2 to 4 hours in children, adolescents, and adults. It is slightly longer in infants and neonates and is longer still in premature neonates.[1] Compared across age groups, pharmacokinetic (PK) parameter estimates for IV acetaminophen were similar in children, adolescents, and adults, when normalized for body weight.[38] Acetaminophen clearance in adults averaged 0.27 L/h/kg and 0.28 and 0.33 L/h/kg in children and adolescents, respectively.[38] Maturational effects in acetaminophen metabolism in neonates and infants are well characterized and have demonstrated a limited ability to metabolize acetaminophen via glucuronide.[39] Neonates and infants, therefore, predominantly metabolize acetaminophen via the sulfation pathway, which may help explain reduced clearance.[39,40] This maturational effect may result in less production and accumulation of NAPQI and, consequently, a decreased susceptibility to acetaminophen hepatotoxicity in infants and children.[41]

PK considerations indicate that oral doses of acetaminophen are likely to expose the liver to maximal amounts of acetaminophen, due to its near complete absorption in the proximal small intestine, delivery into the portal vein, and first-pass metabolism. Conversely, IV dosing is expected to expose the liver to less acetaminophen, because the dose is distributed in the systemic circulation before being delivered to the liver via the hepatic artery. First-pass PK models have shown that the IV route of administration reduced initial hepatic acetaminophen exposure by approximately 2-fold as compared with the oral route.[42] Thus, the lack of a first-pass effect with IV acetaminophen administration may result in reduced hepatic acetaminophen exposure and an improved safety profile compared with equivalent doses of oral acetaminophen.

CLINICAL EFFICACY IN ADULTS: POSTOPERATIVE PAIN

Many randomized and controlled studies have been conducted outside of the United States demonstrating the efficacy and safety of IV acetaminophen. These studies have been reviewed in great detail by Duggan and Scott[43] and Malaise and colleagues.[3] More recently, and in anticipation of its availability in the United States, the results of several US clinical trials with IV acetaminophen have been completed with favorable results. Although the results of these studies have yet to be formally presented and are pending publication, they have essentially confirmed the favorable findings of the European experience with IV acetaminophen for the treatment of acute pain and fever.

US Studies: Acute Pain After Total Hip or Knee Arthroplasty

The primary evidence for efficacy and safety for IV acetaminophen in the treatment of moderate to severe pain in adults has been found in patients undergoing major orthopedic surgery. Sinatra and colleagues[44] conducted a randomized, double-blind, placebo- and active-controlled, single- and repeated-dose, 24-hour study at nine study centers in the United States. The primary objective of the study was to compare the analgesic efficacy and safety of a single and repeated (every 6 hours) doses of IV acetaminophen (1000 mg) to placebo in the treatment of adults with moderate to severe postoperative pain after total hip or knee replacement. Pain intensity (PI) was measured on a four-point verbal PI categorical scale and a four-point visual analog scale (VAS). The study included 101 patients, 49 in the IV acetaminophen group and 52 in the placebo group (an additional 50 patients were included in a propacetamol comparator arm).

Statistically significant differences favoring IV acetaminophen compared with placebo were observed for pain relief at 15 and 30 minutes ($P<.05$) and from 45 minutes to 6 hours ($P<.001$). Statistically significant differences favoring IV acetaminophen compared with placebo were also observed for the mean sum of PI differences from 15 minutes through 6 hours ($P<.05$).

Patients who received IV acetaminophen and required rescue analgesia had a significantly longer elapsed time to first-rescue medication and a significantly lower dose of medication (patient-controlled analgesia [PCA] morphine) over the first 6 hours. The median time to first rescue medication was 3 hours for those receiving IV acetaminophen and 0.8 hours for those in the placebo group ($P<.001$). Mean ($\pm$SD) patient-controlled analgesia (PCA morphine) consumption through 6 hours after the first dose of study medication was significantly lower for the IV acetaminophen group (9.7 $\pm$ 10.0 mg) than for the placebo group (17.8 $\pm$ 16.7 mg, $P<.01$), representing a 46% reduction in opioid consumption during the first 6 hours with IV acetaminophen. This trend was maintained over the 24 hours of evaluation (representing doses of study medication administered every 6 hours): mean ($\pm$SD) PCA morphine consumption was lower in the IV acetaminophen group (38.3 $\pm$ 35.1 mg) than in the placebo group (57.4 $\pm$ 52.3 mg), representing a 33% reduction in opioid consumption.[44]

Patients' global satisfaction at 24 hours was significantly higher in the IV acetaminophen group than in the placebo group ($P<.01$). Fair to excellent ratings were reported by 39 (80%) of 49 patients in the IV acetaminophen group compared with 34 (65%) of 52 placebo patients.[44]

US Studies: Acute Pain After Abdominal Laparoscopic Surgery

A second randomized, double-blind, placebo-controlled, multicenter, acute pain efficacy and safety study was conducted at 17 US sites in adults undergoing abdominal laparoscopic surgery. A total of 244 patients experiencing moderate to acute postsurgical pain (measured by a 4-point PI categorical scale and a VAS score $\geq$40 mm and $\leq$70 mm at rest on a 100-mm scale) were randomized to receive IV acetaminophen (1000 mg every 6 hours or 650 mg every 4 hours or matched placebo over 24 hours).[45]

For weighted sum of PI score differences using VAS 100 mm over 24 hours and weighted sum of PI scores using VAS 100 mm over 24 hours, IV acetaminophen (1000 mg) was significantly better than the combined placebo group at reducing pain ($P = .0068$). Statistically significant differences in weighted sum of pain relief scores and subject global evaluation scores favoring IV acetaminophen (1000 mg) over the combined placebo group ($P = .0006$ and $P = .0004$, respectively) were also reported. Time to meaningful pain relief after the first dose was significantly shorter in subjects who received IV acetaminophen (1000 mg) (<25 minutes) compared with subjects in the combined placebo group ($P = .0028$). The time to rescue medication and amount of rescue medication consumption favored IV acetaminophen but did not achieve statistical significance. Of all patients in both study arms, 40% to 50% required no rescue medication during the 24-hour treatment period, and this may have contributed to a reduced chance of demonstrating statistical significance. Results with the 650-mg dose were consistent with the 1000-mg dose; however, not all comparisons to placebo reached statistical significance.[45]

The preliminary summary results of these two multicenter US postoperative pain studies reveal the rapid and sustained pain relief provided by IV acetaminophen after surgical procedures and are significant additions to the already large body of clinical studies performed with IV acetaminophen. Single- and repeated-dose IV acetaminophen efficacy has been well documented in a variety of postoperative settings and patient populations across PI scores from mild to severe pain for periods up to 72 hours. A comprehensive list of published IV acetaminophen studies conducted in adults can be found in **Table 1**. In summary, these studies demonstrate the efficacy of IV acetaminophen across a broad range of pain types and intensities. In many studies, the onset of analgesic action for IV acetaminophen has been documented to occur just before or at the end of the 15-minute infusion. The peak effect as measured by PI or pain relief (PR) endpoints for the IV acetaminophen comparison with placebo has been shown in multiple studies not only statistically significant but also clinically meaningful. The opioid-sparing effect of IV acetaminophen remains somewhat controversial, however. Some, but not all, studies show a statistically significant reduction in opioid consumption. Certain studies have even shown that a substantial percentage of patients have been able to avoid the need for opioid rescue altogether.

The efficacy and safety of IV acetaminophen has also been shown in other unpublished but completed double-blind, placebo-controlled studies in a variety of postoperative pain models, including total hip arthroplasty[76,77] and vaginal hysterectomy.[78] In addition to demonstrating clinically relevant pain relief, reductions in opioid usage of up to 64% were observed in the IV acetaminophen groups compared with the placebo groups.[76–78] In those patients requiring rescue treatment, IV acetaminophen patients typically demonstrated a prolonged time to administration of such rescue.

CLINICAL EFFICACY IN ADULTS: FEVER

In addition to the treatment of acute pain, the possible usefulness of a parenteral antipyretic for the urgent treatment of fever/hyperthermia in patients who are unable to receive oral or rectally administered acetaminophen (eg, nothing by mouth status, immunocompromised patients, or immobilized patients) has also been examined.

The efficacy of IV acetaminophen (1000 mg) in the treatment of fever was evaluated in two randomized studies in 141 healthy adult men, 76 of whom received IV acetaminophen: a placebo-controlled trial and a second active-controlled trial versus oral acetaminophen (1000 mg).[79,80] Both trials evaluated the safety and efficacy of a single dose of IV acetaminophen in the treatment of fever induced by reference standard endotoxin.

A single dose of IV acetaminophen (1000 mg) had a superior and sustained antipyretic effect compared with placebo in blunting endotoxin-induced fever over a 6-hour study period (weighted sum of temperature differences over 6 hours, $P = .0001$).[79] The onset of the antipyretic effect was rapid, with a statistically significant difference from placebo detected by 30 minutes ($P = .0085$), 15 minutes after the end of the IV acetaminophen infusion. The durability of the treatment effect with IV acetaminophen was demonstrated by a substantially lower mean temperature compared with placebo at each time point from 30 minutes to 5.5 hours.

When compared with an equivalent dose of oral acetaminophen, a single dose of IV acetaminophen (1000 mg) demonstrated a faster onset of temperature reduction, with a more pronounced blunting of the reference standard endotoxin–induced fever during the first 2 hours compared with oral acetaminophen (1000 mg) (weighted sum of temperature differences over 2 hours, $P = .0039$).[80] The onset of the antipyretic effect was rapid, with a statistically significant difference from oral acetaminophen detected by 30 minutes, 15 minutes after the end of the IV acetaminophen infusion ($P = .0202$). For an hour afterwards, statistically significant reductions in mean temperature in favor of the IV acetaminophen group compared with the oral acetaminophen group were observed.

The antipyretic effect of IV acetaminophen in these two fever studies demonstrates that 1000 mg produces a rapid temperature-reducing effect that begins approximately 15 minutes after completion of the infusion, peaks at approximately 1 hour and may last for up to 6 hours. In addition, the results of several published studies with oral acetaminophen support the antipyretic efficacy of doses ranging from 500 to 1000 mg in fever of infectious origin[81] and in endotoxin-induced fever.[82–84]

CLINICAL EFFICACY IN PEDIATRIC PATIENTS: POSTOPERATIVE PAIN AND FEVER

Acetaminophen has a long history of safe and effective clinical use and is the first-line choice for the treatment of pain and fever in pediatric patients.[85] Despite this, oral delivery may not represent an ideal route of administration, especially in an inpatient setting. Rectally administered acetaminophen has been routinely used in its place, but absorption via this route may be slow and erratic,[1,86] which may produce subtherapeutic plasma levels or expose neonates and infants to potentially toxic levels of the product. Because of the delayed absorption, using higher doses has been suggested when administering acetaminophen by the rectal route in children as well as adults. Higher rectal doses (45 mg/kg), however, may expose some children to the potential risk of drug accumulation and possible toxicity.[87,88]

European studies on IV formulations of acetaminophen have characterized its PK profile and shown its safety in a wide range of pediatric patients.[89–92] A summary of published studies of IV acetaminophen in pediatric patients can be found in **Table 2**. Despite the strict and ethical limitations of pediatric clinical studies, two recent reports highlight the usefulness of IV acetaminophen for the management of acute pain and fever in this population.

Evidence of efficacy and safety of IV acetaminophen in the treatment of acute pain in pediatric subjects has been investigated for patients undergoing unilateral inguinal

Table 1
Published randomized controlled trials supporting the efficacy and safety of IV acetaminophen in adults

Author (Year)	Pain Model Studied	Comparator/Control	Study Medication Regimen	Total No. of Subjects (Completers/Group)	Study Summary
Alhashemi, 2006[46]	Cesarean section	Oral ibuprofen	IV APAP 1000 mg/PO placebo vs PO ibuprofen 400 mg/IV placebo q6h × 48 h	N = 45 IV APAP: 22 PO ibuprofen: 23	IV APAP provided comparable analgesia to PO ibuprofen
Api, 2009[47]	Fractional curettage	Placebo	IV APAP 1000 mg vs placebo, single dose	N = 70 IV APAP: 36 Placebo: 34	No significant differences noted in pain response; however, all patients had mild to moderate pain (<4 on 10-pt VAS)
Arici, 2009[48]	Total abdominal hysterectomy	Placebo	IV APAP 1000 mg before Ind or before EOS vs placebo, single dose	N = 90 IV APAP Ind: 30 IV APAP EOS: 30 Placebo: 30	Pain response and morphine consumption were significantly better for IV APAP than for placebo; placebo group had significantly greater incidence of nausea, vomiting and pruritus; and significantly longer hospital stays
Atef, 2008[49]	Tonsillectomy	Placebo	IV APAP 1000 mg vs placebo q6h × 24 h	N = 76 IV APAP: 38 Placebo: 38	100% of Patients in the placebo group required rescue analgesia over 24 h vs 29% in the IV APAP group

Study	Condition	Comparator	Intervention/Dose	N	Outcome
Bektas, 2009[50]	Renal colic	Morphine and placebo	IV APAP 1000 mg vs IV morphine 0.1 mg/kg vs placebo, single dose	N = 146, IV APAP: 46, IV morphine: 49, Placebo: 51	IV APAP produced comparable pain relief to IV morphine and significantly better pain relief than placebo
Cakan, 2008[51]	Lumbar laminectomy/discectomy	Placebo	IV APAP 1000 mg vs placebo q6h × 24 h	N = 40, IV APAP: 20, Placebo: 20	PI was significantly higher in the placebo group at 12, 18, and 24 h than in the IV APAP group; no significant differences in morphine consumption; reduced vomiting in the IV APAP group
Canbay, 2008[52]	Propofol injection pain	IV lidocaine and placebo	IV APAP 50 mg or IV lidocaine 40 mg in saline vs placebo, single dose	N = 150, IV APAP: 50, Lidocaine: 50, Placebo: 50	Incidence of pain on injection of propofol with IV APAP (22%) and IV lidocaine (8%) was significantly better than with placebo (64%)
Cattabriga, 2007[4]	Cardiac surgery	Placebo	IV APAP 1000 mg vs placebo q6h × 72 h	N = 113, IV APAP: 56, Placebo: 57	At 12, 18, and 24 h after surgery, the IV APAP group had significantly less pain at rest than the placebo group; cumulative morphine consumption was ~ 50% less with IV APAP (not statistically significant)

(continued on next page)

Table 1
(continued)

Author (Year)	Pain Model Studied	Comparator/Control	Study Medication Regimen	Total No. of Subjects (Completers/Group)	Study Summary
Celik, 2009[53]	Hand surgery with IVRA	IVRA lidocaine and placebo	IV APAP 200 mg in the IVRA vs IV APAP 200 mg IV (in nonoperative arm) vs placebo, single dose	N = 90 IVRA/IV APAP: 30 IV APAP: 30 Placebo: 30	IV APAP added to the IVRA produced superior pain relief and significantly reduced morphine consumption compared with placebo or IV APAP infusion in the nonoperative arm
Evron, 2008[54]	Spontaneous labor	CE vs CE + IV PCA remifentanil vs CE + IV APAP vs IV PCA remifentanil alone	CE with 0.2% ropivacaine vs CE + IV remifentanil vs CE + IV APAP 1 g vs IV remifentanil alone	N = 192 CE + IV APAP: 49 CE + remifentanil: 49 CE alone: 50 Remifentanil alone: 44	IV APAP reduced the temperature compared with the other groups; the pain scores were comparable across the groups
Grundmann, 2006[55]	Lumbar microdiscectomy	IV parecoxib, IV metamizol, and placebo	IV APAP 1000 mg vs IV parecoxib 40 mg vs IV metamizol 1000 mg vs placebo, single dose	N = 80 IV APAP: 20 IV parecoxib: 20 IV metamizol: 20 Placebo: 20	IV APAP was comparable to IV parecoxib in terms of pain response
Holmér Pettersson, 2005[56]	CABG/cardiopulmonary bypass	Oral acetaminophen	IV APAP 1000 mg vs oral acetaminophen 1000 mg q6h × 24 h	N = 77 IV APAP: 39 oral APAP: 38	IV APAP produced comparable pain relief to oral, but significantly reduced consumption of rescue medication

Holmér Pettersson, 2006[57]	Cardiac surgery	Rectal acetaminophen	IV APAP 1000 mg vs rectal acetaminophen 1000 mg q6h × 24 h	N = 48 IV APAP: 24 Rectal APAP: 24	Plasma APAP peaked within 40 min of IV administration but after rectal administration, but at 80 min after rectal administration
Hong, 2010[58]	Thyroidectomy	Placebo	IV APAP 1000 mg vs placebo, single dose, before surgery and q6h × 24 h after surgery	N = 124 IV APAP: 63 Placebo: 61	IV APAP patients had significantly lower pain scores over at 1, 3, 6, and 24 h after surgery; significantly fewer required rescue medication; and significantly reduced incidence of nausea and vomiting
Juhl, 2006[59]	Oral surgery: third molar surgery	Placebo	IV APAP 1000 mg vs IV APAP 2000 mg vs placebo, single dose	N=297 IV APAP 1000 mg: 132 IV APAP 2000 mg: 132 Placebo: 33	IV APAP 1000 mg produced increased magnitude of pain relief and duration of analgesia effect vs placebo; IV APAP 2000 mg was associated with better and longer pain relief; there were no significant safety differences among the 3 groups

(continued on next page)

Table 1
(continued)

Author (Year)	Pain Model Studied	Comparator/Control	Study Medication Regimen	Total No. of Subjects (Completers/Group)	Study Summary
Jokela, 2010[60]	Laparoscopic hysterectomy	Placebo, IV APAP + OND	IV APAP 1000 mg vs placebo at the induction of anesthesia and then 6 h × 24 h; in patients who received IV APAP, OND 4 mg or placebo 1× at end of surgery	N = 120 IV APAP + OND: 40 IV APAP + placebo: 40 Placebo + placebo: 40	IV APAP reduces opioid consumption vs placebo; OND (a 5-HT$_3$ antagonist) does not block IV APAP analgesia
Kampe, 2006[61]	Breast cancer surgery	IV metamizol	IV APAP 1000 mg vs IV metamizol 1000 mg q6h × 24 h	N = 40 IV APAP: 20 IV metamizol: 20	IV APAP provided clinically equivalent pain relief to IV metamizol
Kemppainen, 2006[62]	Endoscopic sinus surgery	Placebo	IV APAP 1000 mg vs placebo, single dose	N = 74 IV APAP: 36 Placebo: 38	Significantly fewer patients in the IV APAP group (25%) required rescue medication than in the placebo group (71%); patients in this group had a significantly longer time to rescue medication (126 min vs 70 min with placebo)
Khan, 2007[63]	Knee arthroscopy	IV morphine	IV APAP 1000 mg vs IV morphine 0.1 mg/kg as a bolus, single dose	N = 84 IV APAP: 43 IV morphine: 41	IV APAP produced comparable pain relief to IV morphine 0.1 mg/kg with lower incidence of nausea, vomiting, and dizziness

Study	Surgery	Comparison	Regimen	N	Outcome
Ko, 2010[64]	Hand or forearm surgery with IVRA	IVRA lidocaine and placebo	IV APAP 300 mg vs IV ketorolac 10 mg vs placebo	N = 60 IV APAP: 20 IV ketorolac: 20 Placebo: 20	The addition of APAP to lidocaine for IVRA significantly shortens the onset time of sensory block and delays pain onset time compared with ketorolac and placebo; both treatments are superior to placebo for reducing overall pain and rescue medication consumption
Koppert, 2006[65]	Total hip arthroplasty or surgery of the femoral shaft	IV parecoxib and placebo	IV APAP 1000 mg q6h or parecoxib 40 mg q12h vs placebo × 72 h	N = 75 IV APAP 1 g: 25 IV parecoxib 40 mg: 25 Placebo: 25	IV APAP was not significantly different from IV parecoxib or placebo in reducing pain; IV APAP significantly reduced rescue medication requirements on day 1 compared with placebo
Korkmaz Dilmen, 2010[66]	Lumbar disc surgery	IV metamizol, IV lornoxicam, and placebo	IV APAP 1000 mg q6h or IV metamizol 1000 mg q6h vs IV lornoxicam 8 mg q12h vs placebo q6h × 24 h	N = 77 IV APAP: 20 IV metamizol: 18 IV lornoxicam: 20 Placebo: 19	IV APAP and metamizol significantly reduced pain vs placebo; the rate of morphine consumption with IV APAP decreased significantly over 24 h; total opioid consumption over 24 h did not differ between groups

(continued on next page)

Table 1
(continued)

Author (Year)	Pain Model Studied	Comparator/Control	Study Medication Regimen	Total No. of Subjects (Completers/Group)	Study Summary
Landwehr, 2005[67]	Retinal surgery	IV metamizol and placebo	IV APAP 1000 mg or IV metamizol 1000 mg vs placebo q6h × 24 h	N = 38 IV APAP: 12 IV metamizol: 13 Placebo: 13	IV APAP achieved significantly greater pain relief vs placebo and was comparable to IV metamizol over 24 h
Marty, 2005[68]	Minor gynecologic surgery	IV propacetamol	IV APAP 1000 mg or IV propacetamol 2000 mg, single dose	N = 161 IV APAP: 80 IV propacetamol: 81	IV APAP was associated with better local tolerability, similar analgesic efficacy, and greater patient satisfaction than IV propacetamol
Memis, 2010[69]	Major surgery (ICU patients)	Placebo	IV meperidine AND IV APAP 1000 mg OR placebo q6h × 24 h	N = 40 IV APAP: 20 Placebo: 20	IV APAP produced significantly better pain relief and reduced opioid consumption vs placebo over 24 h; IV APAP achieved significantly reduced mean time to extubation (64 vs 205 min) and significantly lower incidence of nausea and vomiting than placebo

Study	Surgery	Control	Intervention	N	Results
Ohnesorge, 2009[70]	Breast surgery	IV metamizol and placebo	IV APAP 1000 mg or IV metamizol 1000 mg vs placebo 20 min before the end of surgery and at 4, 10, and 16 h post surgery	N = 79 IV APAP: 27 IV metamizol: 26 Placebo: 26	Ambulation was significantly earlier in the IV APAP group compared with IV metamizol and placebo; significantly more patients receiving IV APAP did not require rescue medication (42%, vs 4% for placebo); however, no significant difference in total morphine consumption among groups was detected
Salihoglu, 2009[71]	Laparoscopic cholecystectomy	Placebo	IV APAP 1000 mg vs placebo, single dose	N = 40 IV APAP: 20 Placebo: 20	IV APAP produced superior pain responses and significantly reduced time to first rescue medication and total rescue medication consumption vs placebo; IV APAP had significantly fewer incidents of nausea and vomiting
Salonen, 2009[72]	Tonsillectomy	Placebo	IV ketoprofen 1 mg/kg PLUS IV APAP 1000 mg OR IV APAP 2000 mg OR placebo	N = 114 IV APAP 1 g: 37 IV APAP 2 g: 39 Placebo: 38	Pain scores across groups were comparable, but IV APAP significantly reduced opioid consumption vs placebo

(continued on next page)

Table 1
(continued)

Author (Year)	Pain Model Studied	Comparator/ Control	Study Medication Regimen	Total No. of Subjects (Completers/Group)	Study Summary
Sen, 2009[73]	Hand surgery with IVRA	IVRA lidocaine and placebo	IV APAP 300 mg in the IVRA vs 300-mg IV vs placebo, single dose	N = 60 IV APAP in IVRA: 20 IV APAP + IVRA: 20 Placebo: 20	IV APAP added to the IVRA produced superior and longer pain relief than IVRA with placebo or IVRA + IV APAP IV in the other hand
Sinatra, 2005[44]	Total hip or knee arthroplasty	Placebo	IV APAP 1000 mg vs IV propacetamol 2000 mg vs placebo q6h × 24 h	N = 151 IV APAP: 49 IV propacetamol: 50 Placebo: 52	IV APAP as effective as IV propacetamol and produced significantly superior pain relief compared with placebo over first 6 h; IV APAP reduced total morphine consumption over 24 h by 33% compared with placebo
Tasmacioglu, 2009[74]	Cancer pain	Placebo	IV APAP 1000 mg vs placebo q6h × 24 h	N = 40 IV APAP: 20 Placebo: 20	When added to morphine, IV APAP produced better pain scores than placebo from 4 to 24 h, but the results were not significant
Tiippana, 2008[75]	Laparoscopic cholecystectomy	IV parecoxib + PO valdexocib dexamethasone	IV APAP 1000 mg + PO APAP 1000 mg q6h × 7 d ± dexamethasone vs IV paraceoxib 40 mg + PO valdexocib 40 mg qd × 7 d ± dexamethasone	N = 159 IV/PO APAP: 39 IV/PO APAP + dexamethasone: 40 IV parecoxib/PO valdecoxib: 40 IV parecoxib/PO valdecoxib + dexamethasone: 40	IV APAP followed by PO APAP was as effective for pain as IV parecoxib/PO valdecoxib; IV/PO APAP significantly reduced rescue medication consumption on day 1 compared with IV/PO coxibs

Abbreviations: APAP, acetaminophen; CE, continuous epidural; EOS, end of surgery; IM, intramuscular; Ind, induction; IVRA regional anesthetic; OND, ondansetron; PO, oral.

hernia repair. Murat and colleagues[98] conducted a randomized, active-controlled, double-blind, parallel group, multicenter study in 183 children ranging in age from 1 to 12 years. Patients were randomized 1:1 to receive either a single dose of IV acetaminophen (15 mg/kg) or a bioequivalent dose of IV propacetamol (30 mg/kg) when their postoperative PI as rated by the investigator was greater than 30 on a 0- to 100-mm VAS. Both treatments rapidly reduced pain scores, with a steep reduction from baseline PI during the first 15-minute interval after infusion. The duration of analgesia, measured as the time to first rescue, was more than 4 hours for both groups. Similarly, only approximately 20% of the patients in both groups required rescue medication, and global evaluations of "excellent" were reported for 76% of patients receiving IV acetaminophen.

Evidence for the efficacy of IV acetaminophen in the treatment of fever of infectious origin has been investigated in 67 children ranging in age from 1 month to 12 years.[96] Patients were randomized to receive IV acetaminophen (15 mg/kg) or a bioequivalent dose of IV propacetamol (30 mg/kg). From a baseline mean of 39.4°C, 79% of the IV acetaminophen group had temperature readings below a median of 38°C by 2 hours, reductions that were maintained for a mean of 3.42 hours. In addition, 69.7% of children in the IV acetaminophen group became afebrile by 3 hours, and 72.7% of children were thought to have had a "good" or "excellent" response on the investigator's global evaluation. IV acetaminophen was well tolerated and resulted in significantly fewer injection-site reactions than seen with IV propacetamol (5.7% vs 28.1%; $P = .0134$).

Additional published studies have reported similar positive results for IV acetaminophen in the treatment of pain associated with tonsillectomy in 80 children and adolescents[93] and adenotonsillectomy in 50 children.[95] Finally, Kumpulainen and colleagues[33] studied the CSF penetration of a single dose of IV acetaminophen (15 mg/kg) in 32 children (3 months to 12 years of age, median 55 months) who were undergoing lower body surgery with spinal anesthesia and demonstrated rapid CSF penetration of IV acetaminophen, with time to peak levels in the CSF occurring in under 1 hour.

CLINICAL TOLERABILITY AND SAFETY

IV acetaminophen is well tolerated and shares many safety aspects of the oral and rectal formulations. Like the oral formula, IV acetaminophen is not associated with the potentially serious adverse events that may occur with NSAIDs, COX-2 inhibitors, and opioids, including gastrointestinal complications, sedation, and bleeding risks.[43,44] In contrast to NSAIDs, such as diclofenac and ketorolac, which can significantly impair platelet aggregation,[99,100] acetaminophen has little or no effect on platelet function. Adverse reactions related to the use of IV acetaminophen are rare—less than 1 in 10,000—and are usually mild and transient. It has demonstrated a safety profile similar to that of placebo, with comparable frequency of adverse events in clinical studies.[43] Treatment-emergent adverse events (TEAEs) reported include hypotension, malaise, hypersensitivity reaction, elevated hepatic transaminases, and thrombocytopenia.[43] Recent open-label, multiple-dose US safety studies in both pediatric and adult inpatients have confirmed these tolerability reports.[101,102]

The primary safety concern with acetaminophen is its potential hepatic toxicity when used at higher-than-recommended doses (>4g/d for adult patients).[103] Hepatic toxicity associated with acetaminophen is rare less than 1 in 500,000 treated patients[44] and is primarily associated with unintentional or uncontrolled oral and rectal overdoses. It is likely that hepatic concerns associated with IV acetaminophen would

Table 2
Published studies supporting the efficacy and safety of IV acetaminophen in pediatric patients

Author (Year)	Pain Model Studied	Comparator/Control	Study Medication Regimen	Total No. of Subjects (Completers/Group)	Study Highlights
Alhashemi, 2006[93]	Pediatric tonsillectomy	IM meperidine	IV APAP 15 mg/kg vs IM meperidine 1 mg/kg, single dose	N = 80 IV APAP: 40 IM meperidine: 40	IV APAP was equivalent to IM meperidine with less sedation and pruritus and significantly faster readiness for PACU discharge
Alhashemi, 2007[94]	Pediatric dental restoration	IM meperidine	IV APAP 15 mg/kg vs IM meperidine 1 mg/kg, single dose	N = 40 IV APAP: 20 IM meperidine: 20	IV APAP was equivalent to IM meperidine with significantly less sedation and faster readiness for PACU discharge
Capici, 2008[95]	Pediatric adenoidectomy or adenotonsillectomy	Rectal acetaminophen	IV APAP 15 mg/kg vs rectal acetaminophen 40 mg/kg	N = 50 IV APAP: 25 Rectal acetaminophen: 25	IV APAP produced pain relief similar to a rectal acetaminophen dose 2.67 times higher. The median time to first rescue for IV APAP was 7 h
Duhamel, 2007[96]	Pediatric fever	IV propacetamol	IV APAP 15 mg/kg vs IV propacetamol 30 mg/kg, single dose	N = 67 IV APAP: 35 IV propacetamol: 32	IV APAP was equivalent to IV propacetamol in antipyretic activity; 79% and 75% of subjects achieved temperature goal of 38°C; IV APAP was associated with significantly fewer injection-site reactions

Study	Condition	Comparator	Intervention/Dose	N	Results
Hong, 2010[97]	Pediatric inguinal herniorrhaphy	Placebo	IV APAP 20 mg/kg + IV ketorolac 1 mg/kg vs placebo, single dose	N = 55 IV APAP + IV ketorolac: 28 Placebo: 27	Ketorolac + IV APAP produced superior pain relief and reduced opioid consumption (by 61%) compared with fentanyl alone
Murat, 2005[98]	Pediatric inguinal hernia surgery	IV propacetamol	IV APAP 15 mg/kg or IV propacetamol 30 mg/kg, single dose	N = 183 IV APAP: 95 IV propacetamol: 88	IV APAP was well tolerated and produced comparable pain relief to IV propacetamol with significantly less injection-site pain
Palmer, 2008[40]	Postoperative pain in pediatric neonates	N/A	IV APAP dosed according to PMA: 28-<32 weeks, 10 mg/kg; 32-<36 weeks, 12.5 mg/kg; and ≥36 weeks, 15 mg/kg q6h prn	N = 50 (median PMA 38.6) IV APAP: 50	No evidence of hepatotoxicity with multiple doses of IV APAP in neonates

Abbreviations: APAP, acetaminophen; IM, intramuscular; N/A, not applicable; PACU, post anesthesia care unit; PMA, postmenstrual age.

be further minimized by controlled dosing in the clinical setting. A recent analysis of eight (4 single-dose and 4 multiple-dose studies) multicenter, double-blind, randomized, placebo-controlled studies conducted in the United States (total N = 1064; IV acetaminophen = 649; placebo = 415) was performed to evaluate the safety of IV acetaminophen in a variety of postoperative environments and endotoxin-induced fever for hepatic TEAEs.[104] The placebo group had a slightly higher rate of hepatic TEAEs (26/415; 6.3%) than the IV acetaminophen group (20/649; 3.1%). In one of the trials, in which patients received repeated doses over 48 hours, the placebo group reported a higher rate and greater severity of hepatic enzyme (alanine aminotransferase/aspartate aminotransferase) elevations (6/165; 3.6%) than the IV acetaminophen group (3/166; 1.8%).[104] Therefore, the risk of hepatotoxicity with repeated dosing of IV acetaminophen 1 g every 6 hours up to 48 hours may be no different from placebo. Nonetheless, IV acetaminophen, as with all forms of acetaminophen, should be used with great caution in patients with impaired liver function.

SUMMARY

The efficacy and safety of single and repeated doses of IV acetaminophen have been well documented in a variety of postoperative settings and patient populations across PI scores from mild to severe for periods up to 72 hours. In many studies, the onset of analgesic action for IV acetaminophen has been documented to occur just before or at the end of the 15-minute infusion. The peak effect, as measured by PI or pain relief, compared with placebo has been shown in several studies not only statistically significant but also clinically meaningful. IV acetaminophen (1000 mg) in the treatment of moderate to severe postoperative pain has an efficacy comparable to ketorolac (30 mg), diclofenac (75 mg), metamizol (0.5 g), or morphine (10 mg).[105]

In the perioperative setting, the parenteral form of acetaminophen may be preferred because patients may be unable to tolerate oral medications and/or may have unpredictable gastrointestinal function after surgery. There may also be a need for parenteral alternatives to treat adult patients who have a relative or absolute contraindication to the use of NSAIDs and who may require urgent treatment of fever/hyperthermia. IV administration can achieve effective levels in a shorter time with more predictable drug levels compared with oral and rectal forms. Additionally, it has demonstrated superior analgesia at least in the first hour after it is administered as well as a longer duration of action. It has demonstrated an adverse reaction profile similar to that of placebo and is, therefore, an appropriate analgesic option for adult and pediatric patients undergoing ambulatory surgery. IV acetaminophen is also effective for the treatment of fever in adults and pediatric patients. Parenteral administration results in higher plasma concentrations, which may contribute to enhanced CSF penetration and more rapid and effective antipyresis.

The opioid-sparing effect of IV acetaminophen remains somewhat controversial. In some but not all studies of IV acetaminophen, a statistically significant reduction in opioid consumption has been documented, with some studies showing that a substantial percentage of patients have been able to avoid the need for opioid rescue altogether. Avoiding or even delaying the use of opioids for moderate to acute pain may help avoid undesirable side effects, hyperalgesic responses, and possible dependency issues. Additionally, the use of IV acetaminophen and decreased use of opioids postoperatively may improve overall patient comfort and satisfaction, allow for earlier ambulation, and possibly translate to a shorter hospital stay.

Owing to its broad compatibility characteristics, IV acetaminophen may also be considered as an adjunct to other analgesics where synergy through complementary mechanisms of action[106,107] may be clinically useful, especially in multimodal analgesic regimens. As technical advances have made many surgical procedures less invasive, there has been a concomitant and associated trend to initiate physical therapy sooner to enhance long-term rehabilitation and healing. Therefore, it may be increasingly important to manage pain effectively and with minimal tolerability and safety issues to effectively transition patients to primary rehabilitative services. Although the emerging clinical picture for IV acetaminophen demonstrates its potential in fulfilling the unmet needs and requirements for the treatment of fever and pain in the perioperative setting, future studies should help clearly define its utility and scope of use in multimodal pain management.

ACKNOWLEDGMENTS

The authors thank Cadence Pharmaceuticals and IntraMed Educational Group for their assistance with the preparation of this manuscript.

REFERENCES

1. Bertolini A, Ferrari A, Ottani A, et al. Paracetamol: new vistas of an old drug. CNS Drug Rev 2006;12:250–75.
2. Kaufman DW, Kelly JP, Rosenberg L, et al. Recent patterns of medication use in the ambulatory adult population of the United States: the Slone survey. JAMA 2002;287:337–44.
3. Malaise O, Bruyere O, Reginster J. Intravenous paracetamol: a review of efficacy and safety in therapeutic use. Future Neurol 2007;2:673–88.
4. Cattabriga I, Pacini D, Lamazza G, et al. Intravenous paracetamol as adjunctive treatment for postoperative pain after cardiac surgery: a double blind randomized controlled trial. Eur J Cardiothorac Surg 2007;32:527–31.
5. Remy C, Marret E, Bonnet F. Effects of acetaminophen on morphine side-effects and consumption after major surgery: meta-analysis of randomized controlled trials. Br J Anaesth 2005;94:505–13.
6. Smith HS. Potential analgesic mechanisms of acetaminophen. Pain Physician 2009;12:269–80.
7. Graham GG, Scott KF. Mechanism of action of paracetamol. Am J Ther 2005;12: 46–55.
8. Remy C, Marret E, Bonnet F. State of the art of paracetamol in acute pain therapy. Curr Opin Anaesthesiol 2006;19:562–5.
9. Myles PS, Power I. Clinical update: postoperative analgesia. Lancet 2007;369: 810–2.
10. American Society of Anesthesiologists Task Force on Acute Pain Management. Practice guidelines for acute pain management in the perioperative setting: an updated report by the American Society of Anesthesiologists Task Force on Acute Pain Management. Anesthesiology 2004;100:1573–81.
11. Apfelbaum JL, Chen C, Mehta SS, et al. Postoperative pain experience: results from a national survey suggest postoperative pain continues to be undermanaged. Anesth Analg 2003;97:534–40.
12. Polomano RC, Dunwoody CJ, Krenzischek DA, et al. Perspective on pain management in the 21st century. J Perianesth Nurs 2008;23(Suppl 1):s4–14.
13. DeFrances CJ, Lucas CA, Buie VC, et al. 2006 National Hospital Discharge Survey. Natl Health Stat Report 2008;5:1–20.
14. Perkins FM, Kehlet H. Chronic pain as an outcome of surgery. A review of predictive factors. Anesthesiology 2000;93:1123–33.

15. Nimmo WS, Duthie DJ. Pain relief after surgery. Anaesth Intensive Care 1987;15: 68–71.
16. Pyati S, Gan TJ. Perioperative pain management. CNS Drugs 2007;21:185–211.
17. Dahl JB, Møiniche S. Pre-emptive analgesia. Br Med Bull 2004;71:13–27.
18. Ong CK, Lirk P, Seymour RA, et al. The efficacy of preemptive analgesia for acute postoperative pain management: a meta-analysis. Anesth Analg 2005; 100:757–73.
19. White PF. Multimodal analgesia: its role in preventing postoperative pain. Curr Opin Investig Drugs 2008;9:76–82.
20. Kehlet H, Dahl JB. The value of "multimodal" or "balanced analgesia" in postoperative pain treatment. Anesth Analg 1993;77:1048–56.
21. Crews JC. Multimodal pain management strategies for office-based and ambulatory procedures. JAMA 2002;288:629–32.
22. Buvanendran A, Kroin JS. Multimodal analgesia for controlling acute postoperative pain. Curr Opin Anaesthesiol 2009;22:588–93.
23. Jahr JS, Reynolds LW, Royal MA. A posthoc analysis of a randomized, double-blind, placebo-controlled study of IV acetaminophen for the treatment of postoperative pain after major orthopedic surgery. [2009 Annual Pain Medicine Meeting and Workshops (ASRA)]. Reg Anesth Pain Med 2009;PSI:10.
24. Oscier CD, Milner QJ. Peri-operative use of paracetamol. Anaesthesia 2009;64: 65–72.
25. Ang R, Kupiec TC, Breitmeyer JB, et al. IV Acetaminophen in-use stability and compatibility with common IV fluids and IV medications. [111th Annual Meeting of the American Society for Clinical Pharmacology and Therapeutics, PII-83]. Clin Pharmacol Ther 2010;87:S39–65.
26. Moller PL, Sindet-Pedersen S, Petersen CT, et al. Onset of acetaminophen analgesia: comparison of oral and intravenous routes after third molar surgery. Br J Anaesth 2005;94:642–8.
27. Jarde O, Boccard E. Parenteral versus oral route increases paracetamol efficacy. Clin Drug Invest 1997;14:474–81.
28. Holmér Pettersson P, Öwall A, Jakobsson J. Early bioavailability of paracetamol after oral or intravenous administration. Acta Anaesthesiol Scand 2004;48: 867–70.
29. Schutz R, Fong L, Chang Y, et al. Open-label, 4-period, randomized crossover study to determine the comparative pharmacokinetics of oral and intravenous acetaminophen administration in healthy male volunteers [poster]. 2007 American Society of Regional Anesthesia and Pain Medicine (ASRA) Annual Pain Medicine Meeting and Workshops. Boca Raton (FL), 2007.
30. Flouvat B, Leneveu A, Fitoussi S, et al. Bioequivalence study comparing a new paracetamol solution for injection and propacetamol after single intravenous infusion in healthy subjects. Int J Clin Pharmacol Ther 2004; 42:50–7.
31. Gregoire N, Hovsepian L, Gualano V, et al. Safety and pharmacokinetics of paracetamol following intravenous administration of 5 g during the first 24 h with a 2-g starting dose. Clin Pharmacol Ther 2007;81:401–5.
32. Jensen LL, Handberg G, Schmedes A, et al. Paracetamol concentrations in plasma and cerebrospinal fluid. Eur J Anaesthesiol 2004;21(Suppl 32):193.
33. Kumpulainen E, Kokki H, Halonen T, et al. Paracetamol (acetaminophen) penetrates readily into the cerebrospinal fluid of children after intravenous administration. Pediatrics 2007;119:766–71.

34. Bannwarth B, Netter P, Lapicque F, et al. Plasma and cerebrospinal fluid concentrations of paracetamol after a single intravenous dose of propacetamol. Br J Clin Pharmacol 1992;34:79–81.

35. Pan CP, Breitmeyer JB, Royal M. IV acetaminophen PK/PD correlation following total hip arthroplasty. [111th Annual Meeting of the American Society for Clinical Pharmacology and Therapeutics]. Clin Pharmacol Ther 2010;87:S39–65.

36. Gelotte CK, Auiler JF, Lynch JM, et al. Disposition of acetaminophen at 4, 6, and 8 g/day for 3 days in healthy young adults. Clin Pharmacol Ther 2007;81:840–8.

37. Manyike PT, Kharasch ED, Kalhorn TF, et al. Contribution of CYP2E1 and CYP3A to acetaminophen reactive metabolite formation. Clin Pharmacol Ther 2000;67: 275–82.

38. Marier JF, Mouksassi S, Pan CC, et al. IV acetaminophen pharmacokinetics in children and adolescents is comparable to adults. [111th Annual Meeting of the American Society for Clinical Pharmacology and Therapeutics, PII-72]. Clin Pharmacol Ther 2010;87:S39–65.

39. van Lingen RA, Deinum JT, Quak JM, et al. Pharmacokinetics and metabolism of rectally administered paracetamol in preterm neonates. Arch Dis Child Fetal Neonatal Ed 1999;80:F59–63.

40. Palmer G, Atkins M, Anderson B, et al. IV acetaminophen pharmacokinetics in neonates after multiple doses. Br J Anaesth 2008;101:523–30.

41. van der Marel CD, Anderson BJ, van Lingen RA, et al. Paracetamol and metabolite pharmacokinetics in infants. Eur J Clin Pharmacol 2003;59:243–51.

42. Royal MA, Gosselin NH, Pan CC, et al. Route of administration significantly impacts hepatic acetaminophen exposure: a simulation based on a first pass model. [111th Annual Meeting of the American Society for Clinical Pharmacology and Therapeutics, PII-73]. Clin Pharmacol Ther 2010;87: S39–65.

43. Duggan ST, Scott LJ. Intravenous paracetamol (acetaminophen). Drugs 2009; 69:101–13.

44. Sinatra RS, Jahr JS, Reynolds LW, et al. Efficacy and safety of single and repeated administration of 1 gram intravenous acetaminophen injection (paracetamol) for pain management after major orthopedic surgery. Anesthesiology 2005;102:822–31.

45. Miller H, Minkowitz H, Wininger S, et al. A phase III, multi-center, randomized, double-blind, placebo-controlled 24 hour study of the efficacy and safety of intravenous acetaminophen in abdominal laparoscopic surgery. [34th Annual Regional Anesthesia Meeting and Workshops, 97]. Reg Anesth Pain Med 2009;32:99.

46. Alhashemi JA, Alotaibi QA, Mashaat MS, et al. Intravenous acetaminophen vs oral ibuprofen in combination with morphine PCIA after Cesarean delivery: [L'acetaminophene intraveineux vs l'ibuprofene par voie orale comme \adjuvant de la morphine AICP apres une cesarienne]. Can J Anaesth 2006;53: 1200–6.

47. Api O, Unal O, Ugurel V, et al. Analgesic efficacy of intravenous paracetamol for outpatient fractional curettage: a randomised, controlled trial. Int J Clin Pract 2009;63:105–11.

48. Arici S, Gurbet A, Türker G, et al. Preemptive analgesic effects of intravenous paracetamol in total abdominal hysterectomy. Agri 2009;21:54–61.

49. Atef A, Fawaz AA. Intravenous paracetamol is highly effective in pain treatment after tonsillectomy in adults. Eur Arch Otorhinolaryngol 2008;265:351–5.

50. Bektas F, Eken C, Karadeniz O, et al. Intravenous paracetamol or morphine for the treatment of renal colic: a randomized, placebo-controlled trial. Ann Emerg Med 2009;54:568–74.

51. Cakan T, Inan N, Culhaoglu S, et al. Intravenous paracetamol improves the quality of postoperative analgesia but does not decrease narcotic requirements. J Neurosurg Anesthesiol 2008;20:169–73.

52. Canbay O, Celebi N, Arun O, et al. Efficacy of intravenous acetaminophen and lidocaine on propofol injection pain. Br J Anaesth 2008;100:95–8.

53. Celik M, Saricaoglu F, Canbay O, et al. The analgesic effect of paracetamol when added to lidocaine for intravenous regional anesthesia. Minerva Anestesiol 2009;75:1–6.

54. Evron S, Ezri T, Protianov M, et al. The effects of remifentanil or acetaminophen with epidural ropivacaine on body temperature during labor. J Anesth 2008;22:105–11.

55. Grundmann U, Wörnle C, Biedler A, et al. The efficacy of the non-opioid analgesics parecoxib, paracetamol and metamizol for postoperative pain relief after lumbar microdiscectomy. Anesth Analg 2006;103:217–22.

56. Holmér Pettersson P, Jakobsson J, Öwall A. Intravenous acetaminophen reduced the use of opioids compared with oral administration after coronary artery bypass grafting. J Cardiothorac Vasc Anesth 2005;19:306–9.

57. Holmér Pettersson P, Jakobsson J, Öwall A. Plasma concentrations following repeated rectal or intravenous administration of paracetamol after heart surgery. Acta Anaesthesiol Scand 2006;50:673–7.

58. Hong JY, Kim WO, Chung WY, et al. Paracetamol reduces postoperative pain and rescue analgesic demand after robot-assisted endoscopic thyroidectomy by the transaxillary approach. World J Surg 2010;34:521–6.

59. Juhl GI, Norholt SE, Tonnesen E, et al. Analgesic efficacy and safety of intravenous paracetamol (acetaminophen) administered as a 2 g starting dose following third molar surgery. Eur J Pain 2006;10:371–7.

60. Jokela R, Ahonen J, Seitsonen E, et al. The influence of ondansetron on the analgesic effect of acetaminophen after laparoscopic hysterectomy. Clin Pharmacol Ther 2010;87:672–8.

61. Kampe S, Warm M, Landwehr S, et al. Clinical equivalence of IV paracetamol compared to IV dipyrone for postoperative analgesia after surgery for breast cancer. Curr Med Res Opin 2006;22:1949–54.

62. Kemppainen T, Kokki H, Tuomilehto H, et al. Acetaminophen is highly effective in pain treatment after endoscopic sinus surgery. Laryngoscope 2006;116:2125–8.

63. Khan ZU, Iqbal J, Saleh H, et al. Intravenous paracetamol is as effective as morphine in knee arthroscopic day surgery procedures. Pakistan J Med Sci 2007;23:851–3.

64. Ko MJ, Lee JH, Cheong SH, et al. Comparison of the effects of acetaminophen to ketorolac when added to lidocaine for intravenous regional anesthesia. Korean J Anesthesiol 2010;58:357–61.

65. Koppert W, Frötsch K, Huzurudin N, et al. The effects of paracetamol and parecoxib on kidney function in elderly patients undergoing orthopedic surgery. Anesth Analg 2006;103:1170–6.

66. Korkmaz Dilmen O, Tunali Y, Cakmakkaya OS, et al. Efficacy of intravenous paracetamol, metamizol and lornoxicam on postoperative pain and morphine consumption after lumbar disc surgery. Eur J Anaesthesiol 2010;27:428–32.

67. Landwehr S, Kiencke P, Giesecke T, et al. A comparison between IV paraceta-mol and IV metamizol for postoperative analgesia after retinal surgery. Curr Med Res Opin 2005;21:1569–75.

68. Marty J, Benhamou D, Chassard D, et al. Effects of single-dose injectable parace-tamolversus propacetamol in pain management after minor gynecologic surgery: a multicenter, randomized, double-blind, active-controlled, two-parallel-group study. Curr Ther Res 2005;66:294–306.

69. Memis D, Inal MT, Kavalci G, et al. Intravenous paracetamol reduced the use of opioids, extubation time, and opioid-related adverse effects after major surgery in intensive care unit. J Crit Care 2010;25(3):458–62.

70. Ohnesorge H, Bein B, Hanss R, et al. Paracetamol versus metamizol in the treat-ment of postoperative pain after breast surgery: a randomized, controlled trial. Eur J Anaesthesiol 2009;26:648–53.

71. Salihoglu Z, Yildirim M, Demiroluk S, et al. Evaluation of intravenous paraceta-mol administration on postoperative pain and recovery characteristics in patients undergoing laparoscopic cholecystectomy. Surg Laparosc Endosc Percutan Tech 2009;19:321–3.

72. Salonen A, Silvola J, Kokki H. Does 1 or 2 g paracetamol added to ketoprofen enhance analgesia in adult tonsillectomy patients? Acta Anaesthesiol Scand 2009;53:1200–6.

73. Sen H, Kulahci Y, Bicerer E, et al. The analgesic effect of paracetamol when added to lidocaine for intravenous regional anesthesia. Anesth Analg 2009; 109:1327–30.

74. Tasmacioglu B, Aydinli I, Keskinbora K, et al. Effect of intravenous administration of paracetamol on morphine consumption in cancer pain control. Support Care Cancer 2009;17:1475–81.

75. Tiippana E, Bachmann M, Kalso E, et al. Effect of paracetamol and coxib with or without dexamethasone after laparoscopic cholecystectomy. Acta Anaesthesiol Scand 2008;52:673–80.

76. Viscusi E, Royal M, Leclerc A, et al. Phramacokinetics, efficacy and safety of IV acetaminophen in the treatment of pain following total hip arthroplasty: Results of a double-blind, randomized, placebo-controlled, single-dose study. [24th Annual Meeting of the American Academy of Pain Medicine]. Pain Medicine 2008;9:88–141.

77. Gimbel J, Royal M, Leclerc A, et al. Efficacy and safety of IV acetaminophen in the treatment of pain following primary total hip arthroplasty: Results of a double-blind, randomized, placebo-controlled, multiple-dose, 24 hour study. [24th Annual Meeting of the American Academy of Pain Medicine, 216]. Pain Medicine 2008;9:88–141.

78. Minkowitz H, Royal M, Leclerc A, et al. Efficacy and safety of IV acetaminophen in the treatment of pain following vaginal hysterectomy: Results of a double-blind, randomized, placebo-controlled, multiple-dose, 24 hour study. [24th Annual Meeting of the American Academy of Pain Medicine]. Pain Medicine 2008;9:88–141.

79. Royal M, Fong L, Smith H, et al. Randomized study of the efficacy and safety of IV acetaminophen compared to oral acetaminophen for the treatment of fever. [12th Annual Meeting of the Society of Hospital Medicine, 84]. J Hosp Med 2009;S1:A11–142.

80. Royal M, Fong L, Smith H, et al. Randomized study of the efficacy and safety of IV acetaminophen compared to placebo for the treatment of fever. [12th Annual Meeting of the Society of Hospital Medicine, 85]. J Hosp Med 2009;S1:A11–142.

81. Bachert C, Chuchalin AG, Eisebitt R, et al. Aspirin compared with acetaminophen in the treatment of fever and other symptoms of upper respiratory tract infection in adults: a multicenter, randomized, double-blind, double-dummy, placebo-controlled, parallel-group, single-dose, 6-hour dose-ranging study. Clin Ther 2005;27:993–1003.

82. McMahon FG, Vargas R. A new clinical bioassay for antipyresis. J Clin Pharmacol 1991;31:736–40.

83. Vargas R, Maneatis T, Bynum L, et al. Evaluation of the antipyretic effect of ketorolac, acetaminophen, and placebo in endotoxin-induced fever. J Clin Pharmacol 1994;34:848–53.

84. Pernerstorfer T, Schmid R, Bieglmayer C, et al. Acetaminophen has greater antipyretic efficacy than aspirin in endotoxemia: a randomized, double-blind, placebo-controlled trial. Clin Pharmacol Ther 1999;66:51–7.

85. Cranswick N, Coghlan D. Paracetamol efficacy and safety in children: the first 40 years. Am J Ther 2000;7:135–41.

86. Prins SA, Van DM, Van LP, et al. Pharmacokinetics and analgesic effects of intravenous propacetamol vs rectal paracetamol in children after major craniofacial surgery. Paediatr Anaesth 2008;18:582–92.

87. Montgomery CJ, McCormack JP, Reichert CC, et al. Plasma concentrations after high-dose (45 mg.kg^{-1}) rectal acetaminophen in children. Can J Anaesth 1995; 42:982–6.

88. American Academy of Pediatrics Committee on Drugs. Acetaminophen toxicity in children. Pediatrics 2001;108:1020–4.

89. Autret E, Dutertre JP, Breteau M, et al. Pharmacokinetics of paracetamol in the neonate and infant after administration of propacetamol chlorhydrate. Dev Pharmacol Ther 1993;20:129–34.

90. Granry JC, Rod B, Monrigal JP, et al. The analgesic efficacy of an injectable prodrug of acetaminophen in children after orthopaedic surgery. Paediatr Anaesth 1997;7:445–9.

91. Allegaert K, Anderson BJ, Naulaers G, et al. Intravenous paracetamol (propacetamol) pharmacokinetics in term and preterm neonates. Eur J Clin Pharmacol 2004;60:191–7.

92. Allegaert K, Rayyan M, De RT, et al. Hepatic tolerance of repeated intravenous paracetamol administration in neonates. Paediatr Anaesth 2008;18:388–92.

93. Alhashemi JA, Daghistani MF. Effects of intraoperative i.v. acetaminophen vs i.m. meperidine on post-tonsillectomy pain in children. Br J Anaesth 2006;96: 790–5.

94. Alhashemi JA, Daghistani MF. Effect of intraoperative intravenous acetaminophen vs. intramuscular meperidine on pain and discharge time after paediatric dental restoration. Eur J Anaesthesiol 2007;24:128–33.

95. Capici F, Ingelmo PM, Davidson A, et al. Randomized controlled trial of duration of analgesia following intravenous or rectal acetaminophen after adenotonsillectomy in children. Br J Anaesth 2008;100:251–5.

96. Duhamel JF, Le GE, Dalphin ML, et al. Antipyretic efficacy and safety of a single intravenous administration of 15 mg/kg paracetamol versus 30 mg/kg propacetamol in children with acute fever due to infection. Int J Clin Pharmacol Ther 2007;45:221–9.

97. Hong JY, Won Han S, Kim WO, et al. Fentanyl sparing effects of combined ketorolac and acetaminophen for outpatient inguinal hernia repair in children. J Urol 2010;183:1551–5.

98. Murat I, Baujard C, Foussat C, et al. Tolerance and analgesic efficacy of a new i.v. paracetamol solution in children after inguinal hernia repair. Paediatr Anaesth 2005;15:663–70.

99. Silvanto M, Munsterhjelm E, Savolainen S, et al. Effect of 3 g of intravenous paracetamol on post-operative analgesia, platelet function and liver enzymes in patients undergoing tonsillectomy under local anaesthesia. Acta Anaesthesiol Scand 2007;51:1147–54.

100. Niemi TT, Backman JT, Syrjala MT, et al. Platelet dysfunction after intravenous ketorolac or propacetamol. Acta Anaesthesiol Scand 2000;44:69–74.

101. Krane E, Malviya S, Del Pizzo K, et al. Pediatric safety of repeated doses of intravenous acetaminophen. [34th Annual Regional Anesthesia Meeting, 58]. Reg Anesth Pain Med 2009;32:100.

102. Singla N, Ferber L, Bergese S, et al. A phase III, multi-center, open-label, prospective, repeated dose, randomized, controlled, multi-day study of the safety of intravenous aceaminophen in adult inpatients. [34th Annual Regional Anesthesia Meeting, 96]. Reg Anesth Pain Med 2009;32:100.

103. Food and Drug Administration. Acetaminophen overdose and liver injury—background and options for reducing injury. Available at: http://www.fda.gov/ohrms/dockets/ac/09/briefing/2009-4429b1-01-FDA.pdf. Accessed June 23, 2010.

104. Singla N, Viscusi E, Candiotti K, et al. A review of the intravenous acetaminophen placebo-controlled clinical trial safety experience: a focus on hepatic transaminases. [33rd Annual Regional Anesthesia Meeting, A-114]. Reg Anesth Pain Med 2007;32: A-114.

105. Göröcs TS, Lambert M, Rinne T, et al. Efficacy and tolerability of ready-to-use intravenous paracetamol solution as monotherapy or as an adjunct analgesic therapy for postoperative pain in patients undergoing elective ambulatory surgery: open, prospective study. Int J Clin Pract 2009;63:112–20.

106. Smith AB, Ravikumar TS, Kamin M, et al. Combination tramadol plus acetaminophen for postsurgical pain. Am J Surg 2004;187(4):521–7.

107. Miranda HF, Puig MM, Prieto JC, et al. Synergism between paracetamol and nonsteroidal anti-inflammatory drugs in experimental acute pain. Pain 2006; 121(1–2):22–8.

Advances in Perioperative Pain Management: Use of Medications with Dual Analgesic Mechanisms, Tramadol & Tapentadol

Vaughn E. Nossaman, MS/MS[a], Usha Ramadhyani, MD[b],
Philip J. Kadowitz, PhD[a], Bobby D. Nossaman, MD[a,b],*

KEYWORDS

- Analgesics • Tramadol • Tapentadol
- Mu/agonists/adverse effects/pharmacology/therapeutic use
- Adrenergic uptake inhibitors/adverse effects/pharmacology/
  therapeutic use
- Monoamine oxidase inhibitors/adverse effects/pharmacology/
  therapeutic use

Noradrenergic and serotonergic neurons originate in the brainstem and terminate in the dorsal horn of the spinal cord. This monoaminergic pathway modulates the spinal processing of nociception through the section of norepinephrine and serotonin.[1–10] Drugs that block the reuptake of either or both of these neurotransmitters, such as tricyclic antidepressants, selective-serotonin reuptake inhibitors, and serotonin-norepinephrine reuptake inhibitors, have shown benefit in the treatment of pain.[11–15] Experimental evidence has also shown that brain and spinal cord serotonergic neurons are involved in the analgesic effects of opiates.[4,6–8,16–19]

Recent studies have shown that large numbers of patients suffer from moderate-to-severe pain during the first 24 to 48 hours after surgery.[20–22] The success of ambulatory surgery depends on effective postoperative pain management routines.

Financial and funding disclosures: The authors have nothing to disclose.

[a] Department of Pharmacology, Tulane University Medical Center, 1430 Tulane Avenue, New Orleans, LA 70129, USA
[b] Department of Anesthesiology, Ochsner Medical Center, 1514 Jefferson Highway, New Orleans, LA 70121, USA
* Corresponding author. Department of Anesthesiology, Ochsner Medical Center, 1514 Jefferson Highway, New Orleans, LA 70121.
E-mail address: bnossaman@ochsner.org

Anesthesiology Clin 28 (2010) 647–666
doi:10.1016/j.anclin.2010.08.009   anesthesiology.theclinics.com
1932-2275/10/$ – see front matter © 2010 Elsevier Inc. All rights reserved.

The cost savings from outpatient surgery may be negated by unanticipated hospital admission from inadequate management of this complication and/or medication side effects, such as nausea and emesis.[20,23,24] Depending on the intensity of postoperative pain, current management includes the use of analgesics, such as opiates and/or nonsteroidal anti-inflammatory drugs (NSAIDs), as part of a balanced analgesic regimen. Opiates, when used to achieve effective postoperative pain control, increase the risk of nausea, emesis, and sedation.[22,25–27] NSAIDs are also used in the management of postoperative pain but are not as effective as opiates.[20,22] NSAIDs inhibit enzymes that synthesize inflammatory prostaglandins and the production of algogenic metabolites from the lipoxygenase pathway.[28] However, it is also clear that NSAIDs induce their analgesic effect through other mechanisms, such as the release of serotonin.[28–32]

Studies have identified a novel class of drugs that can provide nociceptive relief through mechanisms of action possessing monoamine-reuptake inhibitor and opiate agonist properties.[33–36] This class of medications has been used in Europe for more than 30 years, but the centrally acting synthetic analgesics, tramadol and tapentadol, are now approved for clinical use in the United States.[37–39] Evidence from animal and clinical studies suggests that tramadol and the new synthetic, tapentadol, produce their antinociceptive effects in animals and humans through a complementary dual mechanism of action.[40,41] This article examines the potential benefits of these drugs that complement their antinociceptive properties with the potential of a low side-effect profile.

TRAMADOL
Early Studies

In 1978, Frankus and colleagues[42] observed that after dividing the compound 1-(m-Methoxyphenyl)-2-(dimethylaminomethyl)-cyclohexan-1-ol (L 201) into *cis*- and *trans*-isomers, the resultant conformers were geometrically similar to the opiate, morphine. However, the *trans*-isomer, tramadol, was more active than the *cis*-isomer in analgesic action (**Fig. 1**). In subsequent studies, the development of mild dependency was observed when tramadol was studied in rats, mice, and monkeys.[43–46] Tramadol is an analogue of codeine and has central nervous system (CNS)-mediated analgesic properties with a low affinity for opioid receptors.[47] However, the metabolite of tramadol produced by liver O-demethylation, (+)-O-des-methyl-tramadol, also demonstrates affinity for mu-opioid receptors, which is higher than the parent compound and hence plays an active role in the analgesic effect of tramadol.[47–49] (+)-Tramadol inhibits serotonin reuptake, (−)-tramadol inhibits norepinephrine reuptake, and both isomers demonstrate inhibitory effects on pain transmission in the spinal cord.[49–51] Nevertheless, the affinity for CNS mu-opiate receptors remains low, reported to be 6000 times lower than observed with morphine.[47] Tramadol is mainly metabolized by O- and N-demethylation and by conjugation reactions forming glucuronides and sulfates.[52–54] The O-demethylation of tramadol to O-desmethyl-tramadol, the main analgesic effective metabolite, is catalyzed by cytochrome P450 (CYP) 2D6.[50,55–57] Tramadol and its metabolites are mainly excreted via the kidneys.[52,58–60] The mean elimination half-life for tramadol is about 6 hours.[61–63] Tramadol provides postoperative pain relief comparable with that of meperidine[64–66] and may prove particularly useful in patients with a risk of poor cardiopulmonary function following surgery on the thorax or upper abdomen and when NSAIDs are contraindicated.[50,67,68] Tramadol is an effective and well-tolerated agent able to reduce pain resulting from trauma, renal or biliary

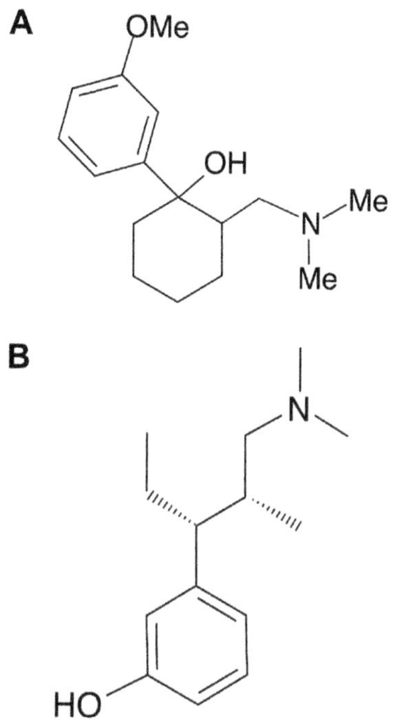

Fig. 1. Chemical structures of tramadol (*A*) and tapentadol (*B*).

colic, and labor.[69–79] Tramadol seems to produce less constipation and emesis than equianalgesic doses of opioids.[50,80–82]

Mechanism of Action: Opioid Activity

Tramadol has been shown to induce antinociception via opioid mechanisms, because tramadol can displace naloxone binding in rat brain suspensions,[33] and the tramadol-induced antinociception in rodents can be blocked by opioid antagonists.[43] Moreover, tramadol-induced antinociception is attenuated in morphine-tolerant rodents, suggesting an antinociceptive cross-tolerance.[83] Finally, in studies with morphine-tolerant animals, tramadol does not precipitate signs of opioid withdrawal,[43] suggesting that tramadol is a pure opioid agonist with little or no antagonist activity. However, despite these preclinical pharmacologic studies that show an opioid mechanism of action, clinical studies with tramadol have not been associated with significant clinical side effects, such as the development of respiratory depression, sedation, or constipation, as observed in other opiate studies.[84–87] The development of analgesic tolerance has not been a significant problem even during repeated administration,[88] nor has the development of psychological dependence or euphoric effects in long-term clinical trials been observed.[84,85,88] Taken together, these clinical studies suggest that tramadol produces antinociception via predominantly, but not only, a mu-opioid receptor mechanism.

Mechanism of Action: Monoaminergic Activity

The analgesic action of tramadol can only be partially inhibited by the opioid antagonist, naloxone; a finding that suggests another mechanism of action.[47,89,90] In 1904, Weber[91] was able to demonstrate that the administration of epinephrine to the spinal cord attenuated thermally evoked withdrawal responses in the cat. Subsequent studies in spinal adrenergic receptors have demonstrated intense antinociceptive activity from various sympathomimetic agents in the mouse, rat, cat, and primate.[92–100] After injury to peripheral nerves, myelinated and unmyelinated afferent nerve fibers become sensitive to sympathetic stimulation and to adrenergic compounds.[101–103] Nociceptive C and A delta fibers are particularly excited by norepinephrine and sympathetic stimulation.[104,105] Moreover, the administration of alpha-2 agonists, such as clonidine, produce antinociception in laboratory animals and analgesia in humans.[106–110] This novel mechanism of analgesic action was clarified by the observation that the antinociceptive activity of tramadol was blocked after administration of yohimbine or ritanserin (adrenergic antagonists).[34,111] Serotoninergic activity in the brain also plays a role in the modulation of beta-endorphin and clonidine analgesia, because the analgesic response can be blocked by specific serotonin antagonists.[112–114] Moreover, the secretion of serotonin can be enhanced and the reuptake of serotonin in the CNS can be inhibited by tramadol.[34,115,116]

Mechanism of Action: CYP2D6 Pathway

In interesting studies on experimental pain, tramadol was studied in volunteers who could or could not metabolize tramadol by way of the CYP2D6 enzymatic pathway.[50,55–57,117–119] The opioid effect of the metabolite of tramadol, O-desmethyl-tramadol, contributed to the analgesic effect of tramadol, but the parent molecule also produced analgesia via a monoaminergic action.[117] In the second study, those volunteers who could metabolize tramadol had increased thresholds to experimental pain than volunteers who could not metabolize tramadol.[118] These studies suggest that formation of the major metabolite of tramadol, O-desmethyl-tramadol, by way of the CYP2D6 enzymatic pathway is important for the effect of tramadol on experimental pain. Moreover, the use of the potent CYP2D6 pathway inhibitor—the selective-serotonin reuptake inhibitor, paroxetine—in healthy volunteers who could metabolize tramadol, the antidepressant was able to reduce, but not abolish, the hypoanalgesic effect of tramadol in opioid-sensitive experimental pain tests.[119]

Human Studies

Early clinical studies were conducted in Europe,[84,88,120,121] with one of the earliest studies including the administration of tramadol to 840 patients by injection (intramuscular or intravenous [IV]) or in suppository form in an open multicenter trial.[85] Tramadol was found to be an effective and well-tolerated analgesic in all 3 forms of administration, with patients rating the therapeutic efficacy at more than 80%. In most cases, the onset of analgesia was within 30 minutes and had a duration of action from 3 to 7 hours. Drowsiness was the most frequent side effect. However, transient hot flushes and outbreaks of sweating occasionally occurred after IV injection.[85] Another early analgesia study was performed in 23 obstetric patients who underwent a comparative study of tramadol versus meperidine during normal delivery.[122] Parenteral administration produced identical levels of analgesia. Moreover, no adverse effects were observed in the parturient after labor or in the newborn.[122] A follow-up study in 40 obstetric patients during labor observed that the efficacy and safety of 100 mg tramadol was comparable to 100 mg meperidine in women asking for pain relief during labor.[65] The duration of labor was slightly shorter in the meperidine group. Onset of analgesia was approximately 10 minutes after administration of tramadol with a duration of approximately 2 hours. Fewer complaints of weariness and less somnolence were observed in the parturients. Moreover, the newborn ventilatory frequency tended to be higher in the tramadol group when compared with the meperidine group.[65]

In an early postoperative clinical study, tramadol was administered to 204 patients who underwent surgery including operations involving the lung, heart, and abdomen.[123] The administration of tramadol provided satisfactory analgesia in patients who underwent lung (approximately 75%), cardiovascular (approximately 77%), abdominal (approximately 89%), and great vessel (approximately 70%) procedures.[123] Respiratory depression and an associated but acceptable sedative effect were observed. In patients who required postoperative mechanical ventilation, tramadol assisted with normalization of ventilatory mechanics with minimal effects on the patient's level of consciousness. Moreover, cessation of muscular shivering was observed after tramadol administration. Finally, adverse effects of tramadol were of no clinical significance and were minimized when it was not rapidly injected into the vein.[123]

An early clinical study examined the role of tramadol when used as a continuous infusion or during patient-controlled analgesia (PCA) administration.[124] The study was performed on 20 American Society of Anesthesiologists (ASA) I or II patients between 20 and 60 years of age who underwent gynecologic procedures under general anesthesia. The patients were randomly allocated to 2 groups. After institution of analgesia regimens, pain scores rapidly decreased in both groups and the analgesia scores were comparable and reported as excellent after 6 hours.[124] Hemodynamic changes were minor and were without clinical significance. PaO_2 and $PaCO_2$ values remained stable. However, a high incidence of nausea and vomiting was observed in the early phase of the study after administration of the loading dose of tramadol.[124] In a parallel study, 40 patients with ASA status I to III who were recovering from major orthopedic or gynecologic operations were investigated to evaluate analgesic efficacy in the early postoperative period using PCA.[87] Analgesia ranged from good to excellent. Side effects were minor and were without clinical concern. The potency of tramadol was judged to be about one-sixth to one-tenth as potent as morphine.[87] In a later study, under double-blind conditions, 135 ASA I and II patients were assigned at random to 2 groups, each receiving a 100 mg bolus of tramadol, with the 2 groups receiving an infusion of 12 mg/h tramadol or saline infusion for 24 hours.[125] The pain relief was reported to be excellent or good by 77% of the tramadol infusion group and less satisfactory (66%) in the saline infusion group. A higher percentage of patients in the saline group required 2 or more tramadol boluses for management of breakthrough pain. Side effects were reported in both groups (25%) but were judged not to be clinically significant.[125]

Epidural Studies

Epidural administration of tramadol has been studied.[126–132] In the first study, 42 surgical patients were given epidural tramadol in doses of 25, 50, and 75 mg for control of postoperative pain.[126] In the 25-mg group, approximately 27% of the patients had significant pain relief but the remainder required at least one additional dose of 25 mg of tramadol. The 50-mg tramadol group had a significant decrease in baseline pain scores with an average duration of pain relief of approximately 12 hours. Similar duration of analgesia and decreases in pain scores were observed in the 75-mg tramadol group, but common side effects, such as dizziness, nausea, and dry mouth, were most frequently found in this group.[126] In a contrasting study, epidural catheter analgesia in 20 patients after surgical correction of scoliosis was studied.[127] At the end of the operation but before closing the fascia, the orthopedic surgeon placed an epidural catheter. After emerging from general anesthesia and endotracheal extubation, evaluation of the motor function of all extremities was performed, followed by epidural administration of 6 to 10 mL 0.25% bupivacaine and continuous administration of 0.25% bupivacaine at a rate of 4 to 8 mL/h. Analgesic level and hemodynamic parameters were monitored. Insufficient analgesia was treated with intravenous tramadol or piritramide (a opiate with a potency 0.65–0.75 times that of morphine).[127] Comparable rates of satisfactory analgesia were obtained in both groups, although in 4 patients, effective analgesia was not achieved with epidural analgesia or systemic opioids. No complications were reported.[127] Epidural analgesia has also been studied with tramadol in the elderly patient population, because this patient group has altered pharmacokinetics and pharmacodynamics and higher rates of perioperative mental dysfunction.[128] Preoperative peridural catheters were placed in 52 patients in a sitting position. The following day, after premedication with atropine, meperidine, or midazolam, 20 to 25 mL of 0.5% bupivacaine was instilled through the peridural catheter and the patients were sedated with small doses of propofol for their operation. Patients were administered peridural morphine or administered tramadol if nausea with emesis developed. Early mobilization of patients was observed and there were no pulmonary complications. Peridural anesthesia with tramadol can provide effective postoperative analgesia in elderly patients with minimal disturbance of pulmonary and mental function.[128] A supportive study examined the role of epidural tramadol in postoperative analgesia when compared with epidural morphine in 20 patients undergoing major abdominal surgery.[129] A balanced technique of general anesthesia combined with lumbar epidural lidocaine was used for surgery, and postoperative analgesia was divided amongst 2 groups of 10 patients receiving 100 mg tramadol diluted in 10 mL normal saline or 4 mg epidural morphine. In all patients, although mean hourly pain scores ranged from 0.2 ± 0.6 to 1.4 ± 2.5, the mean PaO_2 was only postoperatively decreased in the epidural morphine group.[129] The absence of clinically relevant respiratory depression in the epidural tramadol group suggests that epidural tramadol can be used to provide prolonged postoperative analgesia without serious side effects.[129] A contemporary clinical study also examined the efficacy of epidural-administered tramadol in 60 patients undergoing abdominal surgery.[130] Patients were randomly allocated to 3 epidural treatment groups, tramadol 50 mg, tramadol 100 mg, and 10 mL of 0.25% bupivacaine. Pain scores were significantly less in patients receiving tramadol in a dose of 100 mg than in those who had received tramadol 50 mg or only bupivacaine local anesthetic. However, the incidence of nausea and vomiting in the 100-mg tramadol group was significantly higher than that observed in the local anesthetic group.[130] In a thoracotomy study, tramadol was studied to determine its role in providing postoperative pain relief with minimal risk of respiratory depression.[131] In this randomized, double-blind study, a single IV bolus dose of 150 mg of tramadol was compared with the epidural administration of morphine. Both groups obtained adequate pain relief, with no differences in pain scores or PCA morphine consumption between the groups. PaO_2 levels were significantly higher and $PaCO_2$ levels were significantly lower in patients receiving tramadol when compared with morphine. The investigators observed that when compared with epidural morphine, a single dose of 150 mg of tramadol given at the end of surgery could provide effective postoperative analgesia in the initial postoperative period with fewer respiratory complications.[131] Epidural tramadol has been evaluated in patients undergoing caesarean section delivery under epidural anesthesia.[132] Patients received 50 mg of tramadol mixed with 2% lidocaine/epinephrine (1:200,000) or 2% lidocaine/epinephrine (1:200,000) alone. In those patients receiving epidural tramadol, a longer duration (approximately 15 hours) of analgesia was observed when compared with the lidocaine group alone (2.5 hours). Neonatal behavioral assessments were similar in both groups.[132]

Not all studies were able to demonstrate effective postoperative analgesia with epidural administration of tramadol.[133,134] Postoperative analgesia was compared with 2 extradural tramadol regimens in patients undergoing total knee replacement.[133] Extradural anesthesia with light general anesthesia was used for the operative procedure. Patients received a bolus of 50 mg or 100 mg of tramadol followed by a tramadol infusion. A third group received epidural morphine followed by infusion.[133] Visual analogue pain scores were markedly worse and PCA consumption was significantly greater in both tramadol groups when compared with the morphine group. The study was discontinued after recruiting 12 patients.[133] In a second study, tramadol was prospectively studied in a double-blind, randomized trial.[134] Forty patients undergoing knee or hip surgery received anesthesia with epidural lidocaine and epidural tramadol 20, 50, or 100 mg or placebo as a preoperative adjuvant. Although postoperative pain scores were similar in all groups, the interval to first PCA use was shorter, the total dose and duration of PCA use greater, and side effects more common with the 20 mg tramadol group than the 100 mg tramadol or placebo group. Preoperative adjuvant epidural tramadol did not improve the incidence of postoperative analgesia after lidocaine epidural anesthesia; moreover, the administration of 20 mg of tramadol may have resulted in antianalgesia and increased side effects.[134]

Intrathecal Studies

Following intrathecal pharmacodynamic animal studies with tramadol,[34,90,135,136] postoperative analgesia was clinically evaluated.[137–139] In a double-blind, placebo-controlled study, the effect of intrathecal tramadol administration on pain control after transurethral resection of the prostate (TURP) was studied.[137] Sixty-four patients undergoing TURP were randomized to intrathecally receive 3 mL of 0.5% bupivacaine premixed with 25 mg of tramadol or 0.5 mL of saline. There were no differences between the groups with regard to postoperative morphine requirements and sedation scores. Times to first analgesic requirement and length of hospital stay were similar in both groups. Intrathecal tramadol was not different from intrathecal saline in its effect on postoperative morphine requirements after TURP.[137] In subsequent studies, intrathecal administration of tramadol provided improved analgesic profiles.[138] Forty parturients in active labor requesting labor analgesia received a combined spinal/epidural technique and were randomly assigned to receive one of the following intrathecal solutions: 2.5 μg sufentanil in 2.5 mg bupivacaine or 25 mg tramadol in 2.5 mg bupivacaine. Patients who received intrathecal tramadol with 2.5 mg bupivacaine had significantly longer duration of analgesia (114 ± 7 minutes) than those who received intrathecal 2.5 μg sufentanil and 2.5 mg bupivacaine (54 ± 11 minutes).[138] Although no adverse maternal or fetal effects were noted in the sufentanil group, 5 parturients in the tramadol group experienced emesis 10 minutes after administration. There were no observed differences in the time from analgesia to delivery, incidence of operative or assisted delivery, or cervical dilation curves. The administration of 25 mg of intrathecal tramadol with 2.5 mg bupivacaine provides rapid-onset and profound analgesia during the first stage of labor without adverse maternal or fetal effects but with a major side effect of emesis when compared with intrathecal sufentanil.[138] In a third intrathecal tramadol study, the duration of analgesia and/or pain-free period produced by intrathecal tramadol was studied when added to bupivacaine in patients undergoing major gynecologic surgery.[139] Fifty patients (ASA I and II) were randomly allocated to 2 equal groups. Patients received 15 mg of hyperbaric bupivacaine with 20 mg of tramadol or saline. Duration of analgesia or pain-free period in the intrathecal tramadol group was significantly higher (380 ± 12 minutes) when compared with the placebo group (210 ± 10 minutes).[139]

Adverse Events: Dependence

In 1994, the Drug Abuse Advisory Committee of the Food and Drug Administration (FDA) recommended that tramadol could be promoted as an analgesic drug based on extensive preclinical, clinical, and European epidemiologic data.[140] However, to guard against unexpectedly high levels of abuse in the United States, an independent steering committee was appointed to monitor abuse/dependence. In the course of this surveillance project, the committee received reports of withdrawal after abrupt discontinuation of tramadol, and in some instances after dose reductions.[140] With further data collection and analysis, rates of abuse were estimated to be less than one in 100,000 patients.[141] Nevertheless, withdrawal does occur, and in most cases, withdrawal symptoms were comparable to the symptoms seen with opioid withdrawal, but some cases were accompanied by symptoms not normally observed, such as hallucinations, paranoia, extreme anxiety, panic attacks, confusion, and unusual sensory experiences, such as numbness and tingling in one or more extremities.[140] However, tramadol has been recommended as a useful treatment option in patients undergoing opioid detoxification.[142]

Adverse Events: Serotonin Syndrome

Tramadol is a racemic mixture of 2 enantiomers displaying differing affinities for various receptors. (+−) Tramadol is a selective agonist of mu-opiate receptors and preferentially inhibits serotonin reuptake, whereas (−)-tramadol mainly inhibits noradrenaline reuptake.[47] The serotonin syndrome can develop with the use of tramadol and with tapentadol, and the drugs should not be combined with serotonergic drugs, such as selective-serotonin reuptake inhibitors, selective-norepinephrine reuptake inhibitors, triptans, or tricyclic antidepressants.[143–150] The serotonin syndrome can induce mental status changes, and patients have reported hallucinations, tachycardia, and hyperthermia as well as hyperreflexia, muscular incoordination, coma, and death.[143,148,151–155]

TAPENTADOL

Tapentadol 3-[(1R,2R)-3-(dimethylamino)-1-ethyl-2-methylpropyl]phenol (see **Fig. 1**B) is the second clinically approved, centrally acting analgesic with 2 mechanisms of action in a single molecule: mu-opioid agonism and norepinephrine reuptake inhibition.[156] In 2008, the FDA approved tapentadol hydrochloride for oral treatment of moderate-to-severe acute pain in patients older than 18 years.[38,39] The drug has been classified as a schedule II controlled substance.[39] Tapentadol differs from tramadol in several important ways. Tramadol is a racemic mixture of a (+)- and a (−)-enantiomer, whereas tapentadol is a nonracemic compound.[47] Moreover, unlike tramadol, tapentadol has no active metabolites.[156] Tramadol is a prodrug that requires transformation by the cytochrome P450 complex to the metabolically active O-desmethyl-tramadol.[34,157] Caucasians are poor metabolizers of tramadol because of natural variation in this enzymatic system (CYP2D6),[119,158–160] and may not be adequately treated with recommended initial doses.[118] Therefore, tapentadol can be expected to offer advantages over tramadol.[79] Studies published to date (reviewed later) indicate that tapentadol is as effective as oxycodone or morphine, with a lower incidence of gastrointestinal adverse side effects.[161–167]

Initial studies with tapentadol were conducted to characterize the absorption, metabolism, and excretion of the centrally acting oral analgesic in humans.[168] Four healthy male subjects received a single 100-mg oral dose of a radiolabeled 3-[^{14}C]-tapentadol HCl for evaluation of the pharmacokinetics of the drug and the excretion balance of radiocarbon. Oral absorption of tapentadol was rapid; the drug was primarily present in the serum in the form of conjugated metabolites; and excretion of radiocarbon was rapid, within 5 days. Excretion was exclusively renal (99%: 69% conjugates; 27% other metabolites; 3% in unchanged form). No severe adverse events or clinically relevant changes in vital signs, laboratory measurements, or physical examination findings were reported.[168] Tapentadol was also evaluated for induction and inhibition of several cytochrome P450 enzymes in vitro and assayed for protein binding; the conclusion was that no clinically relevant drug-drug interactions were likely to occur through either mechanism.[169]

In clinical studies, tapentadol was compared with standard doses of morphine in patients undergoing mandibular third molar extraction.[161] Patients were randomized to receive single, oral doses of tapentadol (25, 50, 75, 100, or 200 mg), morphine sulfate (60 mg), ibuprofen (400 mg), or placebo. Four hundred patients were randomized to treatment and completed the study. Pain relief scores with morphine sulfate (60 mg) were between those of 100- and 200-mg doses of tapentadol. The incidence of nausea and vomiting was lower with all doses of tapentadol when compared with morphine sulfate (60 mg) but was not statistically significant. An oral dose of tapentadol 75 mg or higher was effective in reducing postoperative dental pain in a dose-related fashion and side effects were well-tolerated when compared with morphine.[161] In a second clinical study, tapentadol was studied as an immediate-release formulation in patients with postsurgical orthopedic pain.[162] In this randomized, double-blind, phase II study in patients with moderate-to-severe pain after bunionectomy surgery, 269 patients were randomly assigned to receive tapentadol (50 or 100 mg), oxycodone (10 mg), or placebo. Although tapentadol provided similar rates of analgesic efficacy, tapentadol (50 mg dose) was associated with lower rates of nausea (46.3% vs 71.6% for oxycodone [10 mg]), dizziness (32.8% vs 56.7%), emesis (16.4% vs 38.8%), and constipation (6.0% vs 17.9%) but with similar rates of somnolence (28.4% vs 26.9%) when compared with oxycodone (10 mg). Both doses of tapentadol were effective in this study for the relief of acute postoperative pain, but an improved rate of gastrointestinal tolerability was observed with the lower dose of tapentadol (50 mg) when compared with oxycodone (10 mg).[162] In another orthopedic population, tapentadol was evaluated for tolerability relative to oxycodone and for incidence of withdrawal symptoms and pain intensity in a phase III, randomized, double-blind study in the management of low back pain or osteoarthritic pain (hip or knee), using a flexible dosing schedule over 90 days.[163] Random assignment of 878 patients was done in a 4:1 ratio to receive tapentadol (50 or 100 mg, every 4–6 hours, by mouth) or oxycodone (10 or 15 mg, every 4–6 hours, by mouth), respectively. In this clinical study, only 391 patients (57.6%) in the tapentadol group and 86 patients (50.6%) in the oxycodone group completed the study. Pain intensity measurements showed similar efficacy for tapentadol and oxycodone. Gastrointestinal events, including nausea (18.4% vs 29.4%), emesis (16.9% vs 30.0%), and constipation (12.8% vs 27.1%), were reported by 44.2% of patients receiving tapentadol and 63.5% of those receiving oxycodone, respectively.[163] Nervous system events, including dizziness (18% vs 17%), headache (12% vs 10%), and somnolence (10% vs 9%), were reported by 37% of patients receiving tapentadol and 37% of patients receiving oxycodone, respectively. Odds ratios (tapentadol/oxycodone) showed that the incidences of somnolence and dizziness were similar; whereas nausea, vomiting, and constipation were significantly less likely to occur with tapentadol. The pattern of withdrawal symptoms suggested that drug tapering may not be necessary after 90-day treatment. In this 90-day study, tapentadol was associated with improved gastrointestinal tolerability when compared with oxycodone.[163] In another orthopedic study, the efficacy and tolerability of tapentadol was studied in patients who were candidates for joint replacement surgery due to end-stage joint disease.[164] In this 10-day, phase III, randomized, double-blind study in patients with uncontrolled osteoarthritis pain who were candidates for primary replacement of the hip or knee as a result of end-stage degenerative joint disease, patients received tapentadol (50 mg or 75 mg), oxycodone (10 mg), or placebo every 4 to 6 hours during waking hours. The sum of pain intensity difference over 5 days was significantly lower in those treated with tapentadol (50 mg and 75 mg) and oxycodone (10 mg) when compared with placebo. Although the efficacy of tapentadol (50 mg and 75 mg) was noninferior to that of oxycodone (10 mg), the incidence of selected gastrointestinal adverse events, such as nausea, emesis, and constipation, were significantly lower for both doses of tapentadol when compared with oxycodone.[164]

Extended release (ER) formulations of tapentadol were studied to evaluate the efficacy and safety of this formulation in the management of moderate-to-severe chronic low back pain.[165] Nine hundred eighty-one patients were randomized (1:1:1) to receive tapentadol ER 100 to 250 mg twice daily; oxycodone HCl controlled release (CR) 20 to 50 mg twice daily, or placebo over a 15-week period after a 3-week titration period into a 12-week maintenance period. Tapentadol ER significantly reduced average pain intensity throughout the maintenance period when compared with placebo. Tapentadol ER was associated with a lower incidence of treatment-emergent adverse events when compared with oxycodone CR. The odds of experiencing constipation or nausea and/or vomiting were significantly lower with tapentadol ER than with oxycodone CR. Tapentadol ER (100–250 mg twice daily) effectively relieved moderate-to-severe chronic low back pain over 15 weeks and had better gastrointestinal tolerability than oxycodone HCl CR (20–50 mg twice daily).[165] In a recently published study, long-term use of tapentadol in a prolonged-release formulation was compared with CR oxycodone in 2968 patients.[166] Although the efficacy of tapentadol was noninferior to oxycodone, tapentadol had superior gastrointestinal tolerability to oxycodone. More patients would discontinue treatment with oxycodone when compared with tapentadol. These data suggest that tapentadol is efficacious and similar to oxycodone but with superior gastrointestinal tolerability and fewer treatment discontinuations.[166]

In the management of pain, it is important to evaluate the effects of other commonly administered analgesics, such as acetaminophen, naproxen, and acetylsalicylic acid, on the pharmacokinetics of tapentadol. A 2-way crossover study in 24 adults and a 3-way crossover study in 38 adults were conducted in the presence of a single dose of immediate-release tapentadol (80 mg) when administered as a single oral dose alone.[167] No clinically relevant changes were noted in serum concentrations of tapentadol in healthy human volunteers, and the investigators recommended that no dosage adjustments for tapentadol were warranted when concomitantly given with the common analgesics, acetaminophen, naproxen, or acetylsalicylic acid.[167]

SUMMARY

Postoperative pain is the most commonly reported complication of ambulatory surgery. Despite ongoing improvements in the management of postoperative pain, patient surveys continue to show poor pain control in the routine clinical setting of outpatient surgery. Although the number of analgesic techniques is more limited in outpatient surgery when compared with inpatient surgery, the use of analgesic regimens with multimodal actions may improve postoperative analgesia and functional outcome after ambulatory surgery. Tramadol and tapentadol hydrochloride are novel in that their analgesic actions occur at multiple sites. Both agents are reported to be mu-opioid receptor agonists and monoamine-reuptake inhibitors. In contrast to pure opioid agonists, both drugs have been demonstrated to have lower risks of respiratory depression, tolerance, and dependence and lower incidence of gastrointestinal adverse side effects when initial bolus dosing is minimized. Caution is warranted when administering these drugs to patients on long-term tricyclic antidepressants, selective-serotonin reuptake inhibitors, and serotonin-norepinephrine reuptake inhibitors; however, no dosage adjustments, at least for tapentadol, are currently warranted when concomitantly given with other common analgesics, acetaminophen, naproxen, or acetylsalicylic acid. The addition of tramadol and tapentadol hydrochloride to the outpatient formulary may improve postoperative analgesia and functional outcome in patients after ambulatory surgery.

REFERENCES

1. Hole K, Berge OG. Regulation of pain sensitivity in the central nervous system. Cephalalgia 1981;1(1):51–9.
2. Akil H, Liebeskind JC. Monoaminergic mechanisms of stimulation-produced analgesia. Brain Res 1975;94(2):279–96.
3. Jensen TS, Smith DF. Monoaminergic mechanisms in stress-induced analgesia. J Neural Transm 1982;53(4):247–55.
4. Yaksh TL, Hammond DL, Tyce GM. Functional aspects of bulbospinal monoaminergic projections in modulating processing of somatosensory information. Fed Proc 1981;40(13):2786–94.
5. Cheng RS, Pomeranz B. Monoaminergic mechanism of electroacupuncture analgesia. Brain Res 1981;215(1–2):77–92.
6. Watkins LR, Johannessen JN, Kinscheck IB, et al. The neurochemical basis of footshock analgesia: the role of spinal cord serotonin and norepinephrine. Brain Res 1984;290(1):107–17.
7. Giordano J, Barr GA. Effects of neonatal spinal cord serotonin depletion on opiate-induced analgesia in tests of thermal and mechanical pain. Brain Res 1988;469(1–2):121–7.
8. Weil-Fugazza J, Godefroy F. Further evidence for the involvement of the diencephalo-dopaminergic system in pain modulation: a neurochemical study on the effect of morphine in the arthritic rat. Int J Tissue React 1991;13(6):305–10.
9. Carruba MO, Nisoli E, Garosi V, et al. Catecholamine and serotonin depletion from rat spinal cord: effects on morphine and footshock induced analgesia. Pharmacol Res 1992;25(2):187–94.
10. Ortega-Alvaro A, Gibert-Rahola J, Mellado-Fernandez ML, et al. The effects of different monoaminergic antidepressants on the analgesia induced by spinal cord adrenal medullary transplants in the formalin test in rats. Anesth Analg 1997;84(4):816–20.
11. Carter GT, Sullivan MD. Antidepressants in pain management. Curr Opin Investig Drugs 2002;3(3):454–8.
12. Vonvoigtlander PF, Lewis RA, Neff GL, et al. Involvement of biogenic amines with the mechanisms of novel analgesics. Prog Neuropsychopharmacol Biol Psychiatry 1983;7(4–6):651–6.
13. Tura B, Tura SM. The analgesic effect of tricyclic antidepressants. Brain Res 1990;518(1–2):19–22.
14. O'Connor AB, Dworkin RH. Treatment of neuropathic pain: an overview of recent guidelines. Am J Med 2009;122(10 Suppl):S22–32.

15. Dworkin RH, O'Connor AB, Audette J, et al. Recommendations for the pharmacological management of neuropathic pain: an overview and literature update. Mayo Clin Proc 2010;85(3 Suppl):S3–14.
16. Messing RB, Lytle LD. Serotonin-containing neurons: their possible role in pain and analgesia. Pain 1977;4(1):1–21.
17. Khachaturian H, Watson SJ. Some perspectives on monoamine-opioid peptide interaction in rat central nervous system. Brain Res Bull 1982;9(1–6):441–62.
18. Tyce GM, Yaksh TL. Monoamine release from cat spinal cord by somatic stimuli: an intrinsic modulatory system. J Physiol 1981;314:513–29.
19. Lipp J. Possible mechanisms of morphine analgesia. Clin Neuropharmacol 1991;14(2):131–47.
20. Rawal N. Postoperative pain treatment for ambulatory surgery. Best Pract Res Clin Anaesthesiol 2007;21(1):129–48.
21. Schecter WP, Bongard FS, Gainor BJ, et al. Pain control in outpatient surgery. J Am Coll Surg 2002;195(1):95–104.
22. Chauvin M. State of the art of pain treatment following ambulatory surgery. Eur J Anaesthesiol Suppl 2003;28:3–6.
23. White PF. The changing role of non-opioid analgesic techniques in the management of postoperative pain. Anesth Analg 2005;101(5 Suppl):S5–22.
24. White PF, Kehlet H, Neal JM, et al. The role of the anesthesiologist in fast-track surgery: from multimodal analgesia to perioperative medical care. Anesth Analg 2007;104(6):1380–96.
25. Power I, Barratt S. Analgesic agents for the postoperative period. Nonopioids. Surg Clin North Am 1999;79(2):275–95.
26. Langford RM. Pain management today – what have we learned? Clin Rheumatol 2006;25(Suppl 1):S2–8.
27. Pyati S, Gan TJ. Perioperative pain management. CNS Drugs 2007;21(3):185–211.
28. Cashman JN. The mechanisms of action of NSAIDs in analgesia. Drugs 1996;52(Suppl 5):13–23.
29. Walker JS. NSAID: an update on their analgesic effects. Clin Exp Pharmacol Physiol 1995;22(11):855–60.
30. Mort JR, Aparasu RR, Baer RK. Interaction between selective serotonin reuptake inhibitors and nonsteroidal antiinflammatory drugs: review of the literature. Pharmacotherapy 2006;26(9):1307–13.
31. Hersh EV, Pinto A, Moore PA. Adverse drug interactions involving common prescription and over-the-counter analgesic agents. Clin Ther 2007;29 Suppl:2477–97.
32. Kaye AD, Baluch A, Kaye AJ, et al. Pharmacology of cyclooxygenase-2 inhibitors and preemptive analgesia in acute pain management. Curr Opin Anaesthesiol 2008;21(4):439–45.
33. Hennies HH, Friderichs E, Wilsmann K, et al. Effect of the opioid analgesic tramadol on inactivation of norepinephrine and serotonin. Biochem Pharmacol 1982;31(8):1654–5.
34. Raffa RB, Friderichs E, Reimann W, et al. Opioid and nonopioid components independently contribute to the mechanism of action of tramadol, an 'atypical' opioid analgesic. J Pharmacol Exp Ther 1992;260(1):275–85.
35. Lee CR, McTavish D, Sorkin EM. A preliminary review of its pharmacodynamic and pharmacokinetic properties, and therapeutic potential in acute and chronic pain states. Drugs 1993;46(2):313–40.

36. Desmeules JA, Piguet V, Collart L, et al. Contribution of monoaminergic modulation to the analgesic effect of tramadol. Br J Clin Pharmacol 1996;41(1):7–12.
37. New oral analgesic, tramadol, gains marketing approval. Am J Health Syst Pharm 1995;52(11):1153–4.
38. Tapentadol (Nucynta)–a new analgesic. Med Lett Drugs Ther 2009;51(1318): 61–2.
39. Drug Enforcement Administration, Department of Justice. Schedules of controlled substances: placement of tapentadol into schedule II. Final rule. Fed Regist 2009;74(97):23790–3.
40. Raffa RB. A novel approach to the pharmacology of analgesics. Am J Med 1996;101(1A):40S–6S.
41. Schroder W, Vry JD, Tzschentke TM, et al. Differential contribution of opioid and noradrenergic mechanisms of tapentadol in rat models of nociceptive and neuropathic pain. Eur J Pain 2010;14(8):814–21.
42. Frankus E, Friderichs E, Kim SM, et al. [On separation of isomeres, structural elucidation and pharmacological characterization of 1-(m-methoxyphenyl)-2-(dimethylaminomethyl)-cyclohexan-1-ol (author's transl)]. Arzneimittelforschung 1978;28(1a):114–21 [in German].
43. Friderichs E, Felgenhauer F, Jongschaap P, et al. [Pharmacological studies on analgesia, dependence on and tolerance of tramadol, a potent analgetic drug (author's transl)]. Arzneimittelforschung 1978;28(1a):122–34 [in German].
44. Murano T, Yamamoto H, Endo N, et al. Studies on dependence on tramadol in rats. Arzneimittelforschung 1978;28(1a):152–8.
45. Osterloh G, Friderichs E, Felgenhauer F, et al. [General pharmacological studies on tramadol, a potent analgetic agent (author's transl)]. Arzneimittelforschung 1978;28(1a):135–51 [in German].
46. Yanagita T. Drug dependence upotential of 1-(m-methoxyphenyl)-2-dimethylaminomethyl)-cyclohexan-1-ol hydrochloride (tramadol) tested in monkeys. Arzneimittelforschung 1978;28(1a):158–63.
47. Dayer P, Desmeules J, Collart L. [Pharmacology of tramadol]. Drugs 1997; 53(Suppl 2):18–24 [in French].
48. Sevcik J, Nieber K, Driessen B, et al. Effects of the central analgesic tramadol and its main metabolite, O-desmethyltramadol, on rat locus coeruleus neurones. Br J Pharmacol 1993;110(1):169–76.
49. Bamigbade TA, Davidson C, Langford RM, et al. Actions of tramadol, its enantiomers and principal metabolite, O-desmethyltramadol, on serotonin (5-HT) efflux and uptake in the rat dorsal raphe nucleus. Br J Anaesth 1997; 79(3):352–6.
50. Grond S, Sablotzki A. Clinical pharmacology of tramadol. Clin Pharmacokinet 2004;43(13):879–923.
51. Reimann W, Hennies HH. Inhibition of spinal noradrenaline uptake in rats by the centrally acting analgesic tramadol. Biochem Pharmacol 1994;47(12):2289–93.
52. Lintz W, Erlacin S, Frankus E, et al. [Biotransformation of tramadol in man and animal (author's transl)]. Arzneimittelforschung 1981;31(11):1932–43 [in German].
53. Paar WD, Frankus P, Dengler HJ. The metabolism of tramadol by human liver microsomes. Clin Investig 1992;70(8):708–10.
54. Paar WD, Frankus P, Dengler HJ. High-performance liquid chromatographic assay for the simultaneous determination of tramadol and its metabolites in microsomal fractions of human liver. J Chromatogr B: Biomed Appl 1996; 686(2):221–7.

55. Abdel-Rahman SM, Leeder JS, Wilson JT, et al. Concordance between tramadol and dextromethorphan parent/metabolite ratios: the influence of CYP2D6 and non-CYP2D6 pathways on biotransformation. J Clin Pharmacol 2002;42(1):24–9.
56. Garrido MJ, Sayar O, Segura C, et al. Pharmacokinetic/pharmacodynamic modeling of the antinociceptive effects of (+)-tramadol in the rat: role of cytochrome P450 2D activity. J Pharmacol Exp Ther 2003;305(2):710–8.
57. Levo A, Koski A, Ojanpera I, et al. Post-mortem SNP analysis of CYP2D6 gene reveals correlation between genotype and opioid drug (tramadol) metabolite ratios in blood. Forensic Sci Int 2003;135(1):9–15.
58. Potyka U, Paar WD, Sauerbruch T, et al. Labelling studies for structure elucidation of a new hydroxymetabolite of tramadol. Isotopes Environ Health Stud 1998; 34(1–2):119–25.
59. Rudaz S, Veuthey JL, Desiderio C, et al. Simultaneous stereoselective analysis by capillary electrophoresis of tramadol enantiomers and their main phase I metabolites in urine. J Chromatogr A 1999;846(1–2):227–37.
60. Ogunleye DS. Investigation of racial variations in the metabolism of tramadol. Eur J Drug Metab Pharmacokinet 2001;26(1–2):95–8.
61. Lintz W, Barth H, Osterloh G, et al. Bioavailability of enteral tramadol formulations. 1st communication: capsules. Arzneimittelforschung 1986;36(8):1278–83.
62. Lintz W, Barth H, Becker R, et al. Pharmacokinetics of tramadol and bioavailability of enteral tramadol formulations. 2nd communication: drops with ethanol. Arzneimittelforschung 1998;48(5):436–45.
63. Lintz W, Barth H, Osterloh G, et al. Pharmacokinetics of tramadol and bioavailability of enteral tramadol formulations. 3rd Communication: suppositories. Arzneimittelforschung 1998;48(9):889–99.
64. Parth P, Madler C, Morawetz RF. [Characterization of the effect of analgesics on the assessment of experimental pain in man. Pethidine and tramadol in a double-blind comparison]. Anaesthesist 1984;33(5):235–9 [in German].
65. Husslein P, Kubista E, Egarter C. [Obstetrical analgesia with tramadol–results of a prospective randomized comparative study with pethidine]. Z Geburtshilfe Perinatol 1987;191(6):234–7 [in German].
66. Chaturachinda K, Tangtrakul S, Pausawasdi S, et al. A comparative study of tramadol and pethidine in laparoscopic interval sterilization. J Med Assoc Thai 1988;71(Suppl 1):55–7.
67. Scott LJ, Perry CM. Tramadol: a review of its use in perioperative pain. Drugs 2000;60(1):139–76.
68. Klotz U. Tramadol–the impact of its pharmacokinetic and pharmacodynamic properties on the clinical management of pain. Arzneimittelforschung 2003; 53(10):681–7.
69. Suvonnakote T, Thitadilok W, Atisook R. Pain relief during labour. J Med Assoc Thai 1986;69(11):575–80.
70. Viegas OA, Khaw B, Ratnam SS. Tramadol in labour pain in primiparous patients. A prospective comparative clinical trial. Eur J Obstet Gynecol Reprod Biol 1993;49(3):131–5.
71. Primus G, Pummer K, Vucsina F, et al. [Tramadol versus metimazole in alleviating pain in ureteral colic]. Urologe A 1989;28(2):103–5 [in German].
72. Bierbach H. [Treatment of acute gastrointestinal pain]. Schmerz 1993;7(3): 154–9 [in German].

73. Schmieder G, Stankov G, Zerle G, et al. Observer-blind study with metamizole versus tramadol and butylscopolamine in acute biliary colic pain. Arzneimittelforschung 1993;43(11):1216–21.

74. Stankov G, Schmieder G, Zerle G, et al. Double-blind study with dipyrone versus tramadol and butylscopolamine in acute renal colic pain. World J Urol 1994;12(3):155–61.

75. Eray O, Cete Y, Oktay C, et al. Intravenous single-dose tramadol versus meperidine for pain relief in renal colic. Eur J Anaesthesiol 2002;19(5):368–70.

76. Mortelmans LJ, Desruelles D, Baert JA, et al. Use of tramadol drip in controlling renal colic pain. J Endourol 2006;20(12):1010–5.

77. Hoogewijs J, Diltoer MW, Hubloue I, et al. A prospective, open, single blind, randomized study comparing four analgesics in the treatment of peripheral injury in the emergency department. Eur J Emerg Med 2000;7(2):119–23.

78. Vergnion M, Degesves S, Garcet L, et al. Tramadol, an alternative to morphine for treating posttraumatic pain in the prehospital situation. Anesth Analg 2001; 92(6):1543–6.

79. Wilder-Smith CH, Hill LT, Laurent S. Postamputation pain and sensory changes in treatment-naive patients: characteristics and responses to treatment with tramadol, amitriptyline, and placebo. Anesthesiology 2005;103(3):619–28.

80. Maurer AH, Krevsky B, Knight LC, et al. Opioid and opioid-like drug effects on whole-gut transit measured by scintigraphy. J Nucl Med 1996;37(5): 818–22.

81. Smith AB, Ravikumar TS, Kamin M, et al. Combination tramadol plus acetaminophen for postsurgical pain. Am J Surg 2004;187(4):521–7.

82. Bourne MH, Rosenthal NR, Xiang J, et al. Tramadol/acetaminophen tablets in the treatment of postsurgical orthopedic pain. Am J Orthop (Belle Mead NJ) 2005;34(12):592–7.

83. Mattia A, Vanderah T, Raffa RB, et al. Tramadol produces antinociception through spinal sites, with minimal tolerance, in mice. FASEB J 1991;5:A473.

84. Arend I, von Arnim B, Nijssen J, et al. [Tramadol and pentazocine in a clinical double-blind crossover comparison]. Arzneimittelforschung 1978;28(1a): 199–208 [in German].

85. Schenck EG, Arend I. [The effect of tramadol in an open clinical trial (author's transl)]. Arzneimittelforschung 1978;28(1a):209–12 [in German].

86. Muller-Limmroth W, Krueger H. [The effect of tramadol on psychic and psychomotor performance in man (author's transl)]. Arzneimittelforschung 1978;28(1a): 179–80 [in German].

87. Lehmann KA, Kratzenberg U, Schroeder-Bark B, et al. Postoperative patient-controlled analgesia with tramadol: analgesic efficacy and minimum effective concentrations. Clin J Pain 1990;6(3):212–20.

88. Flohe L, Arend I, Cogal A, et al. [Clinical study on the development of dependency after long-term treatment with tramadol (author's transl)]. Arzneimittelforschung 1978;28(1a):213–7 [in German].

89. Nickel B. The antinociceptive activity of flupirtine: a structurally new analgesic. Postgrad Med J 1987;63(Suppl 3):19–28.

90. Carlsson KH, Jurna I. Effects of tramadol on motor and sensory responses of the spinal nociceptive system in the rat. Eur J Pharmacol 1987;139(1):1–10.

91. Weber H. Uber Anfisthesie durch Adrenalin. Verh Dtsch Ges Inn Med 1904;21: 616–9.

92. Burrill DY, Goetzl FR, Ivy AC. The pain threshold raising effect of amphetamine. J Dent Res 1944;23:337–44.

93. Kiessig HJ, Orzechowski G. Untersuchungen fiber die wirkungsweise der sympathomometic. Naunyn Schmiedebergs Arch Exp Pathol Pharmacol 1941;197: 391–404.

94. Fairbanks CA, Stone LS, Kitto KF, et al. alpha(2C)-Adrenergic receptors mediate spinal analgesia and adrenergic-opioid synergy. J Pharmacol Exp Ther 2002; 300(1):282–90.

95. Archer T, Jonsson G, Minor BG, et al. Noradrenergic-serotonergic interactions and nociception in the rat. Eur J Pharmacol 1986;120(3):295–307.

96. Loomis CW, Cervenko FW, Jhamandas K, et al. Analgesia and autonomic function following intrathecal administration of morphine and norepinephrine to the rat. Can J Physiol Pharmacol 1985;63(6):656–62.

97. Li X, Zhao Z, Pan HL, et al. Norepinephrine release from spinal synaptosomes: auto-alpha2 -adrenergic receptor modulation. Anesthesiology 2000;93(1): 164–72.

98. Howe JR, Yaksh TL. Changes in sensitivity to intrathecal norepinephrine and serotonin after 6-hydroxydopamine (6-OHDA), 5,6-dihydroxytryptamine (5,6-DHT) or repeated monoamine administration. J Pharmacol Exp Ther 1982; 220(2):311–21.

99. Hayashida K, DeGoes S, Curry R, et al. Gabapentin activates spinal noradrenergic activity in rats and humans and reduces hypersensitivity after surgery. Anesthesiology 2007;106(3):557–62.

100. Eisenach JC, Detweiler DJ, Tong C, et al. Cerebrospinal fluid norepinephrine and acetylcholine concentrations during acute pain. Anesth Analg 1996;82(3): 621–6.

101. Devor M, Janig W. Activation of myelinated afferents ending in a neuroma by stimulation of the sympathetic supply in the rat. Neurosci Lett 1981;24(1): 43–7.

102. Devor M, Janig W, Michaelis M. Modulation of activity in dorsal root ganglion neurons by sympathetic activation in nerve-injured rats. J Neurophysiol 1994; 71(1):38–47.

103. Wall PD, Gutnick M. Properties of afferent nerve impulses originating from a neuroma. Nature 1974;248(5451):740–3.

104. Lu Y, Perl ER. Selective action of noradrenaline and serotonin on neurones of the spinal superficial dorsal horn in the rat. J Physiol 2007;582(Pt 1):127–36.

105. Ren Y, Zou X, Fang L, et al. Sympathetic modulation of activity in Adelta- and C-primary nociceptive afferents after intradermal injection of capsaicin in rats. J Neurophysiol 2005;93(1):365–77.

106. Paalzow L. Analgesia produced by clonidine in mice and rats. J Pharm Pharmacol 1974;26(5):361–3.

107. Yaksh TL, Reddy SV. Studies in the primate on the analgetic effects associated with intrathecal actions of opiates, alpha-adrenergic agonists and baclofen. Anesthesiology 1981;54(6):451–67.

108. Skingle M, Hayes AG, Tyers MB. Antinociceptive activity of clonidine in the mouse, rat and dog. Life Sci 1982;31(11):1123–32.

109. Tamsen A, Gordh T. Epidural clonidine produces analgesia. Lancet 1984; 2(8396):231–2.

110. Coombs DW, Saunders RL, Fratkin JD, et al. Continuous intrathecal hydromorphone and clonidine for intractable cancer pain. J Neurosurg 1986;64(6):890–4.

111. Frink MC, Hennies HH, Englberger W, et al. Influence of tramadol on neurotransmitter systems of the rat brain. Arzneimittelforschung 1996;46(11):1029–36.

112. Yaksh TL, Wilson PR. Spinal serotonin terminal system mediates antinociception. J Pharmacol Exp Ther 1979;208(3):446–53.
113. Lin MT, Chi ML, Chandra A, et al. Serotoninergic mechanisms of beta-endorphin- and clonidine-induced analgesia in rats. Pharmacology 1980;20(6): 323–8.
114. Hylden JL, Wilcox GL. Intrathecal serotonin in mice: analgesia and inhibition of a spinal action of substance P. Life Sci 1983;33(8):789–95.
115. Raffa RB, Friderichs E, Reimann W, et al. Complementary and synergistic antinociceptive interaction between the enantiomers of tramadol. J Pharmacol Exp Ther Oct 1993;267(1):331–40.
116. Driessen B, Reimann W. Interaction of the central analgesic, tramadol, with the uptake and release of 5-hydroxytryptamine in the rat brain in vitro. Br J Pharmacol 1992;105(1):147–51.
117. Enggaard TP, Poulsen L, Arendt-Nielsen L, et al. The analgesic effect of tramadol after intravenous injection in healthy volunteers in relation to CYP2D6. Anesth Analg 2006;102(1):146–50.
118. Poulsen L, Arendt-Nielsen L, Brosen K, et al. The hypoalgesic effect of tramadol in relation to CYP2D6. Clin Pharmacol Ther 1996;60(6):636–44.
119. Laugesen S, Enggaard TP, Pedersen RS, et al. Paroxetine, a cytochrome P450 2D6 inhibitor, diminishes the stereoselective O-demethylation and reduces the hypoalgesic effect of tramadol. Clin Pharmacol Ther 2005;77(4):312–23.
120. Huber HP. [Examination of psychic effects of a new analgesic agent of the cyclohexanols series. A contribution to a possible psychic dependence potential of tramadol (author's transl)]. Arzneimittelforschung 1978;28(1a):189–91 [in German].
121. Rost A, Schenck EG. [The effect of tramadol and other analgesics on the pain threshold in human dental pulp (author's transl)]. Arzneimittelforschung 1978; 28(1a):181–3 [in German].
122. Bitsch M, Emmrich J, Hary J, et al. [Obstetrical analgesia with tramadol]. Fortschr Med 1980;98(16):632–4 [in German].
123. Lebedeva RN, Bondarenko AV, Abbakumov VV, et al. [Clinical use of tramal in patients in the early postoperative period]. Anesteziol Reanimatol 1989;5:50–4 [in Russian].
124. Jellinek H, Haumer H, Grubhofer G, et al. [Tramadol in postoperative pain therapy. Patient-controlled analgesia versus continuous infusion]. Anaesthesist 1990;39(10):513–20 [in German].
125. Rud U, Fischer MV, Mewes R, et al. [Postoperative analgesia with tramadol. Continuous infusion versus repetitive bolus administration]. Anaesthesist 1994; 43(5):316–21 [in German].
126. Fu YP, Chan KH, Lee TK, Chang JC, Daiy YP, Lee TY. Epidural tramadol for postoperative pain relief. Ma Zui Xue Za Zhi 1991;29(3):648–52.
127. Otto S, Dietz C, Kuleszynski P, et al. [Postoperative analgesia following spondylodesis using a peridural catheter placed during surgery. Results of a pilot study]. Anaesthesist 1991;40(4):235–7 [in German].
128. Fuchs C. [Continuous peridural anesthesia in abdominal surgery. An alternative for elderly patients]. Anaesthesist 1992;41(10):634–8 [in German].
129. Baraka A, Jabbour S, Ghabash M, et al. A comparison of epidural tramadol and epidural morphine for postoperative analgesia. Can J Anaesth 1993;40(4): 308–13.
130. Delilkan AE, Vijayan R. Epidural tramadol for postoperative pain relief. Anaesthesia 1993;48(4):328–31.

131. James MF, Heijke SA, Gordon PC. Intravenous tramadol versus epidural morphine for postthoracotomy pain relief: a placebo-controlled double-blind trial. Anesth Analg 1996;83(1):87–91.

132. Pan AK, Mukherjee P, Rudra A. Role of epidural tramadol hydrochloride on postoperative pain relief in caesarean section delivery. J Indian Med Assoc 1997; 95(4):105–6.

133. Grace D, Fee JP. Ineffective analgesia after extradural tramadol hydrochloride in patients undergoing total knee replacement. Anaesthesia 1995;50(6): 555–8.

134. Wilder-Smith CH, Wilder-Smith OH, Farschtschian M, et al. Preoperative adjuvant epidural tramadol: the effect of different doses on postoperative analgesia and pain processing. Acta Anaesthesiol Scand 1998;42(3):299–305.

135. Bernatzky G, Jurna I. Intrathecal injection of codeine, buprenorphine, tilidine, tramadol and nefopam depresses the tail-flick response in rats. Eur J Pharmacol 1986;120(1):75–80.

136. Selve N, Englberger W, Friderichs E, et al. Galanin receptor antagonists attenuate spinal antinociceptive effects of DAMGO, tramadol and non-opioid drugs in rats. Brain Res 1996;735(2):177–87.

137. Alhashemi JA, Kaki AM. Effect of intrathecal tramadol administration on postoperative pain after transurethral resection of prostate. Br J Anaesth 2003;91(4): 536–40.

138. Frikha N, Ellachtar M, Mebazaa MS, et al. Combined spinal-epidural analgesia in labor–comparison of sufentanil vs tramadol. Middle East J Anesthesiol 2007; 19(1):87–96.

139. Chakraborty S, Chakrabarti J, Bhattacharya D. Intrathecal tramadol added to bupivacaine as spinal anesthetic increases analgesic effect of the spinal blockade after major gynecological surgeries. Indian J Pharmacol 2008;40(4): 180–2.

140. Senay EC, Adams EH, Geller A, et al. Physical dependence on Ultram (tramadol hydrochloride): both opioid-like and atypical withdrawal symptoms occur. Drug Alcohol Depend 2003;69(3):233–41.

141. Cicero TJ, Adams EH, Geller A, et al. A postmarketing surveillance program to monitor Ultram (tramadol hydrochloride) abuse in the United States. Drug Alcohol Depend 1999;57(1):7–22.

142. Lanier RK, Lofwall MR, Mintzer MZ, et al. Physical dependence potential of daily tramadol dosing in humans. Psychopharmacology (Berl) 2010;211(4):457–66.

143. Egberts AC, ter Borgh J, Brodie-Meijer CC. Serotonin syndrome attributed to tramadol addition to paroxetine therapy. Int Clin Psychopharmacol 1997;12(3): 181–2.

144. Kitson R, Carr B. Tramadol and severe serotonin syndrome. Anaesthesia 2005; 60(9):934–5.

145. Vizcaychipi MP, Walker S, Palazzo M. Serotonin syndrome triggered by tramadol. Br J Anaesth 2007;99(6):919.

146. Takeshita J, Litzinger MH. Serotonin syndrome associated with tramadol. Prim Care Companion J Clin Psychiatry 2009;11(5):273.

147. Tashakori A, Afshari R. Tramadol overdose as a cause of serotonin syndrome: a case series. Clin Toxicol (Phila) 2010;48(4):337–41.

148. Lantz MS, Buchalter EN, Giambanco V. Serotonin syndrome following the administration of tramadol with paroxetine. Int J Geriatr Psychiatry 1998;13(5):343–5.

149. Lange-Asschenfeldt C, Weigmann H, Hiemke C, et al. Serotonin syndrome as a result of fluoxetine in a patient with tramadol abuse: plasma level-correlated symptomatology. J Clin Psychopharmacol 2002;22(4):440–1.
150. Nayyar N. Serotonin syndrome associated with sertraline, trazodone and tramadol abuse. Indian J Psychiatry 2009;51(1):68.
151. Vadivelu N, Mitra S, Narayan D. Recent advances in postoperative pain management. Yale J Biol Med 2010;83(1):11–25.
152. Devulder J, De Laat M, Dumoulin K, et al. Nightmares and hallucinations after long-term intake of tramadol combined with antidepressants. Acta Clin Belg 1996;51(3):184–6.
153. John AP, Koloth R. Severe serotonin toxicity and manic switch induced by combined use of tramadol and paroxetine. Aust N Z J Psychiatry 2007;41(2):192–3.
154. Pilgrim JL, Gerostamoulos D, Drummer OH. Deaths involving serotonergic drugs. Forensic Sci Int 2010;198(1–3):110–7.
155. Shadnia S, Soltaninejad K, Heydari K, et al. Tramadol intoxication: a review of 114 cases. Hum Exp Toxicol 2008;27(3):201–5.
156. Tzschentke TM, Jahnel U, Kogel B, et al. Tapentadol hydrochloride: a next-generation, centrally acting analgesic with two mechanisms of action in a single molecule. Drugs Today (Barc) 2009;45(7):483–96.
157. Wu WN, McKown LA, Codd EE, et al. In vitro metabolism of the analgesic agent, tramadol-N-oxide, in mouse, rat, and human. Eur J Drug Metab Pharmacokinet 2002;27(3):193–7.
158. Lotsch J, Skarke C, Liefhold J, et al. Genetic predictors of the clinical response to opioid analgesics: clinical utility and future perspectives. Clin Pharmacokinet 2004;43(14):983–1013.
159. Pedersen RS, Damkier P, Brosen K. Tramadol as a new probe for cytochrome P450 2D6 phenotyping: a population study. Clin Pharmacol Ther 2005;77(6):458–67.
160. Zhou SF. Polymorphism of human cytochrome P450 2D6 and its clinical significance: part I. Clin Pharmacokinet 2009;48(11):689–723.
161. Kleinert R, Lange C, Steup A, et al. Single dose analgesic efficacy of tapentadol in postsurgical dental pain: the results of a randomized, double-blind, placebo-controlled study. Anesth Analg 2008;107(6):2048–55.
162. Stegmann JU, Weber H, Steup A, et al. The efficacy and tolerability of multiple-dose tapentadol immediate release for the relief of acute pain following orthopedic (bunionectomy) surgery. Curr Med Res Opin 2008;24:3185–96.
163. Hale M, Upmalis D, Okamoto A, et al. Tolerability of tapentadol immediate release in patients with lower back pain or osteoarthritis of the hip or knee over 90 days: a randomized, double-blind study. Curr Med Res Opin 2009; 25(5):1095–104.
164. Hartrick C, Van Hove I, Stegmann JU, et al. Efficacy and tolerability of tapentadol immediate release and oxycodone HCl immediate release in patients awaiting primary joint replacement surgery for end-stage joint disease: a 10-day, phase III, randomized, double-blind, active- and placebo-controlled study. Clin Ther 2009;31(2):260–71.
165. Buynak R, Shapiro DY, Okamoto A, et al. Efficacy and safety of tapentadol extended release for the management of chronic low back pain: results of a prospective, randomized, double-blind, placebo- and active-controlled Phase III study. Expert Opin Pharmacother 2010;11(11):1787–804.

166. Lange B, Kuperwasser B, Okamoto A, et al. Efficacy and safety of tapentadol prolonged release for chronic osteoarthritis pain and low back pain. Adv Ther 2010;27(6):381–99.

167. Smit JW, Oh C, Rengelshausen J, et al. Effects of acetaminophen, naproxen, and acetylsalicylic acid on tapentadol pharmacokinetics: results of two randomized, open-label, crossover, drug-drug interaction studies. Pharmacotherapy 2010;30(1):25–34.

168. Terlinden R, Ossig J, Fliegert F, et al. Absorption, metabolism, and excretion of 14C-labeled tapentadol HCl in healthy male subjects. Eur J Drug Metab Pharmacokinet 2007;32(3):163–9.

169. Kneip C, Terlinden R, Beier H, et al. Investigations into the drug-drug interaction potential of tapentadol in human liver microsomes and fresh human hepatocytes. Drug Metab Lett 2008;2(1):67–75.

Anticoagulants: Newer Ones, Mechanisms, and Perioperative Updates

Julie A. Gayle, MD[a],*, Alan D. Kaye, MD, PhD[b],
Adam M. Kaye, PharmD[c], Rinoo Shah, MD[d]

KEYWORDS

- New anticoagulants • Anesthetic concerns
- Herbal medications • Perioperative anticoagulation

The ongoing research and development of new anticoagulant/antiplatelet drugs deserves special attention in the evaluation and management of patients presenting for surgery. As part of the development of the ideal anticoagulant, the newer drugs aim to provide safe, effective, and predictable anticoagulant activity with ease of use (ie, oral administration or minimal number of daily injections) and no need for monitoring.[1] Anesthesiologists must be familiar with the newly developed anticoagulants because their use in the perioperative setting will likely increase. Mechanisms of action of these newer anticoagulants warrant consideration as do the risks and benefits of discontinuation or reversal of the drugs before surgery.[2] Of equal importance are the recommendations by the American Society of Regional Anesthesia and Pain Medicine (ASRA) pertaining to regional anesthesia in patients receiving these new anticoagulants.

The use of herbal medications and certain vitamin supplements has dramatically increased in recent years. Some of these alternative medicines enhance the effects of anticoagulant drugs. Therefore, it is important to elicit a history of use to avoid exaggerated effects, specifically bleeding.[3]

[a] Department of Anesthesiology, Louisiana State University Health Sciences Center, New Orleans, LA, USA
[b] Departments of Anesthesiology and Pharmacology, Louisiana State University School of Medicine, 1542 Tulane Avenue, Room 656, New Orleans, LA, USA
[c] Department of Pharmacy Practice, Thomas J. Long School of Pharmacy and Health Sciences, University of the Pacific, Stockton, CA, USA
[d] Department of Anesthesiology, Guthrie Clinic-Big Flats, Horseheads, NY, USA
* Corresponding author.
E-mail address: Jgayle477@cox.net

Anesthesiology Clin 28 (2010) 667–679
doi:10.1016/j.anclin.2010.08.013
1932-2275/10/$ – see front matter © 2010 Elsevier Inc. All rights reserved.

NEW ANTICOAGULANTS

The development of newer anticoagulants and their emergence into clinical practice is a result of the demand for more efficacious anticoagulation therapy with a better safety profile than the older anticoagulants, such as heparin and warfarin.[4] Anticoagulants are the agents of choice for prevention and treatment of venous thromboembolism (VTE). Venous thrombi develop under low shear conditions and are made of fibrin and trapped red cells. These thrombi contain few platelets.[4,5] Anticoagulants inhibit specific targets in the coagulation pathway (**Fig. 1**). This article focuses on the newer anticoagulants and their mechanisms of action.

Factor Xa Inhibitors

New factor Xa inhibitors block factor Xa either directly or indirectly (**Table 1**). Fondaparinux (Arixtra), an indirect factor Xa inhibitor, is a synthetic pentasaccharide that selectively binds to antithrombin III, potentiating factor Xa neutralization and inhibiting thrombin formation. Fondaparinux, a parenteral agent, is approved for prevention of VTE in high-risk orthopedic surgeries and as a substitute for heparin or low-molecular-weight heparin for the initial treatment of VTE.[2,5] The plasma half-life of fondaparinux is 21 hours; therefore, it is dosed once a day with the first dose given 6 hours postoperatively.[6] Compared with unfractionated heparin, fondaparinux has excellent bioavailability and should not cause heparin-induced thrombocytopenia (HIT).

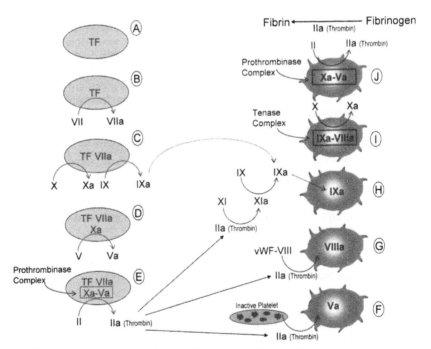

Fig. 1. The coagulation mechanism. A through F represent the complex mechanisms of interaction amongst the factors in the coagulation pathway. TF, membrane-bound tissue factor on a extravascular cell surface; vWF, von Willebrand factor. (*From* Drummond JC, Petrovitch CT. Hemotherapy and hemostasis. In: Barash PG, Cullen BF, Stoelting RK, editors. Clinical anesthesia. 5th edition. Philadelphia: Lippincott Williams & Wilkins; 2006. p. 223; with permission.)

Table 1
Summary of factor Xa inhibitors

	Fondaparinux	Rivaroxaban	Apixaban
Action	Inhibits fXa	Inhibits fXa	Inhibits fXa
Route of administration	Subcutaneous	Oral	Oral
Indication	VTE/PE8 prophylaxis	VTE/PE prophylaxis	VTE/PE prophylaxis
Half-life	17–21 hours	5–10 hours	10–14 hours
Elimination	Renal	Renal	Renal
Monitoring	Anti-Xa assay	Anti-Xa assay	Anti-Xa assay

Abbreviation: PE, pulmonary embolism.

A specific anti-Xa assay is needed to measure its anticoagulant effects. Major bleeding complications are less likely to be associated with fondaparinux compared with heparin. Anti-Xa activity of antithrombin from fondaparinux, however, is not reversed with protamine sulfate.[7] Recombinant factor VIIa can partially reverse the anticoagulant effect of fondaparinux.[8]

A Food and Drug Administration (FDA) black box warning is similar to that of the low-molecular-weight heparin warning of the risk of epidural/spinal hematoma in patients who are or will be anticoagulated with fondaparinux. The ARSA evidence-based guidelines state the actual risk of spinal hematoma with fondaparinux is unknown. Until further clinical experience is available, neuraxial techniques in patients who receive fondaparinux prophylaxis should occur under the strict parameters used in clinical trials (single-needle pass, atraumatic needle placement, and avoidance of indwelling neuraxial catheters). Other forms of prophylaxis may be more feasible.[6] In patients with severe renal insufficiency, elimination of fondaparinux is prolonged and the risk of bleeding is increased. It is, therefore, contraindicated in this setting.[5,9]

Direct factor Xa inhibitors bind directly to the active site of Xa and block its interaction with substrates, thereby inhibiting both free and platelet-bound (bound in the prothrominase complex) factor Xa.[5] Rivaroxaban (Xarelto) is the first available oral direct factor Xa inhibitor. The drug has completed phase III clinical trials and is reported to have a favorable benefit-to-risk ratio for thromboprophylaxis after elective hip and knee arthroplasty. In patients undergoing major orthopedic surgery, rivaroxaban demonstrated comparable safety and superior efficacy compared with enoxaparin.[10,11] Rivaroxaban inhibits factor Xa in a concentration-dependant manner and binds rapidly and reversibly.[12] Rivaroxaban's oral bioavailability is 80%; half-life is approximately 9 hours and is cleared by the kidneys and gut.[5] Maximum inhibitory effect is between 1 and 4 hours after dosing and inhibition is maintained for 12 hours. Once daily dosing is possible because factor Xa activity does not return to normal within 24 hours. Dosing adjustments should be made for patients with renal insufficiency. The drug is contraindicated in patients with severe liver disease. The antithrombotic effect of rivaroxaban may be monitored with prothrombin time, activated partial thromboplastin time (aPTT), and Heptest. These all show linear dose effects.[6] Because the accuracy of these laboratory assays to measure the anticoagulant effects of rivaroxaban is uncertain, assessment of these assays continues.[13] ASRA recommends a "cautious approach" in performing regional anesthesia in light of the lack of information regarding the specifics of block performance during clinical trials and the prolonged half-life of rivaroxaban.[6]

Like rivaroxaban, apixaban is direct inhibitor of factor Xa administered orally. Apixaban has a bioavailability greater than 50% and reaches peak plasma concentration

3 to 4 hours after dosing. With repeated dosing, the terminal half-life of apixaban is 10 to 14 hours. The drug is partially metabolized in the liver and is cleared via the renal and fecal route. At present, it is undetermined if apixaban can safely be used in patients with mild to moderate hepatic or renal impairment.[14] Trials evaluating apixaban for the prevention of VTE are ongoing. When compared with enoxaparin for thromboprophylaxis after knee replacement, apixaban was associated with lower rates of clinically relevant bleeding. It did not meet the prespecified statistical criteria for noninferiority, however.[15] The Apixaban Versus Acetylsalicylic Acid to Prevent Strokes (AVERROES) trial compared the safety and effectiveness of apixaban and aspirin in patients with atrial fibrillation. Recently, the trial was stopped early due to reports of clear evidence of a clinically important reduction in stroke and systemic embolism.

Direct Thrombin Inhibitors

Thrombin converts fibrinogen to fibrin and can be inhibited directly or indirectly (**Table 2**). The direct inhibitors of thrombin work by binding to thrombin and blocking its interaction with substrates. Currently, there are three parenteral direct thrombin inhibitors and one oral direct thrombin inhibitor licensed in North America for limited indications. Hirudin and argatroban are used for treatment of HIT. Bivalirudin is approved for use as an alternative to heparin in percutaneous coronary intervention (PCI) patients with or without HIT.[5] Hirudin is a natural anticoagulant originally isolated from the salivary gland of the medicinal leech. Hirudin, bivalirudin, and lepirudin exhibit bivalent binding. Hirudin and its recombinant analogs block the substrate recognition and the catalytic site on thrombin responsible for fibrinogen cleavage. Hirudin acts only on thrombin and has no effect on other components of the clotting pathway.[16] Desirudin (Iprivask) for injection is a new direct thrombin inhibitor similar in structure to hirudin. Approved for use by the FDA in 2003, but not immediately marketed, it is indicated for use in preventing deep vein thrombosis in patients undergoing elective hip arthroplasty. Desirudin is a selective inhibitor of free circulating and clot-bound thrombin. Peak plasma concentrations occur between 1 and 3 hours after subcutaneous injection. Terminal elimination half-life of desirudin is 2 to 3 hours. The drug is primarily eliminated and metabolized by the kidney. Patients with moderate to severe renal impairment require dose reductions and monitoring of daily aPTT and serum

Table 2
Summary of direct thrombin inhibitors

	Dabigatran	Hirudin	Bivalirudin	Argatroban	Desirudin
Action	Inhibits thrombin	Inhibits thrombin	Inhibits thrombin	Inhibits thrombin	Inhibits thrombin
Route of administration	Oral	IV	IV	IV	Subcutaneous
Indication	Not yet approved[a]	HIT	PCI	HIT	VTE/PE prophylaxis
Half-life	14–17 hours	1–2 hours	25 minutes	40–50 minutes	2–3 hours
Elimination	Renal	Proteolysis and renal	Plasma/ renal	Hepatic and biliary	Renal
Monitoring	None	aPTT	aPTT	aPTT/ACT	aPTT

Abbreviations: ACT, activated clotting time; IV, intravenous; PE, pulmonary embolism.
  [a] Completed clinical trials for stoke prevention and nonvalvular atrial fibrillation and treatment of acute VTE; currently in clinical trials for treatment and prevention of secondary VTE.

creatnine. Desirudin carries a black box warning like that of the other thrombin inhibitors. There is an increased risk of epidural or spinal hematoma when neuraxial anesthesia is performed on patients who are anticoagulated or scheduled to be anticoagulated with thrombin inhibitors, such as desirudin. The risk may be increased with indwelling catheters or by concomitant use of other medications altering hemostasis, such as nonsteroidal anti-inflammatory medications, platelet inhibitors, or other anticoagulants. Risk of spinal or epidural hematoma formation is further increased by traumatic or repeated epidural or spinal puncture.[17] The ASRA states that there are no case reports of spinal hematoma related to neuraxial anesthesia among patients receiving direct thrombin inhibitors but spontaneous intracranial bleeding has occurred. In general, patients on direct thrombin inhibitors are not good candidates for neuraxial anesthesia due to underlying conditions requiring anticoagulation. ASRA makes no statement regarding risk assessment and patient management in these patients except to recommend identification of cardiac and surgical risk factors associated with bleeding after invasive procedures.[6]

Dabigatran, an oral direct thrombin inhibitor, is being studied for various clinical indications. Dabigatran, like argatroban, is a synthetic small-molecule hirudin analog. It exhibits univalent binding to only one of the two key thrombin sites.[16] Dabigatran etexilate is the prodrug of dabigatran, a reversible inhibitor of the active site of thrombin. The prodrug is rapidly converted to dabigatran after oral ingestion and hepatic processing. Peak plasma concentrations occur approximately 1.5 hours after oral administration. After reaching steady state, dabigatran's half-life is 14 to 17 hours. Bioavailability of dabigatran is 7.2% and it is primarily excreted in feces. Up to 80% of the drug is eliminated by the kidney. Recommendations from countries where dabigatran is already approved suggest renal dosing considerations in patients with moderate renal dysfunction and recommend against its use in patients with severe renal impairment.[14] Dabigatran has been compared with warfarin for stroke prevention in patients with nonvalvular atrial fibrillation and treatment of acute venous thromboembolism.[18,19] Implications of the results of these clinical trials are expected in the near future. Ongoing phase III clinical trials are looking at dabigatran in treatment and prevention of secondary VTE in postoperative orthopedic patients and long-term prophylaxis in acute coronary syndrome. Dabigatran's predictable pharmacokinetic profile would allow for a fixed-dose regimen without the need for routine coagulation monitoring. If an assessment of dabigatran's anticoagulation status were necessary, there is no best method established at present. If available, however, thrombin clotting time and ecarin clotting time determined by thrombin inhibitor assay are reported to be sensitive tests to evaluate dabigatran's anticoagulant effects. Less sensitive but more accessible qualitative methods of anticoagulant effects are aPTT and thrombin clotting time. No antidote is currently available to antagonize dabigatran. It has been suggested that in cases of life-threatening bleeding, recombinant factor activated VII and prothrombin complex concentrate may be considered.[20]

NEW ANTIPLATELET AGENTS

Drugs that block platelet function are vital in the prevention of arterial thrombogenesis. Forming under high shear conditions, arterial thrombi consist of mainly platelet aggregates held together by small amounts of fibrin. Clopidogrel (Plavix) and ticlodipine (Ticlid) are structurally related thienopyridines that inhibit platelet aggregation by selectively and irreversibly inhibiting the adenosine diphosphate (ADP) stimulation of the $P2Y_{12}$ receptor. New antiplatelet drugs include the thromboxane receptor antagonist, PAR-1 antagonists (targets thrombin receptors on platelets), and $P2Y_{12}$ antagonists.[5]

ADP Receptor Antagonists

Of the new antiplatelet agents, the ADP receptor antagonist, prasugrel (Effient), is the only drug currently available in United States. It is indicated to reduce the rate of thrombotic cardiovascular events (including stent thrombosis) in patients with acute coronary syndrome who are to be managed with PCI. These include patients with unstable angina or non-ST–elevation myocardial infarction and patients with ST-elevation myocardial infarction when managed with primary or delayed PCI. Prasugrel is rapidly absorbed from the gastrointestinal tract with mean time to peak plasma concentration of approximately 30 minutes. Prasugrel is a prodrug requiring hepatic conversion to express its antiplatelet activity. Hepatic metabolism results in an active metabolite that irreversibly inhibits the $P2Y_{12}$ receptor. Plasma half-life of the active metabolite is approximately 4 hours and steady state is reached in 3 days. Prasugrel is excreted primarily in the urine.[21] Platelet inhibition is more rapid with prasugrel than with clopidogrel, but both drugs have a delayed offset of action due to the irreversible inhibition of their target receptor.[22] Prasugrel has been shown to have more potent antiplatelet effects, lower interindividual variability in platelet response, and faster onset of activity than clopidogrel. Furthermore, prasugrel is more efficacious in preventing ischemic events in patients with acute coronary syndrome undergoing PCI. Although prasugrel provides more rapid and consistent platelet inhibition than clopidogrel, it also increases the risk of bleeding.[23–25] The manufacturer warns of bleeding risk and recommends discontinuation at least 7 days before any surgery. Although there is no generally accepted test to guide antiplatelet therapy, careful preoperative assessment focusing on alterations in health that might contribute to bleeding is important. Examples include history of easy bruising and/or excessive bleeding, female sex, and increased age. ASRA recommends discontinuation of thienopyridine therapy for 7 days for clopidogrel and 14 days for ticlodipine. Neuraxial techniques should be avoided until platelet function has been recovered.[6] Although not specifically addressed in the ASRA guidelines at this time, the manufacturer recommends stopping prasugrel at least 7 days before planned surgery. Currently, there is no specific reversal agent available for prasugrel. The manufacturer is conducting an open-label trial of ex vivo reversal of platelet inhibition by exogenous platelets at this time.

Cangrelor, an ATP analog, is a direct competitive inhibitor of $P2Y_{12}$ that, unlike prasugrel and clopidogrel, does not require hepatic conversion to an active metabolite. Cangrelor has a short half-life of 3 to 5 minutes and recovery of platelet function occurs within 60 minutes of cessation.[5] Phase III testing of cangrelor in patients undergoing PCI was discontinued by the manufacturer due to evidence that the drug would fail to show a meaningful clinical difference. Cangrelor is currently being evaluated as a bridge therapy for patients who need to discontinue clopidogrel before cardiac surgery.

Glycoprotein IIb/IIIa Antagonists

Although they are not new antiplatelet agents, the use of parenteral glycoprotein IIb/IIIa (GPIIb/IIIa) antagonists is fairly commonplace in preventing thrombotic complications after PCI and in patients with acute coronary syndrome. The GPIIb/IIIa receptor on the platelet surface serves as a base for fibrin cross-linking responsible for platelet aggregation. Platelet antagonists, abciximab (ReoPro), eptifibatide (Integrilin), and tirofiban (Aggrastat), directly block the fibrinogen receptor on platelets, thereby preventing ligand binding and aggregation.[26,27] Based on the success of these parenteral agents, oral GPIIb/IIIa receptor inhibitors were developed for chronic use in patients at high risk for arterial thrombotic events.[28] Results of the first large clinical trials with oral GPIIb/IIIa receptor inhibitors were unfavorable. Oral agents failed to reduce major cardiovascular events and showed a small but significant increase in mortality in patients with acute coronary syndromes.[28,29] Although disappointing, information gleaned for the trials involving the first generation of oral GPIIb/IIIa receptor blockers will perhaps result in another generation's success.

The ASRA guidelines address the GPIIb/IIIa receptor inhibitors by asserting that they have a profound effect on platelet aggregation. Neuraxial techniques should be avoided until platelet function is recovered. After administration of abciximab, time to normal platelet aggregation is 24 to 48 hours. Eptifibatide and tirofiban administration requires 4 to 8 hours for return of normal platelet aggregation. Furthermore, GPIIb/IIIa antagonists are contraindicated within 4 weeks of surgery. ASRA guidelines recommend careful monitoring of neurologic function should one of the GPIIb/IIIa inhibitors be administered in the postoperative period after a neuraxial technique.[6]

HERBAL MEDICATIONS AND DIETARY SUPPLEMENTS

Widespread use of herbal medications and vitamin supplements in the presurgical population necessitates a familiarity with the implications of patient use of alternative medications. Current US regulatory mechanisms for commercial herbal preparations sold in this country do not provide protection against unpredictable effects. Herbal medications and vitamin supplements may pose a concern in the perioperative period by contributing to cardiovascular instability and hypoglycemia, potentiating commonly used anesthetics sedative effects ,and altering metabolism of anesthetic drugs.[30] In addition, some of these alternative medications may result in increased bleeding in the perioperative period, especially in conjunction with other anticoagulants (**Table 3**).

Garlic, ginkgo, and ginseng are three herbal medications that may be commonly encountered in the perioperative setting. Extensive research involving garlic shows the herbal may reduce blood pressure and thrombus formation, thereby modifying risk of atherosclerosis.[30] Also, garlic may lower serum lipid and cholesterol levels.[31] Garlic seem to irreversibly inhibit platelet aggregation in dose-dependant fashion and may potentiate the effect of other platelet inhibitors, such as prostacyclin, indomethacin, and dipyridamole.[30] There is one case report of a spontaneous epidural hematoma attributed to heavy garlic use.[30,32] Insufficient

Table 3
Some commonly used herbal medications and supplements and their anesthetic considerations

Herbal Medication	Adverse Effects	Anesthetic Considerations
Garlic	Prolongation of bleeding time, hypotension	Increased risk of bleeding and hemodynamic instability
Ginger	Prolongation of bleeding time	Increased risk of bleeding and hemodynamic instability
Ginkgo biloba	Platelet dysfunction	Increased risk of bleeding
Kava kava	Platelet dysfunction, hepatotoxicity	Increased risk of bleeding
Fish oil	Platelet dysfunction	Increased risk of bleeding
Vitamin E	Platelet dysfunction	Increased risk of bleeding, may enhance hypertension

pharmacokinetic data preclude development of absolute recommendations regarding discontinuation of garlic before surgery. It has been suggested, however, that given the potential for irreversible inhibition of platelet function, cessation of garlic use 7 days before surgery is warranted.[30] Ginkgo is derived from the leaf of ginkgo biloba. Its common uses include stabilization and/or improvement of cognitive defects in disorders, such as Alzheimer disease and multi-infarct dementia. Ginkgo is also used in patients with peripheral vascular disease, macular degeneration, vertigo, tinnitus, motion sickness, and erectile dysfunction. Terpenoids and flavonoids are the compounds believed to produce its pharmacologic effects. Ginkgo may act as an antioxidant, alter vasoregulation, and modulate neurotransmitter and receptor activity. In addition, ginkgo may inhibit platelet-activating factor and alter platelet function. Study of pharmacokinetic data and bleeding risk suggests that patients should stop taking ginkgo at least 36 hours before surgery.[30] Ginseng, both Asian and American types, is commonly used as an adaptogen, protecting the body from stress and restoring homeostasis. Other uses include lowering postprandial glucose in patients with type 2 diabetes mellitus and without diabetes. Although not completely understood, the underlying pharmacologic mechanism seems similar to that of steroid hormones. Ginsenosides inhibit platelet aggregation in vitro and prolong coagulation time of thrombin and activated partial thromboplastin in laboratory rats. Findings await confirmation in humans. Because platelet inhibition seems irreversible, it is suggested that patients discontinue use of ginseng at least 7 days before surgery.[30] ASRA guidelines state that there does not seem to be a clinically significant increase in surgical bleeding or spinal hematoma overall in patients taking herbal medications. Because the use of herbal medications alone does not create a level of risk that interferes with neuraxial blockade, ASRA recommends against mandatory discontinuation of herbal medications or avoidance of regional anesthetic techniques in these patients. There is a lack of data, however, pertaining to patients taking herbal medications with other forms of anticoagulation. Concurrent use of medications, such as oral anticoagulants or heparin, may increase the risk of bleeding in patients taking herbal medications.[6]

Other herbal medications may increase bleeding, especially in patients already taking drugs and/or other herbs or supplements that affect normal clotting function. These include feverfew, ginger, kava kava, clove, and white willow bark. The American Society of Anesthesiologists suggests that patients should be encouraged to discontinue these products 2 weeks before surgery, which is the estimated time for the compounds to be fully metabolized.[33]

Dietary supplements are taken regularly by all patient populations for various reasons. Vitamins E and A have been implicated in increasing risk of bleeding in combination with prescribed anticoagulants. Vitamin E is popular because it is thought to have antioxidant properties, provide protection against environmental pollution, and slow the aging process. Vitamin E supplementation may increase the effects of anticoagulants and antiplatelet drugs, thereby increasing the risk of bleeding perioperatively. Vitamin A is found in two major forms of foods, including retinol and carotenes. Of concern is the risk of increased bleeding in patients taking vitamin A and warfarin. Vitamin A may increase the anticoagulant effects of warfarin. Informing patients of these potential effects may help to avoid perioperative complications. Another dietary supplement with potential to increase the risk of bleeding is fish oil. Evidence suggests that the components of fish oil, docosahexaenoic acid and eicosapentaenoic acid, lower triglycerides, and reduce the risk of death, heart attack, arrhythmias, and stroke in people with known heart disease. At high doses, however, harmful effects, such as increased risk of bleeding, may occur.[34]

NEW ANTICOAGULANTS AND REGIONAL ANESTHESIA

Anticoagulant, antiplatelet, and thrombolytic drugs are commonly used in the prevention and treatment of thromboembolism. In addition, increasingly more potent antithrombotic medications have raised concerns regarding the risk of increased neuraxial bleeding. The incidence of spinal hematoma is estimated to be less than 1 in 220,000. Although the risk of epidural hematoma is estimated to be 1 in 150,000, the risk is increased 15-fold in patients on anticoagulant therapy.[35] Risk factors for clinically significant bleeding increase with age, associated abnormalities of the spinal cord and vertebral column, underlying coagulopathy, difficult needle placement, and indwelling neuraxial catheter during sustained anticoagulation. To optimize neurologic outcome in the face of a complication, it is imperative to promptly diagnose and intervene.[6] The ARSA published its practice advisory in 2009 addressing patient safety issues and the concerns listed previously. The consensus statements represent opinions of recognized experts in the field of neuraxial anesthesia and anticoagulation. The guidelines are based on case reports, clinical series, pharmacology, hematology, and risk factors for surgical bleeding.

European groups have proposed guidelines to improve safety of neuraxial techniques in patients receiving newer anticoagulants. Proposed recommendations suggest the risk-to-benefit ratio needs to be individualized for each patient depending on type and dose of anticoagulant, the type of regional anesthesia, and patient risk factors.

In addition, neuraxial anesthetic management strategies may be based on pharmacokinetic properties of the anticoagulant drug, including time required to reach maximal concentration, half-life, and dose regimen. The time elapsed from the last injection of anticoagulant to performance of a central neuraxial block should be at least two half-lives of the drug. The same amount of time should elapse before removal of an epidural catheter. Renal function plays a role in half-life. After removal of an epidural catheter, timing of the next dose of anticoagulant should be based on time required for the drug to meet maximum activity. Furthermore, both the American and European societies agree that vigilance in monitoring is crucial to allow for early evaluation of neurologic dysfunction and prompt intervention.[4]

Risk of bleeding after peripheral nerve blockade and plexus nerve blockade in the anticoagulated patient is undefined.[6] There are few investigations examining the frequency and severity of hemorrhagic complications from peripheral nerve blockade and plexus nerve blockade in this patient population. Serious complications have been reported after neurovascular sheath cannulation for surgical, radiologic, and cardiac procedures. ASRA states there are insufficient data to make definitive recommendations regarding performing these blocks in anticoagulated patients. The ASRA suggests, however, that significant blood loss, rather than neural defects, may be the most serious complication of non-neuraxial regional techniques. Hemorrhage after deep plexus/peripheral techniques, such as lumbar sympathetic/plexus and paravertebral blocks, in the presence of antithrombotic activity is a serious complication.[6] Therefore, the ASRA states the same recommendations regarding neuraxial techniques be observed for patients undergoing deep plexus or peripheral nerve block.

Interventional pain management procedures carry a minimal, but potentially hazardous, risk of bleeding. Risk is difficult to assess based on available source data. Anesthesiologists must assess bleeding risk based on existing literature and judgment. Most interventional pain procedures are elective; therefore, bleeding risks should be weighed against potential benefits.[36] The ASRA has adapted guidelines that are reflective of the guidelines for neuraxial anesthesia in patients on anticoagulation therapy. Clopidogrel should be withheld for 7 days before a neuraxial procedure. Thienopyridine derivatives have been implicated in bleeding after lumbar sympathetic blockade and cervical steroid injections.[36] GPIIb/IIIa receptor inhibitors should be discontinued 4 weeks before neuraxial blockade. Neuraxial blockade is contraindicated in patients on oral anticoagulants. Bleeding risk factors associated with technique may influence the risk and consequences of bleeding. Assessment and understanding of the above subject matter improves patient safety during interventional pain procedures.[36]

NEW ANTICOAGULANTS: MONITORING, REVERSAL, AND CONTINUATION THROUGH THE PERIOPERTIVE PERIOD

Approved new anticoagulants and those still in clinical trials offer many benefits and advantages when compared with the older vitamin K antagonists and heparin. Oral administration, more predictable pharmacokinetics, and no need for laboratory monitoring of anticoagulant effects are a few of the advantages. Investigations into monitoring capabilities of the anticoagulation effects of direct factor Xa inhibitors and direct thrombin inhibitors thus far have yielded no standard measure of the of these two new drug classes. Lack of standardization and significant variability of results depending on the reagent or test method make currently available tests of anticoagulant effects unreliable in the case of direct factor Xa and direct thrombin inhibitors.[16]

Specific tests to measure platelet inhibitory effects of clopidogrel are available, including ADP-stimulated aggregometry. The time required to perform this test restricts its usefulness during surgery. Currently, there are two platelet function assays commercially available that measure platelet inhibition by the ADP antagonist clopidogrel. Also, accurate measuring of receptor inhibition by GPIIb/IIIa inhibitors in patients undergoing invasive cardiology procedures has been documented. Platelet inhibition measured by a point-of-care monitor, Ultegra, correlates inversely with adverse outcomes after PCI.[26] Whether or not such monitoring devices will become useful in the perioperative setting is uncertain.

Reversal of the anticoagulant effects of new anticoagulants poses potential problems in managing surgical patients. Traditional agents used to reverse bleeding or older anticoagulants include antifibrinolytics, protamine, desmopressin, fibrinogen, purified protein concentrates, and recombinant factor VIIa.[37] Only one of the new anticoagulants, fondaparinux, is partially reversed by one of these agents, recombinant factor VIIa.[8] Transfusion of fresh platelets can effectively reverse the antiplatelet effects of clopidogrel, but circulating platelets already bound with the drug remain inhibited.[26] Transfusion therapies are often used, but data supporting their efficacy are needed.[37]

Recommendations regarding discontinuation of anticoagulants/antiplatelet medications are discussed previously. In certain patient populations, it is strongly advised that anticoagulation or antiplatelet therapy continue throughout the perioperative period. It is recommended that in patients at high risk for development of VTE, such as cancer patients, thromboprophylaxis be started preoperatively. Fondaparinux is an option for these patients. Trauma patients are also at high risk for development of VTE and sudden fatal pulmonary embolism. In these patients, thromboprophylaxis with enoxaparin should be started as soon as it is considered safe to do so.[38]

Perioperative management of patients with coronary artery stents is one of the most important topics involving anticoagulation and surgery. Perioperative stent thrombosis is life threatening and can occur with both bare-metal and drug-eluting stents. Noncardiac surgery increases risk of stent thrombosis, myocardial infarction, and death. These risks are increased if surgery occurs early after stent implantation and if antiplatelet therapy is discontinued preoperatively.[39] Thienopyridine therapy in combination with aspirin is the treatment strategy used to prevent stent thrombosis. Elective procedures with significant risk of perioperative bleeding should be deferred until patients have completed an appropriate course of thienopyridine therapy. Patients with drug-eluting stents who are not at high risk of bleeding require 12 months of dual antiplatelet therapy after stent implantation. Patients with bare-metal stents require a minimum of 1 month of therapy after stent implantation.[40] If surgery cannot be deferred and thienopyridine therapy must be interrupted in patients with new coronary stents, aspirin should be continued if possible and the thienopyridine restarted as soon as possible. In patients with drug-eluting stents and high risk of stent thrombosis, dual antiplatelet therapy with aspirin and the thienopyridine should be considered perioperatively even if the time since implantation is beyond the initial 12 months. After the thienopyridine has been discontinued, serious consideration should be given to continuing perioperative aspirin antiplatelet therapy in any patient with drug-eluting stents.[41]

SUMMARY

With a growing number of new anticoagulant/antiplatelet agents being developed, it is likely that an increasing number of patients taking these drugs will present for surgery and other procedures. A familiarity with mechanisms of action and drug interactions helps to maintain optimal patient safety in the perioperative period. Furthermore, it is crucial for anesthesiologists to remain current on recommendations regarding discontinuation or need to continue the newer anticoagulants/antiplatelet drugs in patients presenting for surgery and/or regional anesthesia. Further studies are needed for monitoring of many of these newer agents and to identify antidotes.

REFERENCES

1. Trujillo T. Emerging anticoagulants for venous thromboembolism prevention. Am J Health Syst Pharm 2010;67:S17–25.
2. Vitin A, Dembo G, Vater Y, et al. Anesthetic implications of the new anticoagulant and antiplatelet drugs. J Clin Anesth 2008;20:228–37.
3. Kaye AD, Clarke R, Sabar R, et al. Herbal medicines: current trends in anesthesiology practice—a hospital survey. J Clin Anesth 2000;12:468–71.
4. Liau J, Ferrandis R. New anticoagulants and regional anesthesia. Curr Opin Anaesthesiol 2009;22:661–6.
5. Weitz J, Hirsch J, Samama M. New antithrombotic drugs: American College of Chest Physicians Evidence-Based Clinical Practice Guidelines (8th Edition). Chest 2008;133:234–256S.
6. Horlocker T, Wedel D, Rowlingson J, et al. Regional anesthesia in the patient receiving antithrombotic or thrombolytic therapy. American Society of Regional Anesthesia and Pain Medicine Evidence-Based Guidelines (3rd Edition). Reg Anesth Pain Med 2010;35:64–101.
7. Tanaka K, Key N, Levy J. Blood coagulation: hemostasis and thrombin regulation. Anesth Analg 2009;108:1433–46.

8. Hirsh J, O'Donnell M, Eikelboom J. Beyond unfractionated heparin and warfarin: current and future advances. Circulation 2007;116:552–60.

9. Haines S, Dager W, Trujillo T. Clinical management of challenges in preventing venous thromboembolism in health systems: a case-based panel discussion. Am J Health Syst Pharm 2010;67:S26–30.

10. Melillo S, Scanlon J, Exter B, et al. Rivaroxaban for thromboprophylaxis in patients undergoing major orthopedic surgery. Ann Pharmacother 2010;44(6): 1061–71.

11. Lassen M, Ageno W, Borris L, et al. Rivaroxaban versus enoxaparin for thromboprophylaxis after total knee arthroplasty. N Engl J Med 2008;358:2776–86.

12. Perzborn E, Roehrig S, Straub A, et al. Rivaroxaban: a new oral factor Xa inhibitor. Arterioscler Thromb Vasc Biol 2010;30:376–81.

13. Garcia D, Libby E, Crowther M. The new oral anticoagulants. Blood 2010;115(1): 15–20.

14. Samama M, Martinoi JL, LaFlem L, et al. Assessment of laboratory assays to measure rivaoxaban-an oral, direct factor Xa inhibitor. Thromb Haemost 2010; 103(4):686–8.

15. Lassen M, Raskob G, Gallus A, et al. Apixaban or enoxaparin for thromboprophylaxis after knee replacement. N Engl J Med 2009;361:594–604.

16. Ng V. Anticoagulation monitoring. Clin Lab Med 2009;29:283–304.

17. Iprivask [package literature]. Aventis Pharmacueticals; April 2003.

18. Connolly S, Ezekowitz M, Yusuf D, et al. Dabigatran versus warfarin in patients with atrial fibrillation. N Engl J Med 2009;361:1139–51.

19. Schulman S, Kearon C, Kakkar A, et al. Dabigatran versus warfarin in the treatment of acute venous thromboembolism. N Engl J Med 2009;361:2342–52.

20. van Ryn J, Stangler J, Haertter S, et al. Dabigatran etexilate—a novel, reversible, oral direct thrombin inhibitor: interpretation of coagulation assays and reversal of anticoagulant activity. Thromb Haemost 2010;103:1116–27.

21. Dobesh P. Pharmacokinetics and pharmacodynamics of prasugrel, a thienopyridine $P2Y_{12}$ inhibitor. Pharmacotherapy 2009;29(9):1089–102.

22. Kam P, Nethery C. The thienopyridine derivatives (platelet adenosine diphosphate receptor antagonists), pharmacology and clinical developments. Anaesthesia 2003;58:28–35.

23. Mousa S, Jeske W, Fareed J. Antiplatelet therapy prasugrel: a novel platelet ADP $P2Y_{12}$ receptor antagonist. Clin Appl Thromb Hemost 2010;16(2):170–6.

24. Eshaghian S. Advances in antiplatelet treatment for acute coronary syndrome. Heart 2010;96(9):656–61.

25. Veverka A, Hammer J. Prasugrel: a new thienopyridine inhibitor. J Pharm Pract 2009;22(2):158–65.

26. Shore-Lesserson L. Platelet inhibitors and monitoring platelet function: implications for bleeding. Hematol Oncol Clin North Am 2007;21:51–63.

27. Kam P, Egan M. Platelet glycoprotein IIb/IIIa antagonists. Anesthesiology 2002; 96:1237–49.

28. Leeber F, Boersma E, Cannon C, et al. Oral glycoprotein IIb/IIIa receptor inhibitors in patients with cardiovascular disease: why were the results so unfavourable. Eur Heart J 2002;23:444–57.

29. Cannon C, McCabe C, Wilcox R, et al. Oral glycoprotein IIb/IIIa receptor inhibition with orbofiban in patients with unstable coronary syndrome (OPUS-TIMI 16) trial. Circulation 2000;101:r23–35.

30. Ang-Lee M, Moss J, Yuan C. Herbal medicines and perioperative care. JAMA 2001;286(2):208–16.

31. Stevinson C, Pittler M, Ernst E. Garlic for treating hypercholesterolemia: a meta-analysis of randomized clinical trials. Ann Intern Med 2000;133:420–9.
32. Rose K, Croissant P, Parliament C, et al. Spontaneous spinal epidural hematoma with associated platelet dysfunction form excessive garlic ingestion: a case report. Neurosurgery 1990;26:880–2.
33. Leak J. Herbal medicines: what do we need to know? ASA Newsletter. February, 2000;64(2).
34. Medline Plus online. Omega-3 fatty acids, fish oil, alpha-linolenic acid. Evidence based Natural Standard Research Collaboration. August 2009.
35. Rosencher N, Bonnet M, Sessler D. Selected new antithrombotic agents and neuraxial anesthesia for major orthopaedic surgery: management strategies. Anaesthesia 2007;62:1154–60.
36. Shah R, Kaye AD. Bleeding risk and interventional pain management. Curr Opin Anaesthesiol 2008;21:433–8.
37. Levy J, Azran M. Anesthetic concerns for patients with coagulopathy. Curr Opin Anaesthesiol 2010;23:400–5.
38. Muntz J, Michota F. Prevention and management of venous thromboembolism in the surgical patient: options by surgery type and individual patient risk factors. Am J Surg 2010;199:s11–20.
39. Newsome L. Coronary artery stents: II. Perioperative considerations and management. Anesth Analg 2008;107(2):570–90.
40. Grines C, Bonow R, Casey D, et al. Prevention of premature discontinuation of dual antiplatelet therapy in patients with coronary artery stents: a science advisory from the American Heart Association, American College of Cardiology, Society for Cardiovascular Angiography and Interventions, American College of Surgeons, and American Dental Association, with representation from the American College of Physicians. J Am Coll Cardiol 2007;49:734–9.
41. Caplan R, Connis R, Nickinovich D, et al. Practice alert for the perioperative management of patients with coronary artery stents. Anesthesiology 2009; 110:22–3.

Recombinant Factor VIIa in Trauma Patients Without Coagulation Disorders

Corey Scher, MD[a],*, Venod Narine, BS[b], Daniel Chien, BS[b]

KEYWORDS

• Recombinant • Coagulapathy • Hemostasis • Combat trauma

DEVELOPMENT

During the 1970s, hemophiliacs with inhibitors against factor VIII (FVIII) or FIX who experienced a major bleed were treated with massive infusions of FVIII/FIX and adsorption of antibodies. For milder bleeds, prothrombin complex concentrates or the activated forms were studied but found to have limited efficacy and unacceptable thromboembolic (TE) complication rates.[1] Recombinant activated factor VIIa (rFVIIa) was developed in the 1980s and approved in Europe in 1996 and the United States in 1999 for this use. During this time, rFVIIa was also investigated for uses in other clinical situations in which major blood loss or coagulopathy may be anticipated, and reports emerged of its ability to facilitate coagulation in such scenarios in supraphysiologic plasma levels.[2]

As its name states, rFVIIa is a recombinant protein. The manufacturers of rFVIIa define recombinant as genetically engineered DNA made without human blood or plasma. The production of a recombinant protein involves the identification and excision of a specific strand of DNA that is then integrated into the DNA of another species to be replicated and mass produced. rFVIIa is specifically produced by the transfer of the DNA gene sequence for plasma human factor VII into cultured hamster cells. The process of transferring DNA (nucleic acid sequences) into cells is known as transfection.

[a] Department of Anesthesiology, Montefiore Medical Center, 111 East 210th Street, Bronx, NY 10467-2490, USA
[b] Department of Anesthesiology, Mount Sinai School of Medicine, KCC 8th Floor, One Gustave L. Levy Place, Box 1010, New York, NY 10029, USA
* Corresponding author.
E-mail address: coreyscher@gmail.com

Anesthesiology Clin 28 (2010) 681–690
doi:10.1016/j.anclin.2010.08.011
1932-2275/10/$ – see front matter © 2010 Elsevier Inc. All rights reserved.

COMBAT TRAUMA

The first report of the successful use of rFVIIa in the setting of massive traumatic hemorrhage occurred in an Israeli solider in 1999.[3] The patient had a high-velocity rifle injury that tore his inferior vena cava, resulting in shock and disseminated intravascular coagulopathy (DIC), with continued bleeding refractory to surgical intervention and transfusion. He was given rFVIIa, after which the bleeding slowed and stopped. Other case reports and series have since showed similar findings in both military and civilian settings.

The use of rFVIIa in combat injuries varies and is not well studied. In 2001, a case series of 7 combat trauma patients, including the first patient, was reported with rFVIIa administered under compassionate-use guidelines, resulting in successful cessation of hemorrhage without TE complications.[4] rFVIIa had just become available in off-label civilian trauma use when the US combat operations in Afghanistan and Iraq began, and it became favored by military hospitals using it as a "universal hemostatic."[5] However, questions about the risk of TE, although difficult to distinguish from background risk, reduced its use more recently.[5] A 2006 survey of a sample of US Army surgeons revealed that this product was available to relatively few surgeons in a forward surgical team, a mobile unit in close proximity to combat areas, whereas most surgeons in combat support hospitals, usually located in areas without active fighting, had access to the product and were using it with variable subjective success.[6] For the most part, rFVIIa was used as an adjunct for hemostasis on a compassionate-use basis.[7] However, only recently have data on the efficacy of such measures become available, with studies pertaining to combat trauma thus far remaining retrospective and controlled trials unlikely. In a study of 124 combat-related trauma patients with severe trauma (Injury Severity Score >15) and massive transfusion (red blood cell count [RBC] >10 units/24 hours), use of rFVIIa was associated with decreased 24-hour and 30-day mortality without an increase in TE risk, although the difference in hemorrhage as a cause of death did not reach statistical significance ($P = 0.12$).[8] Another study showed that although early administration of rFVIIa (ie, before 8 units of blood has been given) can reduce transfusion requirements, there is no change in mortality, including acute respiratory distress syndrome (ARDS), infection, and TE.[9] This finding is supported in another study looking specifically at wartime vascular injuries, which comprise most combat injuries in Iraq and Afghanistan. Although rFVIIa was associated with earlier recovery from acidosis, anemia, and coagulopathy, the authors found no improvement in mortality.[10] More recently, Woodruff and colleagues[11] compared matched controls with 22 battle-injured patients in Operation Iraqi Freedom who received rFVIIa and found no difference in survival.

The efficacy of rFVIIa is being investigated in civilian injuries as well. In 2005, the Israeli Multidisciplinary rFVIIa Task Force published a case series of 36 trauma patients in which the use of rFVIIa controlled hemorrhage and improved international randomized ratio in 72% of the patients. Failure was associated with acidosis but not hypothermia.[12] There has been only 1 randomized controlled trial looking at the use of rFVIIa to control traumatic hemorrhage. Boffard and colleagues[13] published a double-blind placebo-controlled trial with parallel study arms looking at blunt and penetrating trauma treated with or without rFVIIa in addition to standard protocols. They found no difference in mortality but found that rFVIIa decreased transfusion requirements in blunt trauma patients by 2.6 L and reduced the risk of the need for massive transfusion (>20 units packed red blood cells [pRBCs]), with trends toward similar findings in penetrating trauma patients but underpowered to reach statistical significance ($P = 0.10$ and 0.08, respectively). Further analysis of the data revealed a reduction in needs for fresh frozen plasma, platelets, and cryoprecipitate within 48 hours as well as in 30-day risk of ARDS in blunt trauma patients and a trend in the same direction for penetrating trauma.[14] Another group was able to find significance in the reduction of transfusion requirements in penetrating traumas in looking at both civilian and military patients if given within 24 hours[9] and another which found no survival benefit despite a reduction in pRBC count, platelets, and cryoprecipitate used even with doses lower than that used in other studies.[15] The benefit in morbidity has additionally been supported by a retrospective study of 242 trauma patients, 38 of whom received rFVIIa and showed better 24-hour and hospitalization survival rate than the untreated group, despite being more acidotic and requiring more pRBCs initially. This group also found a mortality benefit.[16] However, other groups have not found improvements in measures of morbidity or mortality, including one study of 81 patients that found no survival improvement despite improvement of coagulopathy.[17] The recent CONTROL trial designed to investigate rFVIIa use in trauma patients was halted because of mortality rates that were not high enough to be able to establish any statistical significance in expected results.[18]

OBSTETRICS

Postpartum hemorrhage (PPH) has traditionally been defined as blood loss greater than 500 mL after vaginal delivery or greater than 1000 mL after caesarean delivery. It is a dangerous sequela of pregnancy that the World Health Organization estimates account for nearly 1 quarter of all maternal deaths worldwide. There are many possible underlying causes of PPH; broadly, PPH can be divided into the following 5 groups: placental abnormalities, coagulation disorders, lacerations and trauma, uterine atony, and retained uterine contents. The treatment of PPH may initially involve transfusion therapy, medical management with uterotonic drugs, and conservative surgical procedures, but refractory life threatening cases may ultimately require a hysterectomy. Given the nature of the underlying problem in PPH, intractable bleeding, it follows that rFVIIa may play a role in its management.

Moscardó and colleagues[19] published the first case report of successful treatment of intractable obstetric hemorrhage in a woman without hemophilia using rFVIIa. This paper reported on a woman who was successfully treated with rFVIIa after a caesarean section in which she developed severe DIC. Ahonen and Jokela[20] presented a case series from the Women's Clinic in Helsinki where during a 16-month period rFVIIa was used in the treatment of 12 patients with severe PPH. In their study, 11 women had a partial or good response to rFVIIa in terms of managing bleeding. These findings led Ahonen and Jokela to conclude that in cases of intractable PPH with no other obvious indications for hysterectomy, administration of rFVIIa should be considered before surgery.

Franchini and colleagues'[21] analysis of published data shows that all reports are derived from uncontrolled studies often based on single case reports. The effectiveness of rFVIIa may be overestimated because of paucity of data. Further, the authors recommend particular caution in using rFVIIa in women at higher thrombotic risk, such as those with PPH and DIC or with gynecologic cancers.

In another article by Franchini and colleagues,[22] only case reports describing at least 10 cases in which rFVIIa was used in the treatment of PPH were analyzed. Case reports were again used because of the lack of data in the form of randomized, case control, or interventional cohort studies. Interestingly, the authors cite data from a number of international registries that have been set up since the advent of rFVIIa.

International registries cited included the Northern Europe Factor VIIa in Obstetric Hemorrhage Registry, the Australian and New Zealand Registry, the Italian Registry, and finally an international Internet-based registry. The Northern European Registry presented pooled data from 9 European countries and reported rFVIIa use in treating PPH in 108 patients. Improvement (defined as reduced bleeding) was found in 84% of treated patients and 75% of patients treated with PPH as secondary prophylaxis.[23] The Australian and New Zealand Registry identified 27 cases; 68% of patients were deemed to have shown a decrease (n = 12) or cessation (n = 5) in bleeding, and 85% of patients survived to 28 days.[24] The Italian Registry collected data on 35 cases. An effective response to rFVIIa was defined as a decrease in RBC requirements of at least 30% after rFVIIa administration. This effective response was seen in 89% of the 35 cases presented.[25] In an international Internet-based registry, 25 cases were identified, and rFVIIa use was deemed effective in 24 of these cases.

Franchini and colleagues conclude that rFVIIa may have a beneficial role in the management of PPH. They proposed the following algorithm: (1) consider the use of rFVIIa for treatment of PPH only after the failure of medical, blood component transfusion, and conservative surgical therapies; (2) administer rFVIIa 90 µg/kg as an intravenous bolus over 3 to 5 minutes. Before the rFVIIa injection, check that all abnormal parameters influencing rFVIIa efficacy (ie, acidosis, thrombocytopenia, hypofibrinogenemia, hypothermia, and hypocalcemia) have been corrected; (3) if there is no response 20 minutes after the first dose, administer a second dose of rFVIIa; and (4) if bleeding persists after 2 doses of rFVIIa, consider hysterectomy. The authors caution that their model is based on the limited data but acknowledge that the case reports reviewed have shown a potential role for rFVIIa in treating intractable PPH.

NEUROLOGY

Intracerebral hemorrhage (ICH) is the second most common cause of stroke. Compared with the other types, ICH causes a higher mortality rate and worse functional outcomes. At 7 days, the mortality rate is more than 20%, rising to more than 40% at 1 month and 53% at 1 year.[26] There is currently no effective treatment for intracerebral hemorrhage.[27]

The volume of the hematoma is a critical determinant of mortality and functional outcome after intracerebral hemorrhage,[28,29] and early hematoma growth is an important cause of neurologic deterioration.[30–33] Early hematoma growth occurs in the absence of coagulopathy and seems to result from continued bleeding or rebleeding at multiple sites within the first few hours after onset.[34] Mayer and colleagues[35] conducted a double-blind placebo-controlled trial from August 2002 through March 2004 at 73 hospitals in 20 countries to determine whether rFVIIa can effectively reduce hematoma growth in patients with acute intracerebral hemorrhage and thus improve their outcomes.

Mayer and colleagues randomly assigned 399 patients with ICH to receive placebo or 40 µg of rFVIIa per kilogram of body weight, 80 µg/kg, or 160 µg/kg within 1 hour after a baseline scan. Hematoma volume increased more in the placebo group than in the rFVIIa groups. The mean increase was 29% in the placebo group, as compared with 16%, 14%, and 11% in the groups given 40, 80, and 160 µg of rFVIIa per kilogram, respectively ($P = 0.01$ for the comparison of the 3 rFVIIa groups with the placebo group). The authors concluded that treatment with rFVIIa within 4 hours after the onset of ICH limits the growth of the hematoma, reduces mortality, and improves functional outcomes at 90 days, despite a small increase in the frequency of TE adverse events.

Various case series also support rFVIIa having a role in managing ICH. Bartal and colleagues[36] present 15 patients successfully treated at a level 1 trauma center for acute subdural hematomas with rFVIIa. Morenski and colleagues[37] reported the successful use of rFVIIa to stop severe coagulopathy in 3 pediatric patients. In an open-label, uncontrolled, emergency-use study, Arkin and colleagues[38] found that rFVIIa effectively controlled ICH in 10 of 12 patients. Further research is already underway to further establish the therapeutic status of rFVIIa in ICH.[39]

EFFECTIVENESS OF rFVIIa for FVIII and FIX deficiencies

Hemostasis deals with clot formation at the site of blood vessel injury. Initially, platelets are activated to form a platelet plug. Platelets can be activated via multiple routes. Exposed subendothelial elements as well as thrombin can activate platelets. Upon activation, platelets go on to secrete various substances that play a significant role in activating the coagulation cascade. The coagulation cascade can be divided into extrinsic and intrinsic pathways, both of which propagate the clotting process.

In the extrinsic pathway, tissue factor (TF) at the site of vessel injury interacts with FVII to form an activated complex (TF-FVIIa). This complex goes on to activate FIX and FX. FIXa along with FVIIIa goes on to activate more FX. FXa works in concert with FVa to convert prothrombin to thrombin. Thrombin goes on to convert fibrinogen to fibrin, which functions to propagate clot formation.

In the intrinsic pathway, FXIIa works with high–molecular weight kininogen to activate FXI, which activates FIX. As in the extrinsic pathway, FIXa along with FVIIIa goes on to activate FX. At this point the pathways converge and ultimately activate fibrinogen.

One of the proposed mechanisms of actions for rFVIIa postulates that it forms a complex with TF that leads to thrombin production. Another proposed mechanism of action of rFVIIa states that rFVIIa directly activates FX on the surface of activated platelets at the site of injury independent of TF and FVIII and FIX. This activation of the factors results in thrombin production and ultimately fibrin generation via the common pathway, where the intrinsic and extrinsic pathways of the coagulation cascade converges. Both proposed mechanisms of actions of rFVIIa do not require FVIII or FIX for clotting.

Mechanism of Action

Physiologically, FVIIa acts in concert with TF to initiate the extrinsic pathway of the classical coagulation cascade. Given the convergence of the intrinsic and extrinsic pathways of the coagulation cascade, rFVIIa was originally developed to bypass steps requiring FIXa or FVIIIa in hemophiliac patients who could not receive those products. However, given the supraphysiologic doses of rFVIIa necessary in patients to achieve a clinical response, along with the understanding that both pathways are important in the generation and maintenance of coagulation, alternative explanations of the mechanism of action have been proposed as well, with no definitive answer yet.

TF-Dependent Hypotheses

One hypothesis holds that TF is required for rFVIIa to exert its effect on hemostasis. Rao and Rapaport[40] postulated that supraphysiologic doses may be needed to overcome competitive inhibition of the formation of FVIIa-TF complexes by FVII forming inactive FVII-TF complexes. This model is supported by in vitro studies of hemophilia showing that while FVII is able to inhibit thrombin generation, FVIIa is able to overcome this and promote a procoagulant state.[41] Further, Butenas and colleagues[42,43] showed that in in vitro models, the effect of rFVIIa in promoting thrombin generation is dependent on TF. However, 1 group found that this effect is saturated after rFVIIa reaches a level of 10 nM in vitro, which is below the concentration achieved in therapeutic doses of rFVIIa.[44] Another theory based on a study showing a reduction in bleeding in hemophilia patients receiving daily dosing of rFVIIa despite a half-life of 2 hours and the finding that FVII can bind extravascular TF, speculates that rFVIIa may diffuse out of the vasculature and bind extravascular TF.[45]

TF-Independent Hypotheses

An alternative theory is based on finding that FVIIa can activate FX independent of TF on the negatively charged surface of activated platelets.[46] Studies in in vitro models of hemophilia initially found that this mechanism increases thrombin generation and that the effect plateaued after reaching levels of 250 nM.[44] Specifically, rFVIIa may bind to the phosphatidylserine on the surface of activated platelets.[47] Because platelets are activated at the site of vascular injury, it is theorized that this helps promote local hemostasis without greatly increasing the risk of systemic thrombosis. Another proposed mechanism of action involves inhibiting the fibrinolytic pathway with the finding that rFVIIa enhances the activity of thrombin-activatable fibrinolysis inhibitor.[48]

DOSING AND TIMING

The dosing of rFVIIa in patients with hemophilias or other coagulopathies such as Glanzmann disease is recommended at 90 µg/kg.[49,50] This dosage corresponds to an approximately 25 to 35 nM concentration in plasma.[51] However, the therapeutic dose in nonhemophilia patients has not been established because of lapses in data comparing efficacy, safety, and cost,[52] with doses found in studies and anecdotally varying widely.

The half-life of rFVIIa is approximately 2.5 hours in adults, and it does not seem to be dose-dependent or affected by the presence or absence of hemophilias or liver disease.[53] Thus, current guidelines are to dose it every 2 hours in patients with hemophilias. In a recent study in trauma patients, wide intra- and interpatient variability of pharmacokinetic properties was found in a 2-compartment model, which the authors found was related to transfusion requirements and blood loss.[54] Nonetheless, the authors found that even in these circumstances, using the regimen described by Boffard and colleagues[13] there was still adequate plasma FVIIa coagulant activity. In patients without hemophilias, beneficial effects have been found with doses varying from 20 to 120 µg/kg.[55,56] Boffard and colleagues' study of rFVIIa use in blunt trauma patients used an initial bolus dose of 200 µg/kg, followed by doses of 100 µg/kg at 1 and 3 hours after the first dose,[13] resulting in some experts recommending such a regimen for use in blunt trauma patients.[55,57] Another group using case series recommended up to 3 doses of about 120 µg/kg (100–140 µg/kg) intravenously over 2 to 5 minutes.[12] One group advocates the use of one 4.8-mg vial (now discontinued, replaced by a 5-mg vial) per dose for an adult, which would correspond to a dose of 50 to 100 µg/kg.[56]

However, a meta-analysis of 22 randomized controlled trials of usage for any indication in patients without hemophilia showed a significant reduction in the number of patients requiring transfusion (odds ratio [OR], 0.42; 0.19–0.93) but not if the dose exceeded 90 µg/kg (OR, 0.62; 0.34–1.14).[58] This is the same dose given to hemophilia patients. Interestingly, the reduction in transfusion rates occurred when rFVIIa was administered only once (OR, 0.33; 0.11–0.96) but not with repeated boluses (OR, 0.66; 0.39–1.09).[58] An earlier Cochrane review looking at a cutoff value of 80 µg/kg between low versus high dose found no difference in bleeding of transfusions in patients receiving low-dose versus high-dose rFVIIa in 5 randomized controlled trials.[57] These findings are consistent with a recent dose-escalation study looking at 5 doses between 40 and 200 μg/kg for trauma patients with intracranial hemorrhage which found reduced hematoma progression for groups above 80 μg/kg, although the authors noted a limitation in assessing outcomes in this group.[59]

The report that higher doses do not improve mortality or decrease the units of blood products transfused is significant especially in light of the finding that higher doses may be associated with an increased risk of arterial thrombus[58,60] and resultant cardiac events in high-risk patients.[60] This is especially concerning if physicians are underreporting TE events.[61]

The optimal timing of administration of the medication is also unclear. Although 1 group found that early administration was associated with improved survival,[8] another found that early versus late administration (before the patient receiving 8 units of blood) resulted in no difference in survival, although the number of transfused blood products was decreased.[9] In practice, because of unresolved issues in optimal administration, it is often given as a last resort after other therapies have failed.[62]

Other factors that may affect the efficacy and thus the appropriateness and timing of administration of rFVIIa include fibrinogen levels, platelet levels, pH, and body temperature, which should be corrected as much as possible before administration of rFVIIA.[12] An in vitro study found that a pH of 7.2 or below decreased FVIIa and FVIIa/TF activity, with a reduction in greater than 90% and 60% of activity at a pH of 7.0, respectively, whereas temperature has only a more modest effect, only decreasing FVIIa/TF activity by 20% and having no effect on FVIIa.[63] Because clot generation and therapeutic rFVIIa activity depend on the presence of fibrinogen and activated platelets, some groups have suggested correction of fibrinogen to 50 mg/dL and platelets to at least 50,000 per μL.[12] One group also suggests frequent monitoring of ionized calcium levels with possible intravenous calcium supplementation.[62]

In summary, rFVIIa has many clinical applications for patients with congenital bleeding disorders and in a variety of clinical settings. Additional studies in the future are ongoing and should provide the clinical anesthesiologist an additional option during certain bleeding states. Specific recommendations as to timing of administration and frequent monitoring of ionized calcium status are suggested at this time. Optimization of fibrinogen levels, platelet levels, pH, and body temperature will enhance efficacy of rFVIIa.

REFERENCES

1. Hedner U. History of rFVIIa therapy. Thromb Res 2010;125(Suppl 1):S4–6.
2. Bishop P, Lawson J. Recombinant biologics for treatment of bleeding disorders. Nat Rev Drug Discov 2004;3(8):684–94.
3. Kenet G, Walden R, Eldad A, et al. Treatment of traumatic bleeding with recombinant factor VIIa. Lancet 1999;354(9193):1879.
4. Martinowitz U, Kenet G, Segal E, et al. Recombinant activated factor VII for adjunctive hemorrhage control in trauma. J Trauma 2001;51(3):431–8.
5. D'Alleyrand JC, Dutton RP, Pollak AN. Extrapolation of battlefield resuscitative care to the civilian setting. J Surg Orthop Adv 2010;19(1):62–9.
6. Kembro RJ, Horton JD, Wagner M. Use of recombinant factor VILa in operation Iraqi freedom and operation enduring freedom: survey of army surgeons. Mil Med 2008;173(11):1057–9.
7. Holcomb JB. Treatment of an acquired coagulopathy and recombinant activated factor VII in a damage-control patient. Mil Med 2005;170:287–90.

8. Spinella PC, Perkins JG, McLaughlin DF, et al. The effect of recombinant activated factor VII on mortality in combat-related casualties with severe trauma and massive transfusion. J Trauma 2008;64(2):286–93.

9. Perkins JG, Schreiber MA, Wade CE, et al. Early versus late recombinant factor VIIa in combat trauma patients requiring massive transfusion. J Trauma 2007; 62(5):1095–9.

10. Fox CJ, Mehta SG, Cox ED, et al. Effect of recombinant factor VIIa as an adjunctive therapy in damage control for wartime vascular injuries: a case control study. J Trauma 2009;66(4 Suppl):S112–9.

11. Woodruff SI, Dougherty AL, Dye JL, et al. Use of recombinant factor VIIA for control of combat-related haemorrhage. Emerg Med J 2010;27(2):121–4.

12. Martinowitz U, Michaelson M. Israeli Multidisciplinary rFVIIa Task Force. Guidelines for the use of recombinant activated factor VII (rFVIIa) in uncontrolled bleeding: a report by the israeli multidisciplinary rfviia task force. J Thromb Haemost 2005;3(4):640–8.

13. Boffard KD, Riou B, Warren B, et al. NovoSeven Trauma Study Group. Recombinant factor VIIa as adjunctive therapy for bleeding control in severely injured trauma patients: two parallel randomized, placebo-controlled, double-blind clinical trials. J Trauma 2005;59(1):8–15 [discussion: 15–8].

14. Boffard KD, Choong PI, Kluger Y, et al, Novoseven trauma study group. The treatment of bleeding is to stop the bleeding! treatment of trauma-related hemorrhage. Transfusion 2009;49(Suppl 5):240S–7S.

15. Harrison TD, Laskosky J, Jazaeri O, et al. "Low-dose" recombinant activated factor VII results in less blood and blood product use in traumatic hemorrhage. J Trauma 2005;59(1):150–4.

16. Rizoli SB, Nascimento B Jr, Osman F, et al. Recombinant activated coagulation factor VII and bleeding trauma patients. J Trauma 2006;61(6):1419–25.

17. Dutton RP, McCunn M, Hyder M, et al. Factor VIIa for correction of traumatic coagulopathy. J Trauma 2004;57:709–18.

18. Dutton R, Hauser C, Boffard K, et al, CONTROL Steering Committee. Scientific and logistical challenges in designing the CONTROL trial: recombinant factor VIIa in severe trauma patients with refractory bleeding. Clin Trials 2009;6(5): 467–79.

19. Moscardó F, Pérez F, de la Rubia J, et al. Successful treatment of severe intra-abdominal bleeding associated with disseminated intravascular coagulation using recombinant activated factor VII. Br J Haematol 2001;114(1):174–6.

20. Ahonen J, Jokela R. Recombinant factor VIIa for life-threatening post-partum haemorrhage. Br J Anaesth 2005;94(5):592–5.

21. Franchini M, Lippi G, Franchi M. The use of recombinant activated factor VII in obstetric and gynaecological haemorrhage. BJOG 2007;114(1):8–15.

22. Franchini M, Franchi M, Bergamini V, et al. The use of recombinant activated FVII in postpartum hemorrhage. Clin Obstet Gynecol 2010;53(1):219–27.

23. Alfirevic Z, Elbourne D, Pavord S, et al. Use of recombinant activated factor VII in primary postpartum hemorrhage: the Northern European registry 2000-2004. Obstet Gynecol 2007;110(6):1270–8.

24. Isbister J, Phillips L, Dunkley S, et al. Recombinant activated factor VII in critical bleeding: experience from the australian and new zealand haemostasis register. Intern Med J 2008;38(3):156–65.

25. Barillari G, Frigo M, Malacarne S, et al. Recombinant activated factor VII in the treatment of acute post partum hemorrhage: the italian registry [abstract]. J Thromb Haemost 2007;5(Suppl 2):162.

26. Broderick JP. Advances in the treatment of hemorrhagic stroke: a possible new treatment. Cleve Clin J Med 2005;72(4):341–4.

27. Broderick JP, Adams HP Jr, Barsan W, et al. Guidelines for the management of spontaneous intracerebral hemorrhage: a statement for healthcare professionals from a special writing group of the stroke council, american heart association. Stroke 1999;30:905–15.

28. Broderick JP, Brott TG, Duldner JE, et al. Volume of intracerebral hemorrhage: a powerful and easy-to-use predictor of 30-day mortality. Stroke 1993;24:987–93.

29. Hemphill JC III, Bonovich DC, Besmertis L, et al. The ICH score: a simple, reliable grading scale for intracerebral hemorrhage. Stroke 2001;32:891–7.

30. Brott T, Broderick J, Kothari R, et al. Early hemorrhage growth in patients with intracerebral hemorrhage. Stroke 1997;28:1–5.

31. Fujii Y, Tanaka R, Takeuchi S, et al. Hematoma enlargement in spontaneous intracerebral hemorrhage. J Neurosurg 1994;80:51–7.

32. Fujitsu K, Muramoto M, Ikeda Y, et al. Indications for surgical treatment of putaminal hemorrhage: comparative study based on serial CT and time course analysis. J Neurosurg 1990;73:518–25.

33. Kazui S, Naritomi H, Yamamoto H, et al. Enlargement of spontaneous intracerebral hemorrhage: incidence and time course. Stroke 1996;27:1783–7.

34. Mayer SA. Ultra-early hemostatic therapy for intracerebral hemorrhage. Stroke 2003;34:224–9.

35. Mayer SA, Brun NC, Begtrup K, et al. Recombinant Activated Factor VII Intracerebral Hemorrhage trial investigators. recombinant activated factor VII for acute intracerebral hemorrhage. N Engl J Med 2005;352(8):777–85.

36. Bartal C, Freedman J, Bowman K, et al. Coagulopathic patients with traumatic intracranial bleeding: defining the role of recombinant factor VIIa. J Trauma 2007;63(4):725–32.

37. Morenski JD, Tobias JD, Jimenez DF. Recombinant activated factor VII for cerebral injury-induced coagulopathy in pediatric patients. J Neurosurg 2003;98:611–3.

38. Arkin S, Cooper HA, Hutter JJ, et al. Activated recombinant human coagulation factor VII therapy for intracranial hemorrhage in patients with hemophilia A or B with inhibitors. Results of the novoseven emergency-use program. Haemostasis 1998;28(2):93–8.

39. Kumar S, Badrinath HR. Early recombinant factor VIIa therapy in acute intracerebral hemorrhage: promising approach. Neurol India 2006;54(1):24–7.

40. Rao LV, Rapaport SI. Cells and the activation of factor VII. Haemostasis 1996;26(Suppl 1):1–5.

41. van't Veer C, Mann KG. The regulation of the factor VII-dependent coagulation pathway: rationale for the effectiveness of recombinant factor VIIa in refractory bleeding disorders. Semin Thromb Hemost 2000;26(4):367–72.

42. Butenas S, Brummel KE, Branda RF, et al. Mechanism of factor VIIa-dependent coagulation in hemophilia blood. Blood 2002;99(3):923–30.

43. Butenas S, Brummel KE, Bouchard BA, et al. How factor VIIa works in hemophilia. J Thromb Haemost 2003;1(6):1158–60.

44. Monroe DM, Hoffman M, Oliver JA, et al. Platelet activity of high-dose factor VIIa is independent of tissue factor. Br J Haematol 1997;99(3):542–7.

45. Mackman N. The role of tissue factor and factor VIIa in hemostasis. Anesth Analg 2009;108(5):1447–52.

46. Bom VJ, Bertina RM. The contributions of $Ca2+$, phospholipids and tissue-factor apoprotein to the activation of human blood-coagulation factor X by activated factor VII. Biochem J 1990;265(2):327–36.

47. Hoffman M. A cell-based model of coagulation and the role of factor VIIa. Blood Rev 2003;17(Suppl 1):S1–5.
48. Lisman T, Mosnier LO, Lambert T, et al. Inhibition of fibrinolysis by recombinant factor VIIa in plasma from patients with severe hemophilia A. Blood 2002;99(1): 175–9.
49. Steiner ME, Key NS, Levy JH. Activated recombinant factor VII in cardiac surgery. Curr Opin Anaesthesiol 2005;18(1):89–92.
50. Heuer L, Blumenberg D. Management of bleeding in a multi-transfused patient with positive HLA class I alloantibodies and thrombocytopenia associated with platelet dysfunction refractory to transfusion of cross-matched platelets. Blood Coagul Fibrinolysis 2005;16(4):287–90.
51. Hedner U. Factor VIIa and its potential therapeutic use in bleeding-associated pathologies. Thromb Haemost 2008;100(4):557–62.
52. Levy JH, Azran M. Anesthetic concerns for patients with coagulopathy. Curr Opin Anaesthesiol 2010;23(3):400–5.
53. Erhardtsen E. Pharmacokinetics of recombinant activated factor VII (rFVIIa). Semin Thromb Hemost 2000;26(4):385–91.
54. Klitgaard T, Tabanera Y, Palacios R, et al, NovoSeven Trauma Study Group. Pharmacokinetics of recombinant activated factor VII in trauma patients with severe bleeding. Crit Care 2006;10(4):R104.
55. Vincent JL, Rossaint R, Riou B, et al. Recommendations on the use of recombinant activated factor VII as an adjunctive treatment for massive bleeding–a european perspective. Crit Care 2006;10(4):R120.
56. Goodnough LT, Lublin DM, Zhang L, et al. Transfusion medicine service policies for recombinant factor VIIa administration. Transfusion 2004;44(9):1325–31.
57. Stanworth SJ, Birchall J, Doree CJ, et al. Recombinant factor VIIa for the prevention and treatment of bleeding in patients without haemophilia. Cochrane Database Syst Rev 2007;2:CD005011.
58. Hsia CC, Chin-Yee IH, McAlister VC. Use of recombinant activated factor VII in patients without hemophilia: a meta-analysis of randomized control trials. Ann Surg 2008;248(1):61–8.
59. Narayan RK, Maas AI, Marshall LF, et al. Recombinant factor VIIA in traumatic intracerebral hemorrhage: results of a dose-escalation clinical trial. Neurosurgery 2008;62:776–86.
60. Diringer MN, Skolnick BE, Mayer SA, et al. Thromboembolic events with recombinant activated factor VII in spontaneous intracerebral hemorrhage: results from the factor seven for acute hemorrhagic stroke (FAST) trial. Stroke 2010;41(1): 48–53.
61. Hsia CC, Zurawska JH, Tong MZ, et al. Recombinant activated factor VII in the treatment of non-haemophilia patients: physician under-reporting of thromboembolic adverse events. Transfus Med 2009;19(1):43–9.
62. Spahn DR, Cerny V, Coats TJ, et al. Management of bleeding following major trauma: a european guideline. Crit Care 2007;11:R17.
63. Meng ZH, Wolberg AS, Monroe DM 3rd, et al. The effect of temperature and pH on the activity of factor VIIa: implications for the efficacy of high-dose factor VIIa in hypothermic and acidotic patients. J Trauma 2003;55:886–91.

Sugammadex: Cyclodextrins, Development of Selective Binding Agents, Pharmacology, Clinical Development, and Future Directions

Arezou Sadighi Akha, MD, MS[a], Joseph Rosa III, MD[b],
Jonathan S. Jahr, MD[b],*, Alvin Li[c], Kianusch Kiai, MD, MS[b]

KEYWORDS

- Sugammadex • Cyclodextrins • Selective binding agents
- Neuromuscular blocking agents and reversal

HISTORY OF MUSCLE RELAXANTS

Neuromuscular blocking agents (NMBAs) are widely used in perioperative medicine to aid in endotracheal intubation, facilitate surgery, and in critical care/emergency medicine settings. Muscle relaxants have profound clinical uses in current surgical and intensive care and emergency medical therapy.

A brief history of the first use of muscle relaxants includes European explorers who discovered natives in the Amazon River Basin using poison-tipped arrows. These seventeenth century investigators discovered that this poison, also known

Disclosures: Dr Jahr served as Principal Investigator on two Sugammadex Phase III studies funded by Organon/Schering-Plough/Merck and served on the Speaker's Bureau from 1999–2000 and 2006–2009.

[a] UCLA JCCC Clinical Research Unit, 10945 Le Conte Avenue, 3360 PVUB, Los Angeles, CA 90095, USA

[b] Department of Anesthesiology, David Geffen School of Medicine at UCLA, Ronald Reagan UCLA Medical Center, 757 Westwood Plaza, Suite 3325, Los Angeles, CA 90095, USA

[c] College of Letters and Science, University of California Los Angeles, 310 De Neve Drive, Rieber Terrace 658a, Los Angeles, CA 90024, USA

* Corresponding author. UCLA Anesthesiology, RRUMC, 757 Westwood Plaza, Suite 3325, Los Angeles, CA 90095.

E-mail address: jsjahr@mednet.ucla.edu

Anesthesiology Clin 28 (2010) 691–708
doi:10.1016/j.anclin.2010.08.014
1932-2275/10/$ – see front matter © 2010 Elsevier Inc. All rights reserved.

as *flying death* from the rubber plant Chondrodendron tomentosum, killed animals by skeletal muscle paralysis.[1] Hakluyt published his account of Sir Walter Raleigh's voyage up the Amazon in 1595.[2] Three centuries later, Dale in 1914, used a derivative of the poison, now called tubocurarine, to determine that acetylcholine (ACh) was the neurochemical transmitter at the neuromuscular junction (NMJ). Pal, a physiologist in Vienna, in 1900 experimented on paralyzed dogs administered curare to evaluate the pharmacologic of physostigmine on peristalsis. Pal observed return to spontaneous ventilation and a marked increase in peristalsis after the administration of physostigmine. Pal surmised that physostigmine might be an antidote to curare. In 1912, Lawen demonstrated the clinical usefulness of curare by injecting it intramuscularly to achieve abdominal relaxation for peritoneal surgery.[1] In 1942 in Montreal, Griffith and Johnson introduced curare into clinical anesthesia. Griffith and Johnson administered 5 mL of a curare preparation to a 20-year-old man undergoing general anesthesia by facemask delivered cyclopropane for an appendectomy.[3] By 1946, the use of neuromuscular blocking agents had become established in Great Britain. In his initial report, Gray only recommended pyridostigmine as a reversal drug, but reports of incomplete recovery (recurarization) were published. Neostigmine (5 mg) soon became part of the Liverpool anesthesia technique.[1]

The reversal of the neuromuscular block may pose a safety challenge. Two basic pharmacologic mechanisms are currently in use. One is to allow the NMBA effect to dissipate either by dilution or metabolism, and neuromuscular activity will resume. This option will require time because the half-lives of some muscle relaxants are long. It also mandates that health care professionals be vigilant to examine patients for complete reversal of the NMBAs.

The second option is to reverse the activity of the NMBA through a reversal drug. The only available strategy is the administration of acetylcholinesterase inhibitors. These agents may cause excess parasympathetic activity and require a second agent to ameliorate these side effects. The practitioner must be vigilant because the half-life of acetylcholinesterase may be shorter that the NMBA and the recurarization and weakness may become a serious issue.

Sugammadex is the first of the cyclodextrins to be used as a therapeutic agent. It is a selective inhibitor of steroidal NMBA agents by encapsulating them and thereby rendering them inactive. This medication quickly binds neuromuscular blocking agents and reverses their block.[4] The safety and efficacy of sugammadex is documented in a following section of this review.

This article reviews cyclodextrins, development of selective binding agents, clinical development, and future directions of sugammadex. As this is a review of existing literature, no new information will be presented. All statements are referenced and the source documentation can be found as the listed references.

CYCLODEXTRIN

Cyclodextrins (CD) are a group of compounds composed of sugar molecules bound together in a ring. Cyclodextrins are produced from starch by enzymatic conversion. They are used in multiple different industries, including the food, pharmaceutical, chemical, and environmental industries.[5]

Cyclodextrins are composed of 5 or more alpha-D-glucopyranoside units linked 1 to 4. Typical cyclodextrins contain 6 to 8 glucose members in a ring creating a cone shape: α-cyclodextrin (6-membered sugar ring molecule), β-cyclodextrin (7), and γ-cyclodextrin (8).[6]

Cyclodextrins were initially described as cellulosine in 1891 by A. Villiers when he detected the α, β CD as a product of digestion of starch by bacillus amylobacter. Schardinger identified 2 naturally occurring cyclodextrins (α, β) that were referred to as *Schardinger sugars*. In the 1930s, work by Freudenberg laid the foundation for more cyclodextrin research. Freudenberg and colleagues identified gamma CD. Cramer and coworkers were responsible for the important finding that CDs would form inclusion complexes and also were useful in solubilizing drugs. By the mid 1970s, extensive work has been conducted by Szejtli and others exploring encapsulation by cyclodextrins for industrial and pharmacologic uses.[5,7]

Cyclodextrin synthesis involves treatment of starch with enzymes. Cyclodextrin glycosyltransferase (CGTase) is used along with α-amylase. Ordinary starch is liquefied with heat or α-amylase. The CGTase is added for enzymatic conversion. This process results in a mixture of the 3 types of cyclodextrin molecules mentioned earlier: α, β, and γ. Separation of the 3 types of cyclodextrins is based on water solubility.[6,8]

The cyclodextrin may be imagined as a cone with an open end, the interior of which is not hydrophobic but lipophilic, and is able to host other hydrophobic molecules. The exterior is hydrophilic, thus making the molecule water soluble. The formation of inclusion compounds modifies both the physical and chemical properties of the molecule in terms of water solubility. The host-guest complex is then formed by these ionic interactions.[9,10]

Cyclodextrins are able to form host-guest complexes with hydrophobic molecules. These molecules can be used in environmental protection as they may effectively immobilize toxic compounds inside their rings, such as heavy metals and trichloroethane. They are used in the food industry in the preparation of cholesterol-free products, as weight loss adjuncts, to stabilize volatile compounds, as well as in the fragrance and cleaning industry.[6,8]

DEVELOPMENT OF THE SELECTIVE RELAXANT BINDING AGENTS

Selective relaxant binding agents (SRBAs) are a class of drugs that selectively encapsulates and binds neuromuscular blocking agents. The first drug to be introduced as an SRBA is sugammadex. Sugammadex, originally known as Org 25969,[3] is a modified gamma cyclodextrin that specifically encapsulates and binds the following aminosteroid NMBAs: rocuronium, vecuronium, and pancuronium. SRBAs exert a chelating action that effectively terminates the ability of a NMBA to bind to acetylcholine receptors at the neuromuscular junction.[4,11]

The discovery of sugammadex as an agent to terminate the effect of NMBA is the result of work done at Organon Laboratories in Scotland. Cyclodextrins were explored as a means to solubilize rocuronium bromide (a steroidal NMBA) in a neutral aqueous solution.

The chemical formula for sugammadex is per -6 –(2-carboxyethylthio) – per -6-deoxy-gamma c cyclodextrin sodium salt, and is a modified gamma cyclodextrin with a lipophilic core and a hydrophilic exterior. Gamma cyclodextrin has been altered by placing 8 carboxyl thio-ether groups at the sixth carbon positions. These additions enlarge the cavity size allowing greater encapsulation of the rocuronium molecule. The molecular weight is 2178 g/mol, and the chemical formula is $C_{72}H_{104}Na_8O_{48}S_8$. These carboxyl groups that are negatively charged electrostatically bind to the positive charged ammonium group and help stabilize the cyclodextrin.[12] The rocuronium molecule that is a modified steroid bound within, sugammadex's lipophilic core is unable bind to the ACh receptor. The result of this is termination of action neuromuscular blockade is the lack of need for inhibition of ACh and its inherent muscarinic side effects. Iatrogenic cardiovascular instability at the time of reversal is thus much less of a concern.[3] **Figs. 1–5** provide a graphic visualization of the sugammadex molecule and its chemical interaction with the steroid-based neuromuscular blocking drugs.

Recurarization has been reported with sugammadex but only when insufficient doses were used. The mechanism may be caused by redistribution of relaxant from peripheral to the central compartment, and tends to occur when lower doses of sugammadex are used.[13] Sugammadex has some affinity for other aminosteroidal NMBAs, such as vecuronium and pancuronium, but considerably less than for rocuronium.

PHARMACOLOGY

Sugammadex is the generic name of the modified gamma cyclodextrin: *SU* (sugar molecule), *GAMMA* (gamma core of 8 glucose units), and *DEX* (cyclodextrin).[14]

Of the 3 naturally occurring cyclodextrins (α, β, and γ) it was determined that γ (gamma) cyclodextrins, would have the most appropriate cavity size to encapsulate the aminosteroid muscle relaxant. It was also discovered that the gamma cyclodextrin molecule could be modified to have a high affinity for rocuronium, and thus it might be effective to inactivate by encapsulating aminosteroid-based neuromuscular blocking drugs. Although this modified (gamma) cyclodextrin would have much greater affinity for rocuronium, it has some effect on vecuronium and pancuronium.[12,14]

Sugammadex has a lipophilic inner cavity that was enlarged by adding lipophilic groups (acidic functional groups COO-) to increase the hydrophobic interior and to

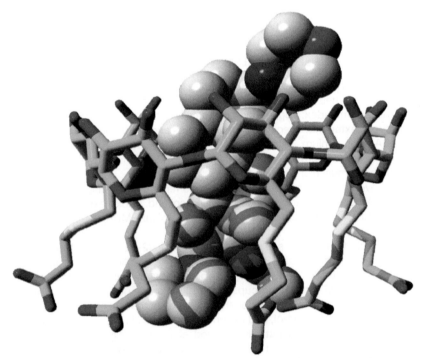

Fig. 1. Sugammadex. (*From* Bom A, Bradley M, Cameron K, et al. A novel concept of reversing neuromuscular block: chemical encapsulation of rocuronium bromide by a cyclodextrin based synthetic host. Angew Chem Int Ed Engl 2002;41:266–70; with permission.)

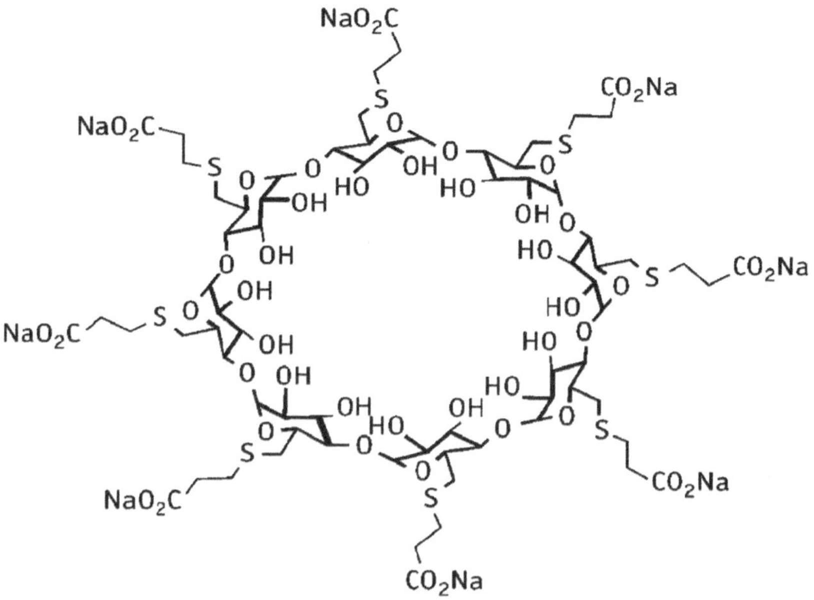

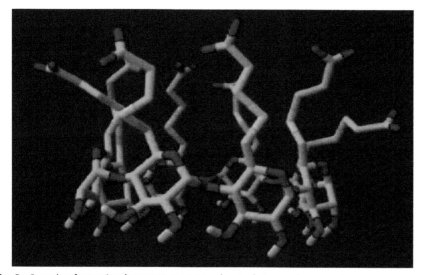

Fig. 2. Cyclodextrin ring structure of Sugammadex. (*From* Epemolu O, et al. Reversal of neuromuscular blockade and simultaneous increase in plasma rocuronium concentration after the intravenous infusion of the Novel Reversal Agent Org 25969. Anesthesiology 2003;99(3):632–7; with permission.)

form electrostatic bond interactions with the positively charged nitrogen of the aminosteroid molecule. Through mutual repulsion, these acidic functional groups keep the central core of the cyclodextrin molecule open. As the steroid nucleus of the vecuronium molecule is inside the core of the sugammadex molecule, the negative bonds of

Fig. 3. Complex formation between sugammadex and rocuronium.

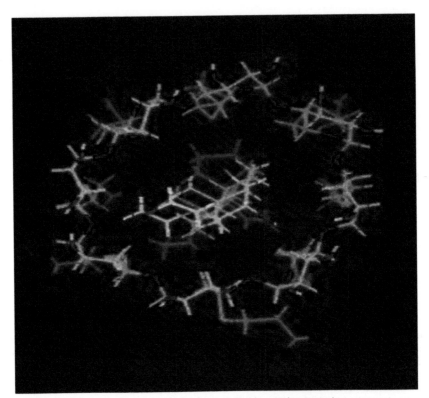

Fig. 4. The radiograph crystal structure of Sugammadex and rocuronium.

the carboxyl groups close as the diverting repulsion is interrupted by the presence of the sugammadex molecule, and these bond tightly to the positively charged nitrogen molecule of rocuronium.[12,14]

Sugammadex cannot distinguish between the aminosteroid NMBAs rocuronium, vecuronium, and pancuronium. However, the differences in affinity are such that sugammadex prefers rocuronium. Sugammadex has 2.5 times the affinity for rocuronium versus vecuronium and little affinity for pancuronium. Importantly, sugammadex has no affinity for succinylcholine or the benzylisoquinoline nonsteroidal muscle relaxants, such as cisatracurium, atracurium, or mivacurium.[3,15]

Sugammadex forms a 1:1 tight noncovalent complex with steroid based neuromuscular blocking agents and functions as a chelating agent. The stability of the rocuronium-sugammadex complex is a result of intermolecular (van der Waals) forces, hydrogen bonds, and hydrophobic interactions. The vecuronium-sugammadex complex exists in equilibrium with a high association rate (association constant of 10^7 M^{-1}) and a low dissociation rate, which favors a stable tight complex. Sugammadex has greater affinity for rocuronium than vecuronium, but to induce a degree of neuromuscular block, fewer molecules of vecuronium are required than for rocuronium. The effective dose (ED50) of vecuronium is approximately 10 times higher than for rocuronium, which results in a reduction of sugammadex molecules necessary for encapsulation.[4]

Sugammadex rapidly reverses NMBAs by removing rocuronium from NMJs as free rocuronium transfers to the central compartment, where it is encapsulated by

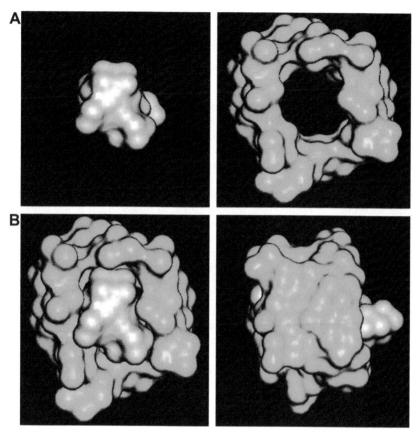

Fig. 5. (*A*) Current Radiograph crystal structure of a rocuronium molecule and a sugamma-dex molecule. (*B*) Synopsis encapsulation of rocuronium molecule (*blue*) by a sugammadex molecule (*green*) at 1:1 ratio. (*From* Cameron KS, Clark JK, Cooper A, et al. Modified gamma-cyclodextrins and their rocuronium complexes. Org Lett 2002;4:3403–6 ©American Chemical Society; with permission.)

sugammadex. This statement is supported by the increase in total plasma concentration of free rocuronium and the rocuronium-sugammadex complex after administration of sugammadex. The concentration of free rocuronium in the plasma decreases more rapidly with the higher sugammadex dose than the lower dose.[4]

The pharmacokinetics of sugammadex shows a dose-dependent linear relationship over the dose range of 0.1 to 8.0 mg kg^{-1}. The elimination half-life is approximately 100 minutes, where 59% to 80% of the administered dose is excreted in the urine over 24 hours and the clearance is 120 L/min, which is similar to normal GFR. The volume of distribution (V_D) is 18 L, which is more than blood volume but less than extracellular volume. Rocuronium is normally cleared permanently by biliary excretion. With sugammadex, renal excretion increases and biliary excretion decreases. The alteration in the method of excretion and thus the pharmacokinetics of an NMBA from primarily hepatic to renal is unprecedented. With administration of 8 mg kg^{-1} at 3 minutes after an intubating dose of rocuronium, renal excretion of rocuronium with 0 to 24 hours increases from 14% to 39% to 68%.[4]

Sugammadex also changes rocuronium V_D from 50 to 15 L, similar to that of sugam-madex. The clearance of sugammadex is 3 times lower than that of rocuronium. The overall pharmacokinetics of sugammadex, rocuronium and the complex of the two is favorable clinically in that there is rapid recovery from NMBAs and lack of recurarization when sugammadex is given at appropriate doses.[4]

CLINICAL DEVELOPMENT

The clinical development of sugammadex will be divided into important preclinical studies, phase I, II, and IIIa studies, leading to European Union approval, and setting the stage for phase IIIb studies to be performed.

The results of several animal studies have shown that sugammadex reverses rocuronium-induced neuromuscular blockade in vitro and in vivo.[12,16,17] In addition, phase I and II trials have demonstrated that sugammadex is effective and safe at reversing rocuronium-induced neuromuscular blockade in healthy volunteers and surgical subjects.[16,18] Additionally, sugammadex, at doses of 2.0 to 4.0 mg/kg, has been shown to reverse safely moderate neuromuscular block induced by rocuronium in a dose-dependent manner in surgical patients.[19,20]

These potential positive effects of sugammadex as a useful SRBA encouraged the investigators to perform different clinical trials to assess and evaluate the efficacy and safety of this novel product as an effective reversal of moderate and profound rocuronium-induced neuromuscular block.

The following studies are phase II and phase III studies from well-respected international centers looking at the efficacy, dosing, and safety of sugammadex. The studies are presented with phase II first followed by the phase III studies. Each group is organized in a chronologic fashion with the oldest study presented first. All studies are multicenter studies. Each has recruited a significant number of subjects (27–172 subjects), all adult with American Society of Anesthesiologists Physical Status (ASA) classification I to III.

A 2-center, partially randomized, safety assessor-blinded, phase II dose-finding study was conducted between March 2003 and September 2004 at 2 centers in Belgium to investigate the dose-response relation of sugammadex administered as a reversal agent at reappearance of the second muscle twitch (T2) in response to train-of-four stimulation after administration of either vecuronium (Norcuron, NV Organon, Oss,) or rocuronium (Esmeron, NV Organon, Oss, Netherlands), and to evaluate the safety of single doses of sugammadex.[21] Eighty subjects were recruited, all older than 18 years with ASA classification I or II, scheduled to undergo surgery of at least 60 minutes duration that required general anesthesia and muscle relaxation only for intubation of the trachea. The primary study endpoint was the time from the start of administration of sugammadex or placebo to recovery of the T4/T1 ratio to 0.9 after rocuronium or vecuronium-induced neuromuscular block, and the secondary endpoints were the times from the start of administration of sugammadex or placebo to recovery of the T4/T1 ratio to 0.8 and 0.7 after rocuronium or vecuronium-induced neuromuscular block.[21]

Subjects were treated in parallel treatment groups and randomly assigned to receive either rocuronium (0.60 mg/kg) or vecuronium (0.10 mg/kg). There was no randomization for sugammadex, but instead, a step-up/step-down design was used. The rocuronium and vecuronium dose groups were enrolled in 5 sequential blocks. Each subject received a single intravenous bolus intubation dose of rocuronium (0.60 mg/kg) or vecuronium (0.10 mg/kg). At the reappearance of T2, sugammadex (1.0 mg/kg) was administered as a single bolus injection to subjects in the first rocuronium and vecuronium groups. The dose of sugammadex administered in each subsequent dose group was determined after evaluation of the primary endpoint in the previous dose groups. The doses were selected in such a way that at least 2 doses of sugammadex would result in a recovery time on the plateau of the exponential curve and at least 2 sugammadex doses would result in a recovery time on the plateau of the dose-response curve. In this way, the dose-response relationship could be determined over a range from placebo (spontaneous recovery) to recovery on the plateau of the dose-response curve (fastest recovery possible).[21] Neuromuscular transmission was monitored by the acceleromyographic response of the adductor pollicis muscle to repetitive train-of-four stimulation of the ulnar nerve every 15 seconds using surface electrodes TOF-Watch SX.[21]

The results showed that compared with the placebo, sugammadex produced dose-dependent decreases in meantime to recovery for all T4/T1 ratios in the rocuronium and vecuronium groups. The mean time for recovery of the T4/T1 ratio to 0.9 in the rocuronium group was 31.8 minutes after placebo compared with 3.7 and 1.1 minutes after 0.5 and 4.0 mg/kg sugammadex, respectively. The mean time for recovery of the T4/T1 ratio to 0.9 in the vecuronium group was 48.8 minutes after placebo, compared with 2.5 and 1.4 minutes after 1.0 and 8.0 mg/kg sugammadex, respectively. In summary, sugammadex, in a dose-dependent manner, decreased the time from the start of administration to recovery of T4/T1 ratio to 0.9, 0.8 and 0.7 in both groups.[21] Additionally, the safety data indicated that sugammadex was safe and well tolerated when used to reverse the neuromuscular block induced either by rocuronium or by vecuronium, and no evidence of recurarization was observed in any subjects. Four of the adverse effects (AEs) that occurred during the trial (tachycardia, prolonged awakening from anesthesia, erythema, and abdominal discomfort) were considered to be related to the study drug; whereas, none of the severe adverse effects (SAEs) (hematoma, perforation of the small intestine, hemorrhage at the incision site, constipation, and muscle hemorrhage) were considered to be treatment related.[21]

Another similar phase II randomized, placebo-controlled, safety assessor-blinded trial was conducted at 2 centers in Denmark in which 27 male subjects aged 18 to 64 years, with physical status class ASA I or II, scheduled to undergo surgery in which anesthesia was anticipated to last for 60 minutes or longer, were randomly assigned to receive placebo or sugammadex (0.5, 1.0, 2.0, 3.0, or 4.0 mg/kg) for reversal of 0.6 mg/kg rocuronium-induced neuromuscular block. Neuromuscular function was monitored using the TOF-Watch SX and train of four (TOF) nerve stimulation. The primary efficacy variable in this study was the time from the start of administration of sugammadex or placebo to the recovery of the TOF ratio (T4/T1) to 0.9, and the secondary efficacy variables were the time from the start of administration of sugammadex or placebo to the recovery of the TOF ratio to 0.8 and 0.7.[19] Urine and blood samples were also collected for safety assessment before administration of rocuronium and at 20 minutes (blood only) and at 4 to 6 hours (blood and urine) after administration of sugammadex or placebo.[19]

Based on the results of this study, sugammadex decreased the median recovery time in a dose-dependent manner from 21.0 minutes in the placebo group to 1.1 minute in the group receiving 4.0 mg/kg sugammadex. Doses of sugammadex of 2.0 mg/kg or greater reversed rocuronium-induced neuromuscular block within 3 minutes. In the placebo group, the rocuronium plasma concentration declined with time after dosing, however, rocuronium plasma concentration at 20 minutes after administration of sugammadex (all doses) were increased compared with those at the corresponding time point in the placebo group, and were still increased at 4 to 6 hours in the highest sugammadex dose group compared with placebo.[19] A median of 59% to 77% of sugammadex was excreted unchanged in the urine within 16 hours, mostly in the first 8 hours. Sugammadex also increased the proportion of the rocuronium dose excreted unchanged in the urine. Three subjects had AEs that were categorized as severe and possibly, probably, or definitely related to treatment (coughing, movement, and hypotension), and 1 subject (in the 3.0 mg/kg dose group) experienced an SAE, possibly related to sugammadex (hypotension beginning 10 minutes after administration of sugammadex and lasting for 5 minutes). In conclusion, the safety data from this study indicated that sugammadex was well tolerated, all subjects' issues recovered without clinical consequences and no evidence of recurarization was observed in any subject.[19]

In maintenance of anesthesia, propofol and sevoflurane are widely used. Other studies have shown that in contrast to propofol, sevoflurane enhances the effects of some NMBAs, including rocuronium.[22,23] A randomized, multicenter, safety assessor-blinded, phase II, parallel group comparative trial was conducted at 3 centers in Belgium, to demonstrate that sugammadex (2.0 mg/kg) is equally effective at reversing rocuronium-induced block, regardless of whether the maintenance anesthetic regimen is propofol or sevoflurane. A total of 42 subjects (ASA physical status I–III) were enrolled in this trial.

The primary endpoint in this study was time from start of sugammadex administration to recovery of the T4/T1 ratio to 0.9. Secondary endpoints were the time from the start of administration of sugammadex to recovery of the TOF ratio (T4/T1) to 0.7 and 0.8. Neuromuscular block was monitored and recorded by acceleromyography TOF Watch SX.[24]

Anesthesia was induced with an intravenous opioid followed by propofol, then subjects were randomized to receive maintenance anesthesia with either propofol (>6.0 mg/kg/h by continuous infusion) or sevoflurane (target minimum alveolar concentration 1.5, adjusted for age). No nitrous oxide was used. After the stabilization period for TOF Watch SX (at least 5 minutes), each subject received a single intravenous (IV) bolus dose of rocuronium 0.6 mg/kg for tracheal intubation. When the second twitch (T2) of the TOF reappeared, a single IV bolus dose of sugammadex 2.0 mg/kg was administered. Adverse events were recorded from administration of sugammadex until the postanesthetic visit that took place at least 10 hours after administration of sugammadex.[24]

Based on the results, the mean recovery time from rocuronium administration to reappearance of T2 was 33.0 minutes in the propofol group and 51.8 minutes in the sevoflurane group. The mean time from start of administration of sugammadex to recovery of the TOF ratio (T4/T1) to 0.9 was 1.8 minutes in both propofol and sevoflurane groups. The meantime from start of administration of sugammadex to recovery of the TOF ratios to 0.8 and 0.7 were 1.5 and 1.3 minutes, respectively, in both the propofol and sevoflurane groups.[24] Four AEs related to treatment were observed during this study (hypotension in sevoflurane group; and bradycardia, nausea, vomiting, hypotension, and hiccups in the propofol group). All AEs were of mild to moderate intensity, except in 1 subject in the sevoflurane group, who reported severe nausea. Eight subjects in the sevoflurane group experienced QTc prolongation that met the criteria for a SAE. None of these subjects had values placing them at risk of arrhythmia and the events were considered unlikely to be related to sugammadex.[24]

In this trial, sugammadex reversed neuromuscular block within 3 minutes of administration in the majority of subjects in both treatment groups. This finding represents a substantial improvement versus conventional cholinesterase inhibitors, which take much longer. Additionally, sugammadex was well tolerated with minimal side effects with both propofol and sevoflorane.[24]

Another similar phase II, randomized, assessor-blinded, parallel group, dose-finding clinical trial was conducted at 4 sites in the United States to explore the dose-response relationship of sugammadex in reversing profound rocuronium-induced NMBA.[25] Fifty subjects aged 18 years or older with ASA physical status I to III, scheduled to undergo an elective surgical procedure anticipated to last at least 45 minutes and requiring endotracheal intubation and the use of the nondepolarizing NMBA were eligible for inclusion. Before the surgical procedure, subjects were randomized to 1 of 2 doses of rocuronium (0.6 or 1.2 mg/kg) and to 1 of 5 doses of sugammadex (0.5, 1.0, 2.0, 4.0, and 8.0 mg/kg) that was administered during profound block. Neuromuscular function was monitored using the TOF Watch SX acceleromyograph.[25] The primary efficacy variable was the time from the start of administration of sugammadex to recovery of the TOF ratio to 0.9, and the secondary efficacy variables were the time from the start of administration of sugammadex to recovery of the TOF ratio to 0.7 and 0.8.[25]

Based on the results, reversal of neuromuscular block was obtained after administration of sugammadex in all but the lowest dose groups (0.5–1.0 mg/kg) where several subjects could not be adequately reversed. At the highest dose (8.0 mg/kg), mean recovery time was 1.2 minutes (range 0.8–2.1 minutes). In both rocuronium dose groups, there was a substantial decrease in time to recovery of the TOF ratio to 0.9 with increasing dose of sugammadex. The investigators identified 4 SAEs during the study, none of which were thought to be related to the study medication, and all 4 subjects made full recoveries. The most common AEs observed in this study were postprocedural pain, nausea, vomiting, hypertension, hypotension, and a brief period of oxygen desaturation. No subject complained of weakness or diplopia during the postanesthesia care unit stay, and no evidence of muscle weakness was seen. In general, sugammadex was well tolerated and effective in rapidly reversing profound rocuronium-induced neuromuscular block at doses greater than or equal to 2 mg/kg.[25]

To support the hypothesis that sugammadex may be used to rescue at 5 minutes after administration of a high dose of rocuronium (1.2 mg/kg), and to evaluate the safety of single doses of sugammadex up to 16.0 mg/kg, a multicenter, randomized, assessor-blinded and placebo-controlled, dose-finding phase II study was conducted at 4 centers in the Netherlands from November 2003 until July 2004.[26] Forty-five subjects of ASA status I and II, aged 18 to 64 years, scheduled to undergo a surgical procedure in the supine position with an anticipated duration of anesthesia of 90 minutes or greater, were randomized to participate in this study, but just 43 of the subjects were treated with either sugammadex or placebo. Profound neuromuscular blockade was induced with 1.2 mg/kg rocuronium bromide, and sugammadex (2.0, 4.0, 8.0, 12.0, or 16.0 mg/kg) or placebo (0.9% saline) was then administered 5 minutes after the administration of rocuronium. Neuromuscular monitoring was performed using the TOF Watch SX by measuring the effect of the stimulation of the ulnar nerve on activity of the adductor pollicis muscle. The primary efficacy variable was defined as the time from the start of the administration of Sugammadex or placebo to recovery of the TOF ratio to 0.9.[26]

The results showed that increasing doses of sugammadex reduced the mean recovery time from 122 minutes (spontaneous recovery) to less than 2 minutes in a dose-dependent manner. Two subjects receiving sugammadex each experienced 1 AE (diarrhea and light anesthesia) that was regarded as possibly related to sugammadex, both subjects recovered without sequelae. Three SAEs (all QTc prolongation) were reported, and these occurred in the 2 mg/kg and 12 mg/kg sugammadex dose groups, none of them were considered related to sugammadex. Sugammadex was well tolerated and produced rapid and effective reversal of profound rocuronium-induced neuromuscular blockade, without signs of recurrence of neuromuscular blockade.[26]

Between October 2005 and May 2006, a phase II, multicenter, randomized, open-label, parallel, dose-response trial was conducted in 7 centers in Europe to explore the dose-response relationship of sugammadex for the reversal of deep neuromuscular blockade induced by rocuronium or vecuronium under propofol-induced and sevoflurane-maintained anesthesia.[27] A total of 102 subjects aged from 20 years to younger than 65 years were randomized in this study to receive a single bolus dose of rocuronium 0.9 mg/kg (n = 50) or vecuronium 0.1 mg/kg (n = 52), followed by maintenance doses of rocuronium (0.1–0.2 mg/kg), or vecuronium (0.02–0.03 mg/kg) as needed.[27] The primary efficacy variable was the time from the start of administration of sugammadex to recovery of T4/T1 ratio to 0.9, then to 0.8 and to 0.7. Subjects were also monitored for AEs and SAEs from the time of administration of vecuronium or rocuronium up to the end of the seventh postoperative day. After induction of anesthesia with IV propofol and an opioid and a maintenance using sevoflurane and an opioid, and before administration of vecuronium or rocuronium, monitoring of neuromuscular transmission at the adductor pollicis muscle was initiated using acceleromyography (TOF Watch SX) and was continued until the end of anesthesia and at least until recovery of the TOF T4/T1 ratio to 0.9.[27]

The results demonstrated that sugammadex provided dose-related reversal of deep rocuronium or vecuronium (induced neuromuscular blockade in surgical patients under sevoflurane maintenance anesthesia). Clear dose-response effects were seen between the sugammadex dose administered after single or multiple doses of rocuronium or vecuronium, and the time to achieve a T4/T1 ratio of 0.9. In the rocuronium group, mean recovery time to a T4/T1 ratio of 0.9 decreased from 79.8 minutes in the sugammadex 0.5 mg/kg group to 3.2 minutes (2.0 mg/kg), 1.7 minutes (4.0 mg/kg) and 1.1 minutes (8.0 mg/kg). In the vecuronium group, mean time to recovery of the T4/T1 ratio to 0.9 decreased from 68.4 minutes in the sugammadex 0.5 mg/kg group to 9.1 minutes (2.0 mg/kg), 3.3 minutes (4.0 mg/kg) , and 1.7 minutes (8.0 mg/kg). Also, the time to recovery of the T4/T1 ratio to 0.7 and 0.8 decreased with increased sugammadex dose in both groups. Neuromuscular monitoring showed recurrent neuromuscular blockade in 5 subjects, all in the rocuronium group (2 given sugammadex 0.5 mg/kg and 3 given 1.0 mg/kg), although there were no clinical events attributable to recurrent or residual neuromuscular blockade. In terms of safety, 28.0% of the subjects in the rocuronium group and 17.6% of the subjects in vecuronium group experienced 1 or more AEs (nausea, procedural complications, and urinary retention) that were considered by the investigators to be possibly, probably or definitely related to the study drug, but there was no relationship observed between the occurrence of drug-related AEs and the dose of sugammadex. Sugammadex at doses of greater than or equal to 4 mg/kg provided rapid reversal of deep rocuronium- and vecuronium-induced neuromuscular blockade under sevoflurane maintenance anesthesia.[27]

To evaluate the dose-response relationship of sugammadex given for reversal of profound neuromuscular blockade induced by high dose rocuronium (1.0 or 1.2 mg/kg) and to investigate the safety profile and tolerability of sugammadex, a total of 176 subjects were randomized in an international, multicenter, dose-finding, safety assessor-blinded phase II trial and were assigned to receive sugammadex (2.0, 4.0, 8.0, 12.0, or 16 mg/kg) or placebo at 3 or 15 minutes after 1.0 or 1.2 mg/kg of rocuronium during propofol anesthesia.[28] Neuromuscular function of the adductor pollicis was monitored on the contralateral arm using the TOF Watch SX acceleromyograph.[28] The primary efficacy variable was the time from the start of administration of sugammadex or placebo to recovery of the TOF ratio (T4/T1) to 0.9. Secondary efficacy variables included time from the start of administration of sugammadex or placebo to recovery of the TOF ratio to 0.7. The incidence of reoccurrence of neuromuscular blockade (a decrease in the TOF ratio to less than 0.8 for 3 consecutive measurements within 30 minutes of achieving sufficient recovery to a TOF ratio of 0.9 first) was also included as an additional efficacy parameter.[28]

Based on the results, all administered doses of sugammadex resulted in a marked reduction in time to recovery of the TOF ratio to 0.9 compared with placebo. Sugammadex administered 3 or 15 minutes after injection of 1 mg/kg rocuronium decreased the median recovery of the TOF ratio (T4/T1) to 0.9 in a dose-dependent manner from 111.1 minutes and 91.0 minutes (placebo) to 1.6 minutes and 0.9 minutes (16 mg/kg sugammadex), respectively. After 1.2 mg/kg rocuronium, sugammadex decreased time to recovery of TOF ratio from 124.3 minutes (3-minute group) and 94.2 minutes (15-minute group) to 1.3 minutes and 1.9 minutes with 16.0 mg/kg sugammadex.[28]

A multicenter, randomized, safety assessor-blinded, parallel-group, active-controlled phase IIIa trial, named the Spectrum study, was conducted in 11 centers in United States and Canada between February and August 2006, to compare the time of sugammadex reversal of profound rocuronium-induced neuromuscular block with time to spontaneous recovery from succinylcholine.[29] A total of 115 subjects aged 18 to 65 years, ASA class I or II, who had a body mass index less than 30 kg/m^2, and were scheduled to undergo an elective surgical procedure under general anesthesia in a supine position requiring a short duration of neuromuscular relaxation for which rocuronium or succinylcholine was indicated, were randomized to receive either 1.2 mg/kg rocuronium or 1.0 mg/kg succinylcholine. Sugammadex (16 mg/kg) was administered 3 minutes after rocuronium administration. Anesthesia was induced and maintained with an intravenous opioid and propofol, and neuromuscular monitoring was performed using the TOF Watch SX. The primary efficacy endpoint was the time from the start of relaxant administration to recovery of the first train-of-four twitch (T1) to 10%.[29]

At the doses tested, the findings in this study showed that with sugammadex, the mean times to recovery from profound rocuronium-induced neuromuscular block were 4.4 minutes (T1 to 10%) and 6.2 minutes (T1 to 90%), significantly shorter than the respective times to spontaneous recovery from succinylcholine-induced block (7.1 and 10.9 minutes). Timed from sugammadex administration, the mean time to recovery of T1 to 10%, T1 to 90%, and the T4/T1 ratio to 0.9 was 1.2, 2.9, and 2.2 minutes, respectively. **Fig. 6** and **Tables 1** and **2** provide graphic representation of some of the results of this study. Both treatments were well tolerated. The most common AEs in these groups were procedural pain and nausea, no reoccurrence of the block was observed and no serious adverse event related to the study drug was reported.[29]

A total of 22 of 157 subjects in the sugammadex group had at least 1 AE that was considered to be possibly, probably, or definitely drug related (nausea, vomiting, QTc prolongation), but the incidence of subjects with drug-related AEs in the dose groups do not indicate a dose-response relation. Twelve subjects (11 in sugammadex group and 1 in placebo group) experienced an SAE (QTc prolongation, postprocedural bleeding, asystole); however, only the QTc prolongation in one of the subjects in the 4 mg/kg sugammadex group was considered by the investigator to be possibly related to sugammadex.[29] Although the number of AEs in this study was high (64.0%), there was no clinical evidence of neuromuscular blockade or residual neuromuscular blockade. Sugammadex provided a rapid and dose-dependent reversal of profound neuromuscular blockade induced by high-dose rocuronium in adult surgical subjects.[29]

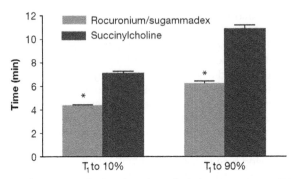

Fig. 6. Results: time from start of administration of NMBA to recover to T1 to 10 and 90%. (*Data from* Lee C, Jahr JS, Candiotti KA, et al. Reversal of profound neuromuscular block by sugammadex administered three minutes after rocuronium. Anesthesiology 2009; 110:1020–5.)

To examine the clinical effects of sugammadex for neuromuscular blockade induced by continuous rocuronium infusion in adults undergoing surgery under maintenance anesthesia with sevoflurane or propofol, 52 subjects aged 20 to 65 years, ASA class I to III, scheduled to undergo surgery under general anesthesia with an expected duration of 2 to 5 hours, were enrolled in a phase III, safety assessor-blinded, comparative, parallel- group study between December 2006 and March 2007, at 4 surgical centers in Germany, to receive maintenance anesthesia with either sevoflurane (n = 26) or propofol (n = 26). Neuromuscular blockade was induced by bolus injection of 0.6 mg/kg rocuronium followed by continuous infusion of 7 mcg/kg/min rocuronium adjusted to maintain a neuromuscular blockade depth of zero response to TOF and a post-tetanic count of no more than 10 responses during a period of at least 90 minutes. At the conclusion of rocuronium infusion, subjects received a single bolus dose of 4.0 mg/kg sugammadex at a target of NMBA of T1 of 3% to 10%. Subjects

Table 1	
Results: time from start of administration of sugammadex to recovery of T1 to 10 and 90%	
	Rocuronium/Sugammadex (n = 55; ITT Population)
T1 to 10%	
n	53
Mean (SD)	1.2 (0.5)
Median	1.0
Range	0.5–3.0
T1 to 90%	
n	53
Mean (SD)	2.9 (1.7)
Median	2.5
Range	1.2–10.3

Abbreviations: IIT, intent to treat; SD, standard deviation.
Data from Lee C, Jahr JS, Candiotti KA, et al. Reversal of profound neuromuscular block by sugammadex administered three minutes after rocuronium. Anesthesiology 2009;110:1020–5.

Table 2
Summary of AEs reported with an incidence of greater than or equal to 10% in either treatment group

AE, n (%)	Rocuronium/Sugammadex (n = 56; Population)	Succinylcholine (n = 54; Population)
Nausea	16 (28.6)	20 (37.0)
Vomiting	9 (16.1)	8 (14.8)
Chills	6 (10.7)	7 (13.0)
Incision-site complication	5 (8.9)	7 (13.0)
Procedural hypertension	7 (12.5)	7 (13.0)
Procedural hypotension	7 (12.5)	13 (24.1)
Procedural pain	32 (57.1)	26 (48.1)
Arthralgia	3 (5.4)	6 (11.1)
Headache	8 (14.3)	2 (3.7)
Pain in extremity	6 (10.7)	7 (13.0)

Data from Lee C, Jahr JS, Candiotti KA, et al. Reversal of profound neuromuscular block by sugammadex administered three minutes after rocuronium. Anesthesiology 2009;110:1020–5.

were not permitted to receive a second dose of sugammadex or an NMBA other than rocuronium during the monitoring of neuromuscular transmission. Neuromuscular function was monitored by acceleromyography at the adductor pollicis muscle using the TOF Watch SX. Two venous blood samples (one before administration of rocuronium and one within 2 minutes before administration of sugammadex) were drawn from each subject for plasma concentration analysis of rocuronium. The main clinical effect variable was time from start of administration of sugammadex to recovery of the TOF ratio to 0.9.[30] The results demonstrated that the median recovery time from start of sugammadex to a T4/T1 ratio of 0.9 in the sevoflurane and propofol groups was 1.3 and 1.2 minutes, respectively. Median plasma rocuronium concentration just before sugammadex administration was 33% lower during maintenance anesthesia with sevoflurane than with propofol. The most frequently reported AEs were procedural pain, constipation, and nausea. No SAEs were reported and no death occurred. Sugammadex was well tolerated and there was just 1 AE (procedural hypotension) in a subject in the sevoflurane group that occurred 2 minutes after administration of sugammadex and was considered by the investigator to be probably related to the sugammadex administration, and there was no clinical evidence of recurrent or residual NMBA in any subject.[30]

In conclusion, and based on the results of the previously mentioned clinical trials, it appears that sugammadex is an effective reversing agent against steroidal neuromuscular NMBA. This reversal is fast and effective in reversing profound blocks in humans. Studies show high safety profile with little adverse reaction to medication. It is safe independent of anesthetic medication used. It is well tolerated during maintenance anesthesia with sevoflurane or propofol, although safety profile is somewhat more favorable under propofol than under sevoflurane anesthesia.[27] The studies suggest that sugammadex is an ideal reversing agent.

FUTURE DIRECTIONS

In 2008, the US Food and Drug Administration (FDA) provided a nonapproval letter for sugammadex in the United States.[31] Despite a positive vote by the ad hoc committee designated to review the application, which included such respected anesthesiologists as Drs Ronald Miller and Terry Monk, the FDA expressed concern regarding allergic reactions and the possibility of interfering with bone and tooth formation and healing.[4] More specifically, the FDA review described the potential of sugammadex to bind to the bone and teeth of developing rats and infers that safety is not well established in pediatric populations and possibly parturients. The FDA also raised concerns regarding immediate and delayed hypersensitivity responses, an adverse event seen only occasionally in clinical trials, but sensitization trials were not reviewed in the submission. Despite these concerns, a comprehensive review of the safety of sugammadex in healthy adult populations found it to be safe compared with neostigmine and placebo.[4] Additionally, the US Clinical Trials Web site in June 2010 reported that the sugammadex hypersensitivity study that was designed to study the potential for hypersensitivity symptoms at the time of initial exposure to sugammadex had been completed; no data or conclusions are yet listed.[32]

Concurrently with the US FDA nonapproval letter, the European Union approved sugammadex in multiple countries.[33] It is likely that there will be significant use of the drug in the European market and Phase IV postmarketing data accumulation and evaluation; however, to the authors' best knowledge, none has been presented to date. This postmarketing data may address the concern of hypersensitivity would address the concern of hypersensitivity and perhaps the issue of bone and tooth modeling, although a single dose of a drug would be unlikely to create any long-lasting effect.

One additional issue is that FDA-sponsored phase IIIb studies were not performed before the original FDA submission. One was recently completed[34] in an outpatient setting. It is probable that more such studies will be required in subset patient populations, such as renal disease/failure; hepatic disease/failure; critically ill patients who are metabolically acidotic, hypothermic, or malnourished; elderly or obese patients; and possibly pediatric patients. These studies may also collect additional information on hypersensitivity reactions that may satisfy the FDA criteria for eventual approval.

ACKNOWLEDGMENTS

The authors would like to thank Suzie Diaz for her administrative assistance.

REFERENCES

1. Srivastava A, Hunter JM. Reversal of NMB. Br J Anaesth 2009;103(1):115–29.
2. Gray TC, Halton J. A milestone in anaesthesia? (d-tubocurarine chloride) [section on anaesthetics]. Proc R Soc Med 1946;39(7):400–8.
3. Naguib M. Sugammadex: another milestone in clinical neuromuscular pharmacology. Anesth Analg. 2007;104(3):575–81.
4. Ren W, Jahr JS. Reversal of neuromuscular block with a selective relaxant binding agent (SRBA). Am J Ther 2009;16(4):295–9.
5. Loftsson T, Masson M. Cyclodextrins in topical drug formulations: theory and practice. Int J Pharm 2001;225(1–2):15–30.
6. Sikharam S, Egan TD, Kern SE. Cyclodextrins as new formulation entitles and therapeutic agents. Curr Opin Anaesthesiol 2005;18(4):392–5.
7. de Boer HD, van Egmond J, van de Pol F, et al. Chemical encapsulation of rocuronium by synthetic cyclodextrin derivatives: reversal of neuromuscular block in anaesthetized Rhesus monkeys. Br J Anaesth 2005;96(2):201–6.
8. Wikipedia. Cyclodextrin. Available at: http://en.wikipedia.org/wiki/Cyclodextrin. Accessed May 2, 2010.

9. Szente L, Szejtli J. Highly soluble cyclodextrin derivatives: chemistry, properties, and trends in development. Adv Drug Deliv Rev 1999;36(1):17–28.

10. Brewster ME, Thorsteinn L. Cyclodextrins as pharmaceutical solubilizers. Adv Drug Deliv Rev 2007;59:645–66.

11. Wikipedia. Selective Relaxant Binding Agents (SRBAs). Available at: http://en.wikipedia.org/wiki/Selective_Relaxant_Binding_Agent. Accessed May 2, 2010.

12. Adam JM, Bennett DJ, Bom A, et al. Cyclodextrin-derived host molecules as reversal agents for the neuromuscular blocker rocuronium bromide: synthesis and structure-activity relationships. J Med Chem 2002;45(9):1806–16.

13. Miller R. Sugammadex, an opportunity to change the practice of anesthesiology? Anesth Analg 2007;104(3):477–8.

14. McDonagh DL, Benedict PE, Kovac AL, et al. Efficacy and safety of sugammadex for reversal of rocuronium induced blockade in elderly patients. Anesthesiology 2007;107:A1583.

15. Nicholson WT, Sprung J, Jankowski CJ. Sugammadex: a novel agent for the reversal of neuromuscular blockade. Pharmacotherapy 2007;27(8):1181–8.

16. Bom A, Bradley M, Cameron K, et al. A novel concept of reversing neuromuscular block: chemical encapsulation of rocuronium bromide by a cyclodextrin based synthetic host. Angew Chem Int Ed Engl 2002;41:266–70.

17. Tarver GJ, Grove SJA, Buchanan K, et al. 2- O- substituted cyclodextrins as reversal agents for the neuromuscular blocker rocuronium bromide. Bioorg Med Chem 2002;10(6):1819–27.

18. Sorgenfrei IF, Norrild K, Larsen PB, et al. Reversal of rocuronium- induced neuromuscular block by the selective relaxant binding agent sugammadex, a dose-finding and safety study. Anesthesiology 2006;104:667–74.

19. Sandman E, Witt H, Olsson R, et al. The incidence and mechanisms of pharyngeal and upper esophageal dysfunction in partially paralyzed humans: pharyngeal videoradiography and simultaneous manometry after atracurium. Anesthesiology 2000;92:977–84.

20. Berg H, Viby- Mogensen J, Roed J, et al. Residual neuromuscular block is a risk factor for postoperative pulmonary complications: a prospective, randomized, and blinded study of postoperative pulmonary complications after atracurium, vecuronium and pancuronium. Acta Anaesthesiol Scand 1997;41:1095–103.

21. Suy K, Morias K, Cammu G, et al. Effective reversal of moderate rocuronium- or vecuronium- induced neuromuscular block with sugammadex, a selective relaxant binding agent. Anesthesiology 2007;106:283–8.

22. Lowry DW, Mirakhur RK, McCarthy GJ, et al. Neuromuscular effects of rocuronium during sevoflurane, isoflurane, and intravenous anesthesia. Anesth Analg 1998;87:936–40.

23. Wulf H, Ledowski T, Lindstedt U, et al. Neuromuscular blocking effects of rocuronium during desflurane, isoflurane, and sevoflurane anesthesia. Can J Anaesth 1998;45:526–32.

24. Vanacker BF, Vermeyen KM, Struys MM, et al. Reversal of rocuronium- induced neuromuscular block with the novel drug sugammadex is equally effective under maintenance anesthesia with propofol or sevoflurane. Anesth Analg 2007;104:563–8.

25. Groudine SB, Soto R, Lien C, et al. A randomized, dose- finding, phase II study of the selective relaxant binding drug, sugammadex, capable of safely reversing profound rocuronium- induced neuromuscular block. Anesth Analg 2007;104:555–62.

26. de Boer HD, Driessen JJ, Marcus MAE, et al. Reversal of rocuronium- induced (1.2 mg/kg) profound neuromuscular block by sugammadex. Anesthesiology 2007;107:239–44.

27. Duvaldestin P, Kuizenga K, Saldien V, et al. A randomized, dose-response study of sugammadex given for the reversal of deep rocuronium- or vecuronium-induced neuromuscular blockade under sevoflurane anesthesia. Anesth Analg 2010;110:74–82.

28. Puhringer K, Rex C, Sielenkamper AW, et al. Reversal of profound, high- dose rocuronium- induced neuromuscular blockade by sugammadex at two different time points. Anesthesiology 2008;109:188–97.

29. Lee C, Jahr JS, Candiotti KA, et al. Reversal of profound neuromuscular block by sugammadex administered three minutes after rocuronium. Anesthesiology 2009; 110:1020–5.

30. Rex C, Wagner S, Spies C, et al. Reversal of neuromuscular blockade by sugammadex after continuous infusion of rocuronium in patients randomized to sevoflurane or propofol maintenance anesthesia. Anesthesiology 2009;111:30–5.

31. Briefing Document for the Anesthesia and Life Support Drug Advisory Committee Meeting. Bridion_ NDA 22–225. March 11, 2008. Department of Health & Human Services Food & Drug Administration Center for Drug Evaluation & Research Division of Anesthesia, Analgesia and Rheumatology Products. Available at: http://www.fda.gov/ohrms/dockets/ac/08/briefing/2008-4346b1-01-FDA.pdf. Accessed May 16, 2008.

32. Sugammadex Hypersensitivity Study (Study P06042)(COMPLETED) Jun 10, 2010. Available at: clinicaltrials.gov/ct2/show/NCT00988065. Accessed June 16, 2010.

33. Schering-Plough Corp. Bridion® (sugammadex sodium) injection: first and only selective relaxant binding agent approved in European Union [online]. Available at: http://www.scheringplough.com/schering_plough/news/release.jsp?releaseID=1180933. Accessed August 20, 2008.

34. Soto R, Jahr J, Pavlin J, et al. Safety of sugammadex reversal of rocuronium block vs spontaneous recovery from succinylcholine [abstract]. American Society of Anesthesiologists Anesthesiology 2010. San Diego (CA); 2010.

Dexmedetomidine: Clinical Application as an Adjunct for Intravenous Regional Anesthesia

Usha Ramadhyani, MD[a], Jason L. Park, MD[a],
Dominic S. Carollo, MS, MD[a], Ruth S. Waterman, MD[b],
Bobby D. Nossaman, MD[a,c],*

KEYWORDS

- Dexmedetomidine • α-2 agonist
- Intravenous regional anesthesia
- Regional anesthesia, complications
- Animal studies • Human studies

Alleviation of pain has become integral in preoperative medicine.[1] Pain pharmacotherapy is directed at peripheral nociceptors, primary and secondary spinal neurons, and pain-processing areas in the central nervous system. Accordingly, three primary pharmacologic strategies have evolved: drugs that activate opioid receptors, drugs that activate α-2 receptors, and drugs that can reduce de novo prostaglandin synthesis.[1]

Inhibition of presynaptic autoreceptors, such as α-2 adrenoceptors present in sympathetic nerve endings and noradrenergic neurons in the central nervous system, can modulate preoperative.[1] Administration of α-2 adrenoceptor agonists has been shown to have several beneficial actions during the perioperative period.[2–13] These agents decrease sympathetic tone, attenuate neuroendocrine responses to injury, reduce intraoperative anesthetic drug and perioperative opiate requirements, and induce dose-dependent sedation and analgesia.[2–13] This reported combination of

Financial and funding disclosures: the authors have nothing to disclose.
[a] Department of Anesthesiology, Ochsner Medical Center, 1514 Jefferson Highway, New Orleans, LA 70121, USA
[b] Department of Anesthesiology, Tulane University Medical Center, 1430 Tulane Avenue, New Orleans, LA 70129, USA
[c] Department of Pharmacology, Tulane University Medical Center, 1430 Tulane Avenue, New Orleans, LA 70129, USA
* Corresponding author. Department of Anesthesiology, Ochsner Medical Center, 1514 Jefferson Highway, New Orleans, LA 70121.
E-mail address: bnossaman@ochsner.org

the beneficial effects of α-2 adrenoceptor agonists might offer additional benefits, not only following systemic during the conduct of intravenous regional anesthesia.[14–20] Hemodynamic side effects of systemic α-2 adrenoceptor agonists consist of mild to moderate cardiovascular depression, with decreases in blood pressure and heart rate.[12,13,21–31] The development of new, more selective α-2 adrenoceptor agonists with an improved side effect profile may provide a novel therapy as an adjunct in the conduct of intravenous regional anesthesia.[16–20] This review examines what is currently known of the properties and applications of the novel α-2 adrenoceptor agonist, dexmedetomidine, when used as an adjunct in intravenous regional anesthesia.

DEXMEDETOMIDINE

In December 1999, dexmedetomidine was approved for clinical practice (**Fig. 1A**).[2,32] Dexmedetomidine is a highly selective α-2 adrenoceptor agonist that has been shown to have both sedative and analgesic effects in adults.[3,13,17,33–39] Dexmedetomidine has an α-2 to α-1 adrenoceptor ratio of approximately 1600:1, which is 7 to 8 times higher than reported for clonidine (see **Fig. 1B**).[40] This ratio favors the sedative/anxiolytic

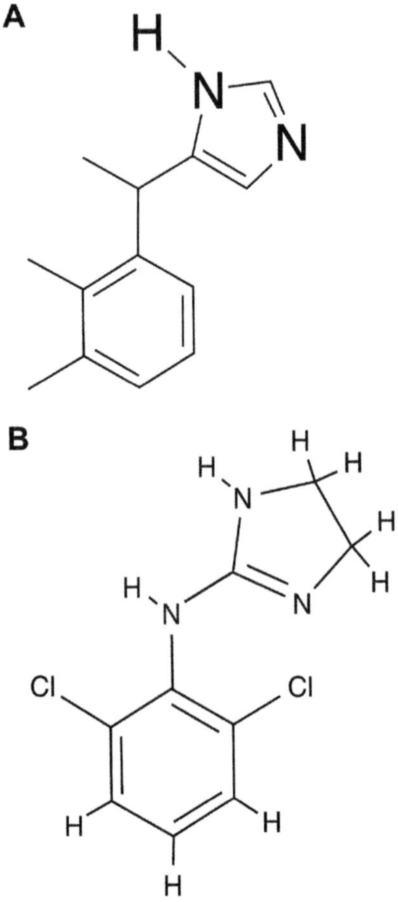

Fig. 1. Chemical structures of dexmedetomidine (A) and clonidine (B).

actions rather than the hemodynamic actions seen in the same class of α-2 adreno-ceptor agonists such as clonidine.[41,42] However, systemic administration of dexmede-tomidine can produce moderate decreases in blood pressure and heart rate.[10,12,13,43] Plasma norepinephrine levels can also be significantly reduced.[10,12,43,44]

Intravenous regional anesthesia is a technically simple and reliable procedure, with reported success rates ranging between 94% and 98%,[45] and has gained in popu-larity.[45–49] This procedure was first described by August Bier in 1908 and he used procaine which was the first injectable local anesthetic synthesized by Einhorn in 1904.[47–49] In 1963, Holmes[50] reported the use of lidocaine as an intravenous local anesthetic, and is the major intravenous local anesthetic agent,[18,51–67] when compared to procaine, prilocaine, or ropivacaine.[62,64–66,68–73]

Modern surgical procedures require fast and effective regional anesthesia techniques, such as intravenous regional anesthesia.[46] Intravenous regional anes-thesia provides safe and effective care for patients undergoing extremity surgery when the surgical procedure lasts less than 1 hour.[74–76] However, the use of this technique is limited by the development of tourniquet pain and by the absence of analgesia following tourniquet release.[74–76] Moreover, the development of compart-ment syndrome following intravenous regional anesthesia has been reported.[77–80] Current clinical research indicates that these limitations can be significantly improved with alteration of the block solution, tourniquet placement, or alteration of the exsanguination technique.[16,46,52,55,58,61,63,67,81–89] In extensive investigations to improve this technique, several medications have been combined with the local anesthetic solutions, such as clonidine, ketorolac, acetaminophen, lysine acetylsalicylate, lormoxicam, tenoxicam, ketamine, sufentanil, alfentanil, tramadol, methylprednisolone, melatonin, and magnesium, with all varying results.[16,19,46,52,53,55,59,60,63,67,70,71,75,82,83,86,90–92]

Following tourniquet deflation, patients frequently complain of a different pain sensation, such as an intense tingling. The nociceptive pain pathways that are most likely stimulated by tourniquet compression are the smaller myelinated AΔ fibers (transmission of fast, sharp pain), and the unmyelinated C fibers (transmission of slow, dull pain). Although larger pain fibers remain blocked and thereby provide adequate motor and sensory anesthesia, the smaller fibers remain relatively unblocked because of the repetitive stimulation from the tourniquet.[93,94] Recent studies have shown that the addition of clonidine can improve the efficacy of lidocaine for intravenous regional anesthesia in decreasing the onset of severe tourniquet pain.[16,75,83,95] The addition of 1 μg/kg of clonidine into 40 mL of 0.5% lidocaine as an adjunct in intravenous regional anesthesia showed a delay in the onset time of tour-niquet pain in healthy, unsedated volunteers.[75] However, the use of clonidine as an adjunct in intravenous regional anesthesia can be associated with significant postop-erative sedation.[83] Nevertheless, these findings, as well those of other studies to be described later, suggest that the addition of α-2 agonists may provide additional bene-fits when compared with plain local anesthetic solutions.[16,70,75,83,86]

DEXMEDETOMIDINE AS A SUPPLEMENT IN INTRAVENOUS REGIONAL ANESTHESIA
Animal Studies

Systemic administration
α-2 adrenergic agonists have direct peripheral cardiovascular effects.[96–100] Systemic administration of dexmedetomidine in open-chest anesthetized dogs can cause immediate, dose-dependent increases in systemic vascular resistance, left ventricular end-diastolic pressure, as well as decreases in mean arterial pressure, cardiac index,

and in heart rate.[101] Moreover, administration of large doses of dexmedetomidine can induce regional coronary vasoconstriction, but without metabolic signs of myocardial ischemia, in young domestic pigs.[102] It has been reported that the endothelial nitric oxide synthase enzyme has a significant role in opposing the vasoconstrictor action of dexmedetomidine when used at drug concentrations within therapeutic ranges.[103] However, the addition of dexmedetomidine (0.5 μg) to a 1.0-mL solution of 0.5% mepivacaine was shown to significantly increase basilar artery blood flow and prolong the duration of vasodilation following stellate ganglion block in dogs.[104]

Intrathecal administration

The intrathecal administration of α-2 adrenergic agonists has been shown to induce antinociception and sedation.[5,105–111] In a neuropathic model of pain, the analgesic potency and site of action of systemic dexmedetomidine administration was investigated in normal and neuropathic rats.[112] Following ligation of the L_5 to L_6 spinal nerves, a chronic mechanical and thermal neuropathic hyperalgesia developed in rats. The systemic administration of dexmedetomidine was able, in a dose-dependent manner, to increase the mechanical and thermal thresholds of injury. There was no difference in sedation.[112] These findings suggest that the analgesic potency of dexmedetomidine was enhanced after nerve injury, with a site of action outside of the central nervous system, and that the administration of α-2 agonists may be useful in the management of neuropathic pain.[112]

Mechanism of action

In a recent study, the effects of α-2 agonists were evaluated on the local anesthetic action of lidocaine.[113] The administration of the α-2 adrenoceptor agonists dexmedetomidine, clonidine, and oxymetazoline were individually combined with lidocaine and intracutaneously injected into the backs of male guinea pigs. All 3 α-2 adrenoceptor agonists were able to enhance the degree of local anesthesia of lidocaine in a dose-dependent manner.[113] The addition of yohimbine, an α-2A, -2B, and -2C adrenoceptor antagonist, inhibited the beneficial effect of dexmedetomidine, whereas prazosin, an α-1, -2B, and -2C adrenoceptor antagonist, did not modulate the analgesic effect. These data suggest that α-2 adrenoceptor agonists are able to enhance the local anesthetic action of lidocaine, and suggest that dexmedetomidine acts specifically via α-2A adrenoceptors.[113]

Cordiotoxicity

In recent studies, the potential benefits of dexmedetomidine in central nervous system or cardiac toxicity induced by local anesthetics have been examined. Following the administration of dexmedetomidine in a central nervous system toxicity model, the α-2 agonist was able to raise the convulsive doses of 2 local anesthetics, bupivacaine and levobupivacaine.[114] In a bupivacaine-induced cardiotoxicity model, pretreatment with dexmedetomidine significantly increased the time of onset to first dysrhythmia and onset time to asystole following administration of the local anesthetic.[115]

Model development

Finally, in a recently published report, a novel model for studying intravenous regional anesthesia and postoperative analgesia has been developed and may hold future promise to further elucidate mechanisms of peripheral anesthesia and analgesia.[116]

Clinical Studies

An early study before the introduction of dexmedetomidine for clinical use analyzed the safety and efficacy of this α-2 agonist as a premedicant when administered before the institution of intravenous regional anesthesia.[17] A group of 30 American Society of Anesthesiologists (ASA) physical status I outpatients who were scheduled for minor hand surgery, conducted with intravenous regional anesthesia, underwent a randomized, double-blinded, placebo-controlled study in 2 parallel groups to study the beneficial effects of dexmedetomidine on perioperative analgesia.[17] Either an infusion of dexmedetomidine (1 μg/kg intravenous) or intravenous saline placebo (n = 15 in each group) was administered for 10 minutes before exsanguination and tourniquet inflation on the operative limb.[17] Intravenous regional blockade was performed using 0.5% lidocaine (3 mg/kg, up to a maximum of 200 mg).[17] Analgesic supplementation, when indicated, consisted of either intraoperative administration of fentanyl (1 μg/kg intravenously) and/or postoperative administration of oxycodone (0.05 mg/kg by mouth). The preoperative administration of dexmedetomidine produced a ~20% decrease in systolic blood pressure as well as decreases in diastolic blood pressure and heart rate that were statistically significant when compared with the control (normal saline infusion) group.[17] These hemodynamic changes returned to preoperative control values within 4 hours in the postoperative period. No clinically significant decreases in arterial oxygen saturation were observed. Although patient-reported intensity of pain during tourniquet inflation was similar in both groups, the intraoperative need for opiates was significantly less in the dexmedetomidine-treated group.[17] Moreover, plasma norepinephrine and the main metabolite of norepinephrine, 3,4-dihydroxyphenylglycol, were significantly decreased. Dexmedetomidine was able to significantly prevent increases in plasma epinephrine levels following tourniquet inflation.[17] Although dexmedetomidine induced subjective sedation ($P = .002$), the Maddox Wing test (a measure of deviation of the visual axes of the eyes) did not show any statistically significant differences between the 2 groups.[17] The effectiveness of dexmedetomidine was rated as superior when compared to control. The investigator concluded that administration of dexmedetomidine is an effective premedicant before institution of intravenous regional anesthesia because the α-2 agonist was able to reduce patient anxiety, decrease sympathoadrenal responses, and modulate the requirements for perioperative opioid analgesics.[17]

In 2 early studies performed during the clinical release of dexmedetomidine, the role of the α-2 adrenoceptor agonist, clonidine, was examined in patients undergoing intravenous regional anesthesia to test the hypothesis that the addition of clonidine as an adjunct may improve the quality of intravenous regional anesthesia.[83,86]

In the first study, 40 patients were randomly allocated in a double-blinded study to receive 40 mL of 0.5% lidocaine and either 1 mL of isotonic saline or clonidine (150 μg). In this study, visual analog scale scores and verbal rating scale scores were significantly lower in the clonidine group 30 and 45 minutes after tourniquet inflation and the tolerance for the tourniquet was also significantly longer in the clonidine group. Although pain assessment were not different in the 2 groups following tourniquet release, the clonidine group experienced a higher degree of sedation.[83]

In the second study using clonidine as a local anesthetic adjuvant, the investigators postulated that using clonidine as a component of intravenous regional anesthesia would enhance postoperative analgesia.[86] In this study 45 patients undergoing ambulatory hand surgery received intravenous regional anesthesia with 0.5% lidocaine alone, a second group received intravenous regional anesthesia with 0.5% lidocaine with coadministration of systemic intravenous clonidine (1 μg/kg), and a third group received intravenous regional anesthesia with 0.5% lidocaine and 1 μg/kg clonidine added as an adjunct to the intravenous regional anesthetic solution.[86] Following surgery, the intravenous regional anesthesia group with coadministration of clonidine in the local anesthetic solution had a significantly longer period of subjective comfort compared with the group receiving local anesthetic alone or the group receiving local anesthetic supplemented with systemic intravenous clonidine. The patients who received intravenous regional anesthesia with coadministration of clonidine reported significantly lower pain scores for 1 and 2 hours after tourniquet deflation compared with the other 2 groups, and required no supplemental opiates in the postanesthesia care unit.[86] No significant episodes of postoperative sedation, hypotension, or bradycardia were observed in any of the groups. The investigators concluded that in patients undergoing ambulatory hand surgery, the coadministration of 1 μg/kg clonidine with 0.5% lidocaine improves postoperative analgesia without causing significant side effects.[86]

Following clinical release of dexmedetomidine, the effects of the α-2 adrenoceptor agonist were evaluated when added to the local anesthetic during the conduct of intravenous regional anesthesia.[16,18,20] In this first clinical study, the onset and duration of sensory and motor blocks, the changes in intra- and postoperative hemodynamic variables, the quality of the anesthetic block, and intra- and postoperative pain and sedation scores were recorded in patients who underwent hand surgery.[16] Thirty patients (n = 15 for each group) received either a mixture of 40 mL of 0.5% lidocaine with 1 mL of isotonic saline or a mixture of 40 mL of 0.5% lidocaine with 0.5 μg/kg of dexmedetomidine. In the group treated with the lidocaine/dexmedetomidine mixture, shorter onset of sensory and motor block times, prolonged sensory and motor block recovery times, prolonged tolerance for the limb tourniquet, and improved quality of anesthesia were observed.[16] Moreover, the intraoperative administration of rescue opiates was also significantly decreased in this group. The visual analgesia pain scale scores were significantly less in the lidocaine/dexmedetomidine group when compared with the saline group, and this analgesia benefit continued the postoperative period for up to 6 hours. There was no statistical difference into sedation at any period. There were no statistical differences in hemodynamic or in oxygen saturation values. The investigators concluded that the addition of dexmedetomidine in the intravenous regional anesthesia solution improved the conduct of regional anesthesia and perioperative analgesia without significant sedative or hemodynamic side effects.[16]

In a second clinical study, the addition of dexmedetomidine to the local anesthetic solution was evaluated in a prospective randomized double-blind study.[20] In patients who were scheduled for elective hand surgery, intravenous regional anesthesia was obtained using lidocaine (3 mg/kg) diluted with saline to a total volume of 40 mL alone; in the second group, the addition of 1 μg/kg of dexmedetomidine to lidocaine (3 mg/kg) was also diluted with saline to a total volume of 40 mL. There were no significant differences between the groups with respect to sensory and motor block onset and regression anesthesia times. However, the quality of anesthesia was statistically better in the lidocaine/dexmedetomidine group than the lidocaine/saline group. Moreover, the intraoperative and postoperative analgesic requirements were greater in the lidocaine/saline group compared with the lidocaine/dexmedetomidine group. The investigators concluded that the addition of dexmedetomidine to the local anesthetic solution was able to improve the quality of intravenous regional anesthesia and decrease intra- and postoperative analgesic requirements, but had no significant effect on the sensory and motor block onset and regression times.[20]

Another clinical study compared the effects of low- and same-dose mixtures of 0.5% lidocaine with and without the addition of dexmedetomidine for intravenous regional anesthesia in patients undergoing outpatient surgery.[18] Forty-five ASA physical status I to II patients who were scheduled to undergo carpal tunnel release as an outpatient procedure were randomized into 3 groups. The onset and recovery times of sensory and motor block, intraoperative and postoperative visual analog scale scores, Ramsay sedation scale scores, analgesic requirements, changes in hemodynamic variables, and side effects were reported. In the first group, following limb exsanguination and tourniquet application, intravenous regional anesthesia was obtained following administration of 40 mL of 0.5% lidocaine. The second and third groups received the reduced dose of 20 mL of 0.5% lidocaine mixed with either dexmedetomidine (0.5 µg/kg) or saline as a placebo.[18] The investigators observed a significant reduction in onset of sensory block in the 40 mL 0.5% lidocaine group and in the 20 mL 0.5% lidocaine/dexmedetomidine group. Moreover, a significant decrease in intraoperative and postoperative visual analog pain scores and the need for rescue analgesics were observed in the 20 mL 0.5% lidocaine/dexmedetomidine group. For hemodynamics, both intraoperative and postoperative heart rates and mean arterial blood pressures were significantly lower in the 20 mL 0.5% lidocaine/dexmedetomidine group compared with the 20 mL 0.5% lidocaine/saline group or in the 40 mL 0.5% lidocaine group, but no adverse effects were observed in any of the 3 groups during the intra- and postoperative periods. The investigators concluded that the addition of dexmedetomidine to the lidocaine solution could significantly improve the quality of anesthesia and the degree of postoperative analgesia without the development of significant side effects.[18]

In one comparative adjunct study, the effects of lornoxicam (a nonsteroidal anti-inflammatory drug with potent analgesic properties that had been shown to be effective in an earlier intravenous regional anesthesia study)[82] or of dexmedetomidine were added to prilocaine in patients who underwent hand or forearm surgery.[18] In this randomized, double-blinded study of 75 patients who were scheduled for hand or forearm surgery, intravenous regional anesthesia was obtained with 2% prilocaine (3 mg/kg); 2% prilocaine (3 mg/kg) plus dexmedetomidine (0.5 µg/kg); or 2% prilocaine (3 mg/kg) plus lornoxicam (8 mg). The onset of sensory block was significantly shorter and sensory block recovery was significantly longer in the prilocaine/dexmedetomidine group when compared with the other 2 groups. Anesthesia quality was better in the prilocaine/dexmedetomidine and prilocaine/lornoxicam groups when compared with the prilocaine alone group. Moreover, the median visual analgesia scores for tourniquet pain in the prilocaine/dexmedetomidine and prilocaine/lornoxicam groups were statistically lower when compared with the prilocaine alone group.[18] Sensory and motor block recovery times and duration of analgesia for tourniquet were significantly prolonged in the prilocaine/dexmedetomidine and prilocaine/lornoxicam groups when compared with the prilocaine alone group. In the postoperative period, the duration of analgesia was statistically longer and median visual analgesia scores were statistically lower during the first 12 hours in the prilocaine/dexmedetomidine and prilocaine/lornoxicam groups when compared with the prilocaine group. Total analgesic consumption in 24 hours was statistically lower in the prilocaine/dexmedetomidine and prilocaine/lornoxicam groups when compared with the prilocaine alone group.[18] No hypotension, bradycardia, or hypoxia requiring treatment was seen in any of the groups. The investigators observed that the addition of dexmedetomidine or lornoxicam to prilocaine during the conduct of intravenous regional anesthesia decreased visual analgesia pain scores, decreased analgesic requirements, and improved anesthesia quality. In this study, the addition of dexmedetomidine had a more potent effect, resulting in a shortening of sensory block onset times and increased sensory block recovery times when compared to those times observed with the nonsteroidal antiinflammatory drug as the additive.[19]

SUMMARY

This article presents a review of the literature on the characteristics and the relevant clinical importance of the adjuvant, dexmedetomidine, when coadministered with local anesthetics for the conduct of intravenous regional anesthesia. When dexmedetomidine was added to intravenous local anesthetics, the regression of sensory and motor block times improved and postoperative analgesia was prolonged. The addition of dexmedetomidine into intravenous regional anesthesia solutions not only improved postoperative analgesia, but was also shown in one study to allow a decrease in the total local anesthetic dose. Intravenous regional anesthesia is a safe technique, and is associated with a low incidence of complications. Animal studies suggest additional dexmedetomidine provides protection from local anesthetic–induced central nervous system and cardiac toxicity.[69]

Changes in hemodynamic values occur when used in this clinical setting, but no major adverse effects were observed. α-2 Adrenoceptor agonists, such as dexmedetomidine, are therefore important as adjuvants to improve the quality of intraoperative anesthesia and postoperative analgesia when used in patients undergoing surgical procedures using intravenous regional anesthesia. Although these recent studies have shown benefits from the coadministration of dexmedetomidine with local anesthetics during the conduct of intravenous regional anesthesia, further investigations are necessary to clarify its role.

REFERENCES

1. Langer SZ. 25 years since the discovery of presynaptic receptors: present knowledge and future perspectives. Trends Pharmacol Sci 1997;18(3):95–9.
2. Gertler R, Brown HC, Mitchell DH, et al. Dexmedetomidine: a novel sedative-analgesic agent. Proc (Bayl Univ Med Cent) 2001;14(1):13–21.
3. Arain SR, Ruehlow RM, Uhrich TD, et al. The efficacy of dexmedetomidine versus morphine for postoperative analgesia after major inpatient surgery. Anesth Analg 2004;98(1):153–8.
4. Venn M, Newman J, Grounds M. A phase II study to evaluate the efficacy of dexmedetomidine for sedation in the medical intensive care unit. Intensive Care Med 2003;29(2):201–7.
5. Guo TZ, Jiang JY, Buttermann AE, et al. Dexmedetomidine injection into the locus ceruleus produces antinociception. Anesthesiology 1996;84(4):873–81.
6. Jaakola ML, Ali-Melkkila T, Kanto J, et al. Dexmedetomidine reduces intraocular pressure, intubation responses and anaesthetic requirements in patients undergoing ophthalmic surgery. Br J Anaesth 1992;68(6):570–5.
7. Weitz JD, Foster SD, Waugaman WR, et al. Anesthetic and hemodynamic effects of dexmedetomidine during isoflurane anesthesia in a canine model. Nurse Anesth 1991;2(1):19–27.
8. Maze M, Regan JW. Role of signal transduction in anesthetic action. Alpha 2 adrenergic agonists. Ann N Y Acad Sci 1991;625:409–22.
9. Zornow MH, Fleischer JE, Scheller MS, et al. Dexmedetomidine, an alpha 2-adrenergic agonist, decreases cerebral blood flow in the isoflurane-anesthetized dog. Anesth Analg 1990;70(6):624–30.
10. Aantaa RE, Kanto JH, Scheinin M, et al. Dexmedetomidine premedication for minor gynecologic surgery. Anesth Analg 1990;70(4):407–13.

11. Segal IS, Vickery RG, Walton JK, et al. Dexmedetomidine diminishes halothane anesthetic requirements in rats through a postsynaptic alpha 2 adrenergic receptor. Anesthesiology 1988;69(6):818–23.
12. Ebert TJ, Hall JE, Barney JA, et al. The effects of increasing plasma concentrations of dexmedetomidine in humans. Anesthesiology 2000;93(2):382–94.
13. Hall JE, Uhrich TD, Barney JA, et al. Sedative, amnestic, and analgesic properties of small-dose dexmedetomidine infusions. Anesth Analg 2000;90(3):699–705.
14. Schneemilch CE, Bachmann H, Ulrich A, et al. Clonidine decreases stress response in patients undergoing carotid endarterectomy under regional anesthesia: a prospective, randomized, double-blinded, placebo-controlled study. Anesth Analg 2006;103(2):297–302.
15. McCutcheon CA, Orme RM, Scott DA, et al. A comparison of dexmedetomidine versus conventional therapy for sedation and hemodynamic control during carotid endarterectomy performed under regional anesthesia. Anesth Analg 2006;102(3):668–75.
16. Memis D, Turan A, Karamanlioglu B, et al. Adding dexmedetomidine to lidocaine for intravenous regional anesthesia. Anesth Analg 2004;98(3):835–40.
17. Jaakola ML. Dexmedetomidine premedication before intravenous regional anesthesia in minor outpatient hand surgery. J Clin Anesth 1994;6(3):204–11.
18. Mizrak A, Gul R, Erkutlu I, et al. Premedication with dexmedetomidine alone or together with 0.5% lidocaine for IVRA. J Surg Res 2009. [Epub ahead of print].
19. Kol IO, Ozturk H, Kaygusuz K, et al. Addition of dexmedetomidine or lornoxicam to prilocaine in intravenous regional anaesthesia for hand or forearm surgery: a randomized controlled study. Clin Drug Investig 2009;29(2):121–9.
20. Esmaoglu A, Mizrak A, Akin A, et al. Addition of dexmedetomidine to lidocaine for intravenous regional anaesthesia. Eur J Anaesthesiol 2005;22(6):447–51.
21. Alhashemi JA. Dexmedetomidine vs midazolam for monitored anaesthesia care during cataract surgery. Br J Anaesth 2006;96(6):722–6.
22. Hogue CW Jr, Talke P, Stein PK, et al. Autonomic nervous system responses during sedative infusions of dexmedetomidine. Anesthesiology 2002;97(3):592–8.
23. Jalonen J, Hynynen M, Kuitunen A, et al. Dexmedetomidine as an anesthetic adjunct in coronary artery bypass grafting. Anesthesiology 1997;86(2):331–45.
24. Talke P, Li J, Jain U, et al. Effects of perioperative dexmedetomidine infusion in patients undergoing vascular surgery. The Study of Perioperative Ischemia Research Group. Anesthesiology 1995;82(3):620–33.
25. Ligier B, Breslow MJ, Clarkson K, et al. Adrenal blood flow and secretory effects of adrenergic receptor stimulation. Am J Physiol 1994;266(1 Pt 2):H220–7.
26. Scheinin H, Jaakola ML, Sjovall S, et al. Intramuscular dexmedetomidine as premedication for general anesthesia. A comparative multicenter study. Anesthesiology 1993;78(6):1065–75.
27. Bloor BC, Frankland M, Alper G, et al. Hemodynamic and sedative effects of dexmedetomidine in dog. J Pharmacol Exp Ther 1992;263(2):690–7.
28. Aho M, Scheinin M, Lehtinen AM, et al. Intramuscularly administered dexmedetomidine attenuates hemodynamic and stress hormone responses to gynecologic laparoscopy. Anesth Analg 1992;75(6):932–9.
29. Karhuvaara S, Kallio A, Salonen M, et al. Rapid reversal of alpha 2-adrenoceptor agonist effects by atipamezole in human volunteers. Br J Clin Pharmacol 1991; 31(2):160–5.
30. Aantaa R, Kanto J, Scheinin M. Intramuscular dexmedetomidine, a novel alpha 2-adrenoceptor agonist, as premedication for minor gynaecological surgery. Acta Anaesthesiol Scand 1991;35(4):283–8.

31. Kallio A, Scheinin M, Koulu M, et al. Effects of dexmedetomidine, a selective alpha 2-adrenoceptor agonist, on hemodynamic control mechanisms. Clin Pharmacol Ther 1989;46(1):33–42.

32. Coursin DB, Maccioli GA. Dexmedetomidine. Curr Opin Crit Care 2001;7(4):221–6.

33. Aantaa R, Kanto J, Scheinin M, et al. Dexmedetomidine, an alpha 2-adrenoceptor agonist, reduces anesthetic requirements for patients undergoing minor gynecologic surgery. Anesthesiology 1990;73(2):230–5.

34. Jaakola ML, Kanto J, Scheinin H, et al. Intramuscular dexmedetomidine premedication–an alternative to midazolam-fentanyl-combination in elective hysterectomy? Acta Anaesthesiol Scand 1994;38(3):238–43.

35. Lawrence CJ, De LS. Effects of a single pre-operative dexmedetomidine dose on isoflurane requirements and peri-operative haemodynamic stability. Anaesthesia 1997;52(8):736–44.

36. Arain SR, Ebert TJ. The efficacy, side effects, and recovery characteristics of dexmedetomidine versus propofol when used for intraoperative sedation. Anesth Analg 2002;95(2):461–6.

37. Alhashemi JA, Kaki AM. Dexmedetomidine in combination with morphine PCA provides superior analgesia for shockwave lithotripsy. Can J Anaesth 2004; 51(4):342–7.

38. Goksu S, Arik H, Demiryurek S, et al. Effects of dexmedetomidine infusion in patients undergoing functional endoscopic sinus surgery under local anaesthesia. Eur J Anaesthesiol 2008;25(1):22–8.

39. Cortinez LI, Hsu YW, Sum-Ping ST, et al. Dexmedetomidine pharmacodynamics: part II: crossover comparison of the analgesic effect of dexmedetomidine and remifentanil in healthy volunteers. Anesthesiology 2004;101(5):1077–83.

40. Paris A, Tonner PH. Dexmedetomidine in anaesthesia. Curr Opin Anaesthesiol 2005;18(4):412–8.

41. Khan ZP, Ferguson CN, Jones RM. Alpha-2 and imidazoline receptor agonists. Their pharmacology and therapeutic role. Anaesthesia Feb 1999; 54(2):146–65.

42. Sanders RD, Maze M. Alpha2-adrenoceptor agonists. Curr Opin Investig Drugs 2007;8(1):25–33.

43. Scheinin H, Aantaa R, Anttila M, et al. Reversal of the sedative and sympatholytic effects of dexmedetomidine with a specific alpha2-adrenoceptor antagonist atipamezole: a pharmacodynamic and kinetic study in healthy volunteers. Anesthesiology 1998;89(3):574–84.

44. Scheinin H, Karhuvaara S, Olkkola KT, et al. Pharmacodynamics and pharmacokinetics of intramuscular dexmedetomidine. Clin Pharmacol Ther 1992;52(5): 537–46.

45. Brown EM, McGriff JT, Malinowski RW. Intravenous regional anaesthesia (Bier block): review of 20 years' experience. Can J Anaesth 1989;36(3 Pt 1):307–10.

46. Choyce A, Peng P. A systematic review of adjuncts for intravenous regional anesthesia for surgical procedures. Can J Anaesth 2002;49(1):32–45.

47. dos Reis A Jr. Eulogy to August Karl Gustav Bier on the 100th anniversary of intravenous regional block and the 110th anniversary of the spinal block. Rev Bras Anestesiol 2008;58(4):409–24.

48. van Zundert A, Helmstadter A, Goerig M, et al. Centennial of intravenous regional anesthesia. Bier's Block (1908–2008). Reg Anesth Pain Med 2008; 33(5):483–9.

49. Brill S, Middleton W, Brill G, et al. Bier's block; 100 years old and still going strong! Acta Anaesthesiol Scand 2004;48(1):117–22.

50. Holmes CM. Intravenous regional analgesia. A useful method of producing analgesia of the limbs. Lancet 1963;1(7275):245–7.
51. Singh R, Bhagwat A, Bhadoria P, et al. Forearm IVRA, using 0.5% lidocaine in a dose of 1.5 mg/kg with ketorolac 0.15 mg/kg for hand and wrist surgeries. Minerva Anestesiol 2010;76(2):109–14.
52. Ko MJ, Lee JH, Cheong SH, et al. Comparison of the effects of acetaminophen to ketorolac when added to lidocaine for intravenous regional anesthesia. Korean J Anesthesiol 2010;58(4):357–61.
53. Viscomi CM, Friend A, Parker C, et al. Ketamine as an adjuvant in lidocaine intravenous regional anesthesia: a randomized, double-blind, systemic control trial. Reg Anesth Pain Med 2009;34(2):130–3.
54. Sen H, Kulahci Y, Bicerer E, et al. The analgesic effect of paracetamol when added to lidocaine for intravenous regional anesthesia. Anesth Analg 2009; 109(4):1327–30.
55. Mowafi HA, Ismail SA. Melatonin improves tourniquet tolerance and enhances postoperative analgesia in patients receiving intravenous regional anesthesia. Anesth Analg 2008;107(4):1422–6.
56. Jankovic RJ, Visnjic MM, Milic DJ, et al. Does the addition of ketorolac and dexamethasone to lidocaine intravenous regional anesthesia improve postoperative analgesia and tourniquet tolerance for ambulatory hand surgery? Minerva Anestesiol 2008;74(10):521–7.
57. Turan A, White PF, Karamanlioglu B, et al. Premedication with gabapentin: the effect on tourniquet pain and quality of intravenous regional anesthesia. Anesth Analg 2007;104(1):97–101.
58. Sen S, Ugur B, Aydin ON, et al. The analgesic effect of nitroglycerin added to lidocaine on intravenous regional anesthesia. Anesth Analg 2006;102(3):916–20.
59. Turan A, Memis D, Karamanlioglu B, et al. Intravenous regional anesthesia using lidocaine and magnesium. Anesth Analg 2005;100(4):1189–92.
60. Taskaynatan MA, Ozgul A, Tan AK, et al. Bier block with methylprednisolone and lidocaine in CRPS type I: a randomized, double-blinded, placebo-controlled study. Reg Anesth Pain Med 2004;29(5):408–12.
61. Perlas A, Peng PW, Plaza MB, et al. Forearm rescue cuff improves tourniquet tolerance during intravenous regional anesthesia. Reg Anesth Pain Med 2003; 28(2):98–102.
62. Hartmannsgruber MW, Plessmann S, Atanassoff PG. Bilateral intravenous regional anesthesia: a new method to test additives to local anesthetic solutions. Anesthesiology 2003;98(6):1427–30.
63. Reuben SS, Steinberg RB, Maciolek H, et al. An evaluation of the analgesic efficacy of intravenous regional anesthesia with lidocaine and ketorolac using a forearm versus upper arm tourniquet. Anesth Analg 2002;95(2):457–60, table of contents.
64. Peng PW, Coleman MM, McCartney CJ, et al. Comparison of anesthetic effect between 0.375% ropivacaine versus 0.5% lidocaine in forearm intravenous regional anesthesia. Reg Anesth Pain Med 2002;27(6):595–9.
65. Atanassoff PG, Ocampo CA, Bande MC, et al. Ropivacaine 0.2% and lidocaine 0.5% for intravenous regional anesthesia in outpatient surgery. Anesthesiology 2001;95(3):627–31.
66. Hartmannsgruber MW, Silverman DG, Halaszynski TM, et al. Comparison of ropivacaine 0.2% and lidocaine 0.5% for intravenous regional anesthesia in volunteers. Anesth Analg 1999;89(3):727–31.
67. Reuben SS, Steinberg RB, Kreitzer JM, et al. Intravenous regional anesthesia using lidocaine and ketorolac. Anesth Analg 1995;81(1):110–3.

68. Nabhan A, Steudel WI, Dedeman L, et al. Subcutaneous local anesthesia versus intravenous regional anesthesia for endoscopic carpal tunnel release: a randomized controlled trial. J Neurosurg 2010. [Epub ahead of print].

69. Guay J. Adverse events associated with intravenous regional anesthesia (Bier block): a systematic review of complications. J Clin Anesth 2009;21(8): 585–94.

70. Hoffmann V, Vercauteren M, Van Steenberge A, et al. Intravenous regional anesthesia. Evaluation of 4 different additives to prilocaine. Acta Anaesthesiol Belg 1997;48(2):71–6.

71. Corpataux JB, Van Gessel EF, Donald FA, et al. Effect on postoperative analgesia of small-dose lysine acetylsalicylate added to prilocaine during intravenous regional anesthesia. Anesth Analg 1997;84(5):1081–5.

72. Marsch SC, Sluga M, Studer W, et al. 0.5% versus 1.0% 2-chloroprocaine for intravenous regional anesthesia: a prospective, randomized, double-blind trial. Anesth Analg 2004;98(6):1789–93.

73. Asik I, Kocum AI, Goktug A, et al. Comparison of ropivacaine 0.2% and 0.25% with lidocaine 0.5% for intravenous regional anesthesia. J Clin Anesth 2009; 21(6):401–7.

74. Estebe JP, Le Naoures A, Chemaly L, et al. Tourniquet pain in a volunteer study: effect of changes in cuff width and pressure. Anaesthesia 2000;55(1):21–6.

75. Lurie SD, Reuben SS, Gibson CS, et al. Effect of clonidine on upper extremity tourniquet pain in healthy volunteers. Reg Anesth Pain Med 2000;25(5):502–5.

76. Tham CH, Lim BH. A modification of the technique for intravenous regional blockade for hand surgery. J Hand Surg Br 2000;25(6):575–7.

77. Ananthanarayan C, Castro C, McKee N, et al. Compartment syndrome following intravenous regional anesthesia. Can J Anaesth 2000;47(11):1094–8.

78. Mabee JR, Bostwick TL, Burke MK. Iatrogenic compartment syndrome from hypertonic saline injection in Bier block. J Emerg Med 1994;12(4):473–6.

79. Maletis GB, Watson RC, Scott S. Compartment syndrome. A complication of intravenous regional anesthesia in the reduction of lower leg shaft fractures. Orthopedics 1989;12(6):841–6.

80. Hastings H 2nd, Misamore G. Compartment syndrome resulting from intravenous regional anesthesia. J Hand Surg Am 1987;12(4):559–62.

81. Johnson CN. Intravenous regional anesthesia: new approaches to an old technique. CRNA 2000;11(2):57–61.

82. Sen S, Ugur B, Aydin ON, et al. The analgesic effect of lornoxicam when added to lidocaine for intravenous regional anaesthesia. Br J Anaesth 2006;97(3):408–13.

83. Gentili M, Bernard JM, Bonnet F. Adding clonidine to lidocaine for intravenous regional anesthesia prevents tourniquet pain. Anesth Analg 1999;88(6): 1327–30.

84. Acalovschi I, Cristea T. Intravenous regional anesthesia with meperidine. Anesth Analg 1995;81(3):539–43.

85. Tan SM, Pay LL, Chan ST. Intravenous regional anaesthesia using lignocaine and tramadol. Ann Acad Med Singapore 2001;30(5):516–9.

86. Reuben SS, Steinberg RB, Klatt JL, et al. Intravenous regional anesthesia using lidocaine and clonidine. Anesthesiology 1999;91(3):654–8.

87. Prieto-Alvarez P, Calas-Guerra A, Fuentes-Bellido J, et al. Comparison of mepivacaine and lidocaine for intravenous regional anaesthesia: pharmacokinetic study and clinical correlation. Br J Anaesth 2002;88(4):516–9.

88. Karalezli N, Karalezli K, Iltar S, et al. Results of intravenous regional anaesthesia with distal forearm application. Acta Orthop Belg 2004;70(5):401–5.

89. Davis R, Keenan J, Meza A, et al. Use of a simple forearm tourniquet as an adjunct to an intravenous regional block. AANA J 2002;70(4):295–8.
90. Arregui-Martinez de Lejarza LM, Vigil MD, Perez Pascual MC, et al. [Evaluation of the analgesic effectiveness of ketorolac in intravenous regional anesthesia induced by lidocaine]. Rev Esp Anestesiol Reanim 1997;44(9):341–4 [in Spanish].
91. Alayurt S, Memis D, Pamukcu Z. The addition of sufentanil, tramadol or clonidine to lignocaine for intravenous regional anaesthesia. Anaesth Intensive Care 2004; 32(1):22–7.
92. Kurt N, Kurt I, Aygunes B, et al. Effects of adding alfentanil or atracurium to lidocaine solution for intravenous regional anaesthesia. Eur J Anaesthesiol 2002; 19(7):522–5.
93. Tetzlaff JE, Yoon HJ, Walsh M. Regional anaesthetic technique and the incidence of tourniquet pain. Can J Anaesth 1993;40(7):591–5.
94. Laursen RJ, Graven-Nielsen T, Jensen TS, et al. The effect of compression and regional anaesthetic block on referred pain intensity in humans. Pain 1999; 80(1–2):257–63.
95. Gorgias NK, Maidatsi PG, Kyriakidis AM, et al. Clonidine versus ketamine to prevent tourniquet pain during intravenous regional anesthesia with lidocaine. Reg Anesth Pain Med 2001;26(6):512–7.
96. Monteiro ER, Campagnol D, Parrilha LR, et al. Evaluation of cardiorespiratory effects of combinations of dexmedetomidine and atropine in cats. J Feline Med Surg 2009;11(10):783–92.
97. Penttila J, Helminen A, Anttila M, et al. Cardiovascular and parasympathetic effects of dexmedetomidine in healthy subjects. Can J Physiol Pharmacol 2004;82(5):359–62.
98. Kuusela E, Vainio O, Kaistinen A, et al. Sedative, analgesic, and cardiovascular effects of levomedetomidine alone and in combination with dexmedetomidine in dogs. Am J Vet Res 2001;62(4):616–21.
99. Pagel PS, Proctor LT, Devcic A, et al. A novel alpha 2-adrenoceptor antagonist attenuates the early, but preserves the late cardiovascular effects of intravenous dexmedetomidine in conscious dogs. J Cardiothorac Vasc Anesth 1998;12(4): 429–34.
100. Savola JM. Cardiovascular actions of medetomidine and their reversal by atipamezole. Acta Vet Scand Suppl 1989;85:39–47.
101. Flacke WE, Flacke JW, Bloor BC, et al. Effects of dexmedetomidine on systemic and coronary hemodynamics in the anesthetized dog. J Cardiothorac Vasc Anesth 1993;7(1):41–9.
102. Jalonen J, Halkola L, Kuttila K, et al. Effects of dexmedetomidine on coronary hemodynamics and myocardial oxygen balance. J Cardiothorac Vasc Anesth 1995;9(5):519–24.
103. Snapir A, Talke P, Posti J, et al. Effects of nitric oxide synthase inhibition on dexmedetomidine-induced vasoconstriction in healthy human volunteers. Br J Anaesth 2009;102(1):38–46.
104. Tezuka M, Kitajima T, Yamaguchi S, et al. Addition of dexmedetomidine prolongs duration of vasodilation induced by sympathetic block with mepivacaine in dogs. Reg Anesth Pain Med 2004;29(4):323–7.
105. Buerkle H, Yaksh TL. Pharmacological evidence for different alpha 2-adrenergic receptor sites mediating analgesia and sedation in the rat. Br J Anaesth 1998; 81(2):208–15.
106. Pertovaara A. Antinociceptive properties of fadolmidine (MPV-2426), a novel alpha2-adrenoceptor agonist. CNS Drug Rev 2004;10(2):117–26.

107. Talke P, Xu M, Paloheimo M, et al. Effects of intrathecally administered dexmedetomidine, MPV-2426 and tizanidine on EMG in rats. Acta Anaesthesiol Scand 2003;47(3):347–54.
108. Xu M, Kontinen VK, Kalso E. Effects of radolmidine, a novel alpha2 -adrenergic agonist compared with dexmedetomidine in different pain models in the rat. Anesthesiology 2000;93(2):473–81.
109. Graham BA, Hammond DL, Proudfit HK. Synergistic interactions between two alpha(2)-adrenoceptor agonists, dexmedetomidine and ST-91, in two substrains of Sprague-Dawley rats. Pain 2000;85(1–2):135–43.
110. Eisenach JC, Lavand'homme P, Tong C, et al. Antinociceptive and hemodynamic effects of a novel alpha2-adrenergic agonist, MPV-2426, in sheep. Anesthesiology 1999;91(5):1425–36.
111. Sabbe MB, Penning JP, Ozaki GT, et al. Spinal and systemic action of the alpha 2 receptor agonist dexmedetomidine in dogs. Antinociception and carbon dioxide response. Anesthesiology 1994;80(5):1057–72.
112. Poree LR, Guo TZ, Kingery WS, et al. The analgesic potency of dexmedetomidine is enhanced after nerve injury: a possible role for peripheral alpha2-adrenoceptors. Anesth Analg 1998;87(4):941–8.
113. Yoshitomi T, Kohjitani A, Maeda S, et al. Dexmedetomidine enhances the local anesthetic action of lidocaine via an alpha-2A adrenoceptor. Anesth Analg 2008;107(1):96–101.
114. Tanaka K, Oda Y, Funao T, et al. Dexmedetomidine decreases the convulsive potency of bupivacaine and levobupivacaine in rats: involvement of alpha2-adrenoceptor for controlling convulsions. Anesth Analg 2005;100(3):687–96.
115. Hanci V, Karakaya K, Yurtlu S, et al. Effects of dexmedetomidine pretreatment on bupivacaine cardiotoxicity in rats. Reg Anesth Pain Med 2009;34(6):565–8.
116. Luo WJ, Chai YF, Liu J, et al. A model of intravenous regional anesthesia in rats. Anesth Analg 2010;110(4):1227–32.

Cardiovascular Pharmacology: An Update

Henry Liu, MD[a,*], Charles J. Fox, MD[a], Shihai Zhang, MD, PhD[b],
Alan D. Kaye, MD, PhD[c]

KEYWORDS

- Cardiovascular • Anesthesia • Levosimendan • Nesiritide
- CK-1827452 • Cardiac myosin activators • Clevedipine

Cardiovascular diseases remain the leading cause of death not only in the United States but also elsewhere in the world. Developing new therapeutic agents for cardiovascular diseases has always been the priority for the pharmaceutical industry because of the huge potential market for these drugs. Some of these newer drugs are frequently used in the practice of cardiovascular anesthesiology. This article reviews the recent advances in cardiovascular medications related to the practice of cardiac anesthesia.

DRUGS FOR THE MANAGEMENT OF HEART FAILURE

Heart failure (HF) is a public health problem and the leading cause of hospitalizations in the United States. It is the most common diagnosis in patients aged 65 years and older, and is associated with significant morbidity, mortality, and resource use. HF-related morbidity and mortality are a significant financial burden on the American health care system. HF is the most expensive disease for Medicare. According to the American Heart Association,[1] in 2006 the prevalence of HF in the United States was 5.7 million people, or 2.5% of the population. In 2005, HF was the primary cause of 58,933 deaths and a contributing factor in an additional 233,281 deaths. That same year, the total direct cost of medical treatment of HF was $33.7 billion. In addition, there were indirect costs of $3.5 billion resulting from HF mortality. Although these expenses represent a substantial burden on the United States health care system and economy, it does not take into account costs derived from lost productivity

The authors have nothing to disclose.
[a] Tulane University Medical Center, 1430 Tulane Avenue, SL-4, New Orleans, LA 70112, USA
[b] Union Hospital of Tongji Medical College, Huazhong University of Science and Technology, 1277 Jie-Fang Da-Dao, Wuhan, Hubei 430022, China
[c] Departments of Anesthesiology and Pharmacology, Louisiana State University School of Medicine, 1542 Tulane Avenue, Room 656, New Orleans, LA 70112, USA
* Corresponding author. Tulane University Medical Center, 29 English Turn Drive, New Orleans, LA 70131.
E-mail address: henryliula@gmail.com

Anesthesiology Clin 28 (2010) 723–738
doi:10.1016/j.anclin.2010.09.001
1932-2275/10/$ – see front matter © 2010 Elsevier Inc. All rights reserved.

caused by HF morbidity. Thus, the combined direct and indirect costs reflect a fraction of the true societal cost of this disease. Moreover, the incidence of HF increases in elderly populations, and, for this reason, the public health burden of HF is predicted to increase proportionally as America ages.

The New York Heart Association (NYHA) classified HF into following 4 categories: class I includes patients without any limitation of physical activities, in whom ordinary physical exercise will not cause undue fatigue, palpitation, or dyspnea; class II indicates that patients may have slight limitation of physical activities. Patients usually feel comfortable at rest, but ordinary physical activities result in fatigue, palpitations, dyspnea, and so forth; class III contains patients with marked limitation of physical activities, but the patient usually feels comfortable at rest; and class IV includes patients who are unable to carry out any physical activities without discomfort and have signs and symptoms of cardiac insufficiency even at rest (**Table 1**).

The NYHA classification is a widely used method for the assessment of disease severity among patients with chronic HF, and is commonly applied to predict response to HF therapy. The NYHA classification has increasingly become a popular eligibility criterion for clinical trial enrollment in patients with chronic systolic and nonsystolic HF. However, Baggish and colleagues[2] recently found that natriuretic peptide testing is a more accurate method of determining prognosis than the NYHA classification among patients with acute decompensated heart failure (ADHF). HF is usually treated with diuretics, vasodilators, and positive inotropes. However, in recent years, only a few new drugs intended to improve either cardiac systolic dysfunction or diastolic dysfunction have been discovered. Those related to the practice of cardiovascular anesthesiology are discussed later.

New Natriuretic Agents: Nesiritide

Cardiomyocytes synthesize natriuretic peptides (NP) in response to increased atrial and ventricular pressure and volume stimuli that occurs during ADHF. There are several different types of NPs (eg, atrial NP, brain NP, C-type NP, D-type NP, V-type NP, and the renal peptide urodilatin) that all share a common amino acid ring structure. Kangwa and colleagues[3] isolated a 28 amino acid peptide in 1984, which has potent natriuretic, diuretic, and vasorelaxant activity. Another natriuretic factor was extracted from porcine brain and it was named brain natriuretic peptide. In recognition of its primary cardiovascular source of production and effect, this peptide was subsequently renamed as B-type natriuretic peptide (BNP). Cardiomyocytes produce a 134 amino acid prepropeptide, following cleavage of a 26 signal peptide, the peptide

Table 1	
NYHA classification of heart failure	
NYHA Class	**Patients' Symptoms**
Class I (mild)	No limitation of physical activity. Ordinary physical activity does not cause undue fatigue, palpitation, or dyspnea
Class II (mild)	Slight limitation of physical activity, comfortable at rest, but ordinary physical activity results in fatigue, palpitation, or dyspnea
Class III (moderate)	Marked limitation of physical activity, comfortable at rest, but less than ordinary activity causes fatigue, palpitation, or dyspnea
Class IV (severe)	Unable to carry out any physical activity without discomfort. Symptoms of cardiac insufficiency at rest. If any physical activity is undertaken, discomfort is increased

becomes a 108 amino acid pro-BNP. In physiologic state, pro-BNP is cleaved by endoproteases into amino-terminal fragments (NT-pro-BNP and the C-terminal portion, BNP).[4] BNP release is triggered by cardiac and noncardiac factors. Cardiac factors include HF, cardiac muscle disease, diastolic dysfunction, ischemia, hypertension, valvular disease, and atrial fibrillation. Noncardiac triggers include acute pulmonary embolization, pulmonary hypertension, septic shock, hyperthyroidism, renal insufficiency, and advanced liver disease.[4]

Nesiritide (Natrecor) is the recombination form of the 32 amino acid human B-type natriuretic peptide (hBNP) (**Fig. 1**). It is produced from *Escherichia coli* using recombinant DNA technology. Nesiritide has the same 32 amino acid sequence as the endogenous peptide produced by ventricular myocardium. It has a molecular weight of 3464 g/mol. Currently, the intravenous formulation is the only available form for clinical application.

Pharmacology

BNP has multiple physiologic effects on cardiovascular, neurohormonal, renal, and pulmonary systems. Nesiritide works to facilitate cardiovascular fluid homeostasis through counter-regulation of the renin-angiotensin-aldosterone system by stimulating cyclic guanosine monophosphate (cGMP) which leads to smooth muscle cell relaxation. Nesiritide is also a venous and arterial vasodilator and may potentiate the effect of concomitant diuretics.

Cardiac effects

Nesiritide reduces transforming growth factor-β–induced cell proliferation and collagen and fibronectin levels. It suppresses excessive fibrosis during cardiac remodeling, which is believed to induce cardiac lusitropy and diastolic dysfunction. Nesiritide also has pulmonary effects, directly inducing bronchodilation and allowing some patients to experience improvement in dyspnea. The neurohormonal effects of nesiritide include endogenously antagonizing the harmful effects of long-term neurohormonal activation. BNP seems to overcome the vasoconstrictive effects of endothelin-1, which leads to both venous and arterial dilation. Furthermore, nesiritide suppresses the activity of the renin-aldosterone-noradrenaline system, and possibly even the levels of the remodeling cytokines tumor necrosis factor-α and interleukin-6.[5] Nesiritide also has renal effects. Significant renal insufficiency often co-exists with HF, and nesiritide might play a role in the maintenance of glomerular filtration rates by enhancing renal vasodilation. Nisiritide can cause vasodilatation by promoting nitric oxide release, increasing intracellular cGMP levels, and activating calcium/potassium channels.[5]

Clinical applications

Nesiritide is used to treat acute severe/decompensated HF with dyspnea at rest or with minimal physical activities. In 2004, Elkayam and colleagues[6] reported an

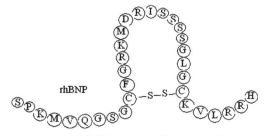

Fig. 1. The 32 amino acid chain of rhBNP (nesiritide). (*Courtesy of* Henry Liu, New Orleans, LA.)

advantage of nesiritide compared with high-dose nitroglycerin in the treatment of patients with decompensated HF. Nesiritide resulted in an early (15 minutes or less) decrease in pulmonary capillary wedge pressure, which was sustained throughout the 24-hour study period without the need for up-titration. Nesiritide is administered intravenously only. The patient is given a bolus dose and placed on a continuous intravenous infusion. Nesiritide is contraindicated in patients with cardiogenic shock or a systolic blood pressure lower than 90 mm Hg. For most adults and elderly patients, a bolus dose of 2 μg/kg is given followed by a continuous IV infusion of 0.01 μg/kg/min. This dosage may be increased every 3 hours to a maximum of 0.03 μg/kg/min. There is limited experience with administration of nesiritide for more than 48 hours. Patients' blood pressure needs to be closely monitored. Nesiritide is physically and/or chemically incompatible with injectable formulations of heparin, insulin, enalaprilat, sodium ethacrynate, hydralazine, bumetanide, and furosemide. Common side effects include hypotension (11% of patients), ventricular dysrhythmia (11%), headache, nausea, abdominal pain, insomnia, and bradycardia. When hypotension occurs, the dose needs to adjusted or discontinued, and aggressive measures to maintain blood pressure applied.

New Inotrope: Cardiac Myosin Activator

Anatomy of cardiac muscle fiber and sarcomeres

Human muscles are categorized into 3 types: skeletal, cardiac, and smooth muscle. Both skeletal and cardiac muscles are striated muscles, both smooth and cardiac muscles are involuntary muscles. The cells that form cardiac muscles are called cardiomyocytes and are sometimes seen as an intermediate between the other 2 types of muscles in terms of appearance, structure, metabolism, excitation coupling, and mechanism of contraction. Cardiac muscle shares some similarities with skeletal muscle in its striated appearance and contraction, and both are multinuclear compared with the mononuclear smooth muscle cells.[7] However, the myofibrils of cardiac muscle cells may be branched instead of linear and longitudinal as in skeletal muscle cells. These branches interlock with those of adjacent fibers by adherens junctions. These strong junctions enable the heart to contract forcefully without ripping the fibers apart. Also, the T-tubules in cardiac muscle are larger, broader, and run along the Z disks. The cardiac muscles contain fewer T-tubules compared with skeletal muscle. In addition, cardiac muscle forms dyads instead of the triads formed between the T-tubules and the sarcoplasmic reticulum in skeletal muscle. T-tubules play a critical role in excitation-contraction coupling (ECC).[7]

The primary structural proteins of cardiac muscle are actin and myosin. As shown in **Fig. 2**, the actin filaments are thin, causing the lighter appearance represented by I bands in striated muscle (see **Fig. 2**A); the thicker myosin filament is represented by a darker appearance to the alternating A bands observed microscopically (see **Fig. 2**B). The A bands are bisected by the H zone, running through the center of which is the M line. The H zone is that portion of the A band where the thick and thin filaments do not overlap. The I bands are bisected by the Z disk. Each myofibril is made up of arrays of parallel filaments. The thin filaments have a diameter of about 5 nm and length of 160 nm (see **Fig. 2**C). They are composed chiefly of the protein actin along with smaller amounts of 2 other proteins, troponin and tropomyosin. The thick filaments have a diameter of about 15 to 20 nm (see **Fig. 2**D). They are composed of the protein myosin. The entire array of thick and thin filaments between the Z disks is called a sarcomere. Molecules of a giant protein, titin (2500 kDa), extend from the M line to the Z disk, and are closely associated with the myosin molecule. They seem to anchor the myosin network to the actin network and maintain the neatly

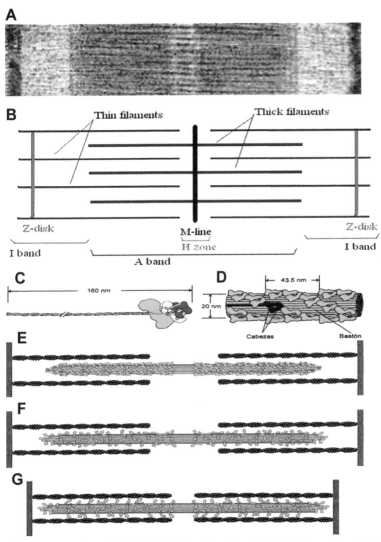

Fig. 2. The structure of myofibril, the basic functional unit of striated muscle. (*A, B*) (*Courtesy of* Henry Liu, New Orleans, LA. Available at http://www.zoology.ubc.ca/~gardner/F18-27A.GIF.) (*C–G*) (*Adapted from* Padrón R. El modelo atómico del filamento de miosina. Investigación y Ciencia 2007; with permission from Prensa Científica.)

ordered striation pattern. One of its functions is to provide a scaffold for the assembly of a precise number of myosin molecules in the thick filament. Titin may also dictate the number of actin molecules in the thin filaments. In a myofibril, shortening of the sarcomeres shortens the myofibril and the muscle fibers. Cardiac myosin is the motor protein directly responsible for converting chemical energy into the mechanical force that results in cardiac contraction. When the muscle is in the state of relaxation, myosin and actin are not engaged (see **Fig. 2**E). However, when the sarcomere is activated and in contraction (see **Fig. 2**F), the myosin and actin are engaged, and the sarcomere is shortened (see **Fig. 2**G). Cardiac contractility is driven by the cardiac sarcomere. This fundamental unit of muscle contraction in the heart is composed of cardiac myosin, actin, and a set of regulatory proteins. The sarcomere also represents one of the most thoroughly characterized protein machines in human biology.

ECC

An action potential (AP) originating in the sinus node depolarizes the cardiomyocyte and calcium ion enters the cytoplasm in phase 2 of the AP through L-type calcium channel located on the sarcolemma. The calcium then triggers the subsequent release of calcium that is stored in sarcoplasmic reticulum (SR) through calcium-releasing channels. This release increases the calcium level in the cytoplasm from 10^{-7} to 10^{-5} M. The binding of free calcium to troponin C (TN-C, part of the regulatory protein complex attached to the thin filaments) induces a conformational change in the regulatory complex such that troponin I (TN-I) exposes a site on the actin molecule that is able to bind to the myosin adenosine triphosphatase (ATPase) located on the myosin head (**Fig. 3**). This binding results in adenosine triphosphate (ATP) hydrolysis, which supplies energy for a conformational change to occur in the actin-myosin complex. The result of these changes is a movement (ratcheting) between the myosin heads and the actin, such that the actin and myosin filaments slide past each other and thereby shorten the sarcomere length. Ratcheting cycles occur as long as the cytosolic calcium remains increased. At the end of phase 2, calcium entry into the cell slows and calcium is sequestered by the SR by an ATP-dependent calcium pump (sarcoendoplasmic reticulum calcium-ATPase), which lowers the cytosolic calcium concentration and removes calcium from the TN-C. To a quantitatively smaller extent, cytosolic calcium is transported out of the cell by the sodium-calcium-exchange pump. The reduced intracellular calcium induces a conformational change in the troponin complex, leading to TN-I inhibition of the actin binding site. This inhibition disengages the myosin head and actin binding site. At the end of the cycle, a new ATP binds to the myosin head, displacing the adenosine diphosphate, and the initial sarcomere length is restored. If the cytosolic calcium level cannot reach the necessary level, cardiac systolic function will be compromised. However, if the cytoplasmic

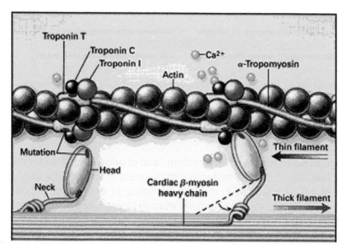

Fig. 3. Sliding filament theory of contraction. (*From* Kamisago M, Sharma SD, DePalma SR, et al. Mutations in sarcomere protein genes as a cause of dilated cardiomyopathy. N Engl J Med 2000;343(23):1688–96; with permission.)

calcium level is unable to reach the lower resting level, cardiac diastolic dysfunction will occur. The calcium ion plays a critically important role in ECC in the myocardium.

Most inotropes used to treat HF increase the intracellular calcium level. β-Adren-ergic receptor agonists or phosphodiesterase inhibitors (PDEI) achieve increased myocardial contractility by increasing the delivery of intracellular calcium to the sarco-meres through increasing the intracellular level of cAMP (**Fig. 4**). However, evidence suggests that this pathway may lead to adverse clinical outcomes. Current inotropic therapy (catecholamines, PDEI) was associated with a twofold increase in the risk of in-hospital mortality compared with treatment with vasodilators. In-hospital mortal-ities were 12.3% and 13.9% in patients receiving milrinone or dobutamine versus 4.7% and 7.1% in those receiving nitrates or nesiritide, respectively.[8] Fellahi and colleagues[9] studied 657 patients, 84 (13%) who received catecholamines, most often dobutamine (76 of 84; 90%). A higher incidence of both major cardiac morbidity (30% vs 9%) and all-cause intrahospital mortality (8% vs 1%) was observed in the catechol-amine group compared with the control group. After adjusting for channeling bias and confounding factors, catecholamine administration was significantly associated with major cardiac morbidity after propensity score stratification, propensity score covari-ance analysis, marginal structural models, and propensity score matching, but not with all-cause intrahospital mortality. The potential mechanism behind these worse-than-expected results in the catecholamine-treated group may be the increased velocity of the cardiac contraction, which shortens systolic ejection time. In contrast with catecholamines, cardiac myosin activators, a new class of inotropes, directly target the kinetics of the myosin head. Myosin activators have been shown to work in the absence of significant increase in intracellular calcium by a novel mechanism that stimulates the activity of the cardiac myosin motor protein. Cardiac myosin acti-vators accelerate the rate-limiting step of the myosin enzymatic cycle and shift the enzymatic cycle in favor of the force-producing state. This inotropic mechanism

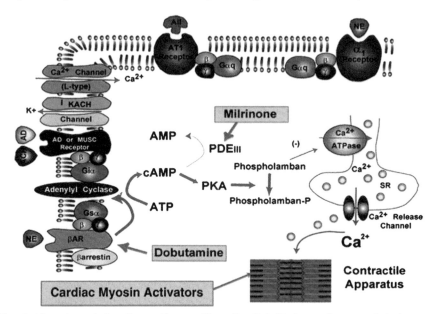

Fig. 4. Myocyte and signaling pathways. (*From* Teerlink JR. A novel approach to improve cardiac performance: cardiac myosin activators. Heart Fail Rev 2009;14:289–98; with permis-sion from Springer Science+Business Media.)

does not increase the velocity of cardiac contraction, but instead lengthens the systolic ejection time, increasing cardiac contractility and cardiac output in a potentially more oxygen-efficient manner, and avoiding oxygen wasting. Myosin activators increase the rate of effective myosin cross-bridge formation, which enhances the duration and quantity of myocyte contraction, and inhibits nonproductive consumption of ATP, potentially improving myocyte energy use, with no effect on intracellular calcium or cAMP.[10]

The most effective currently-available myosin activator is CK-1827452. The phase IIa clinical trials of CK-1827452 were recently completed. The multicenter, double-blind, randomized, and placebo-controlled clinical trials indicated that CK-1827452 was safe and effective for clinical administration in patients with HF. The trials also established a relationship between plasma concentration of CK-1827452 and its pharmacodynamic and pharmacokinetic effects. One of the trials used 45 patients and 151 treatment episodes. The result showed that CK-1827452 increased systolic ejection time, stroke volume, cardiac output, fractional shortening, and ejection fraction in a concentration dependent manner. At 100 ng/mL plasma concentration, systolic ejection time and fractional shortening significantly improved. At 200 ng/mL, stroke volume also improved significantly. At 300 ng/mL, cardiac output improvement was statistically significant. However, at plasma concentrations greater than 400 ng/mL, the increases in stroke volume and cardiac output appeared to plateau in association with concentration. The effects of CK-827452 on systolic ejection time and stroke volume appeared to be persistent over a 24-hour period. With 72 hours of infusion, decreases in ventricular volumes were sustained. The phase II clinical trial concluded that the improvements in cardiac systolic performances accompanied by the declines in left ventricular (LV) volumes observed in this trial may be caused by the decreases in filling pressure.[10] Throughout the clinical trial, continuous intravenous administration of CK-1827452 appeared to be well-tolerated in stable patients with HF over a wide range of plasma concentrations. There was no dose-related increase in the overall incidence of adverse events. At doses greater than the maximal tolerance dose (MTD) that were not tolerated, the CK-1827452 infusions were terminated. The 0.75 mg/kg/h and 1.0 mg/kg/h doses led to early discontinuations in some patients. The most common symptoms were chest tightness, light headedness, palpitations, and feeling hot. Tachycardia, electrocardiogram changes and increased troponin I and T levels were also observed. These symptoms are believed to be related to an excess of the intended pharmacologic effect, resulting in excessive prolongation of the systolic ejection. Other changes induced by myosin activators include ST changes.[11] In this trial, 3 serious adverse events (SAEs) were reported. Only 1 was related to CK-1827452. These SAEs included a non-ST increase myocardial infarction, in the setting of a drug overdose, septicemia, in the setting of a diabetic foot ulcer, and pneumonia. For patients who were tolerant of all study drug infusions, no consistent pattern of adverse events with either dose or duration of infusion emerged. In the patient who experienced the non-ST increased myocardial infarction, the cardiac-specific fraction of the enzyme creatine kinase remained normal. Also, subsequent electrocardiograms and echocardiograms returned to normal in this subject, and cardiac magnetic resonance imaging enhanced by gadolinium, a test for myocardial injury, detected no cardiac abnormality in patients who received CK-1827452.

A first-in-human study in healthy volunteers with the lead cardiac myosin activator, CK-1827452, as well as preliminary results from a study in patients with stable chronic HF, found significant increases in systolic ejection time, fractional shortening, stroke volume, and cardiac output. These studies suggest that cardiac myosin activators may provide a safe and effective treatment of HF. Cytokinetics is developing other compounds that are in the early stages of preclinical trials. These compounds are CK-1122534 (finished second preclinical trial), CK-1213296 (completed third preclinical trial), and CK-2017357. CK-2017357 is directed toward skeletal muscle and may represent a potential treatment of diseases and medical conditions associated with skeletal muscle weakness.[10]

New Inotrope: Calcium Sensitizer Levosimendan

Calcium sensitizers are a new category of inotropes that enhance myocardial performance by increasing the affinity of troponin C to calcium. Levosimendan is a typical calcium sensitizer and K-ATP channel opener that has emerged as an alternative option for inotropic support in patients with decompensated HF. Studies found that the use of levosimendan in severe HF was more favorable than conventional inotropic agents. The prolonged, enhanced contractility during systole (half-life of 80 hours) does not impair ventricular relaxation and it is not cleared by the kidneys. Also, levosimendan does not increase epinephrine or norepinephrine concentrations, thus avoiding resultant vasoconstriction, remodeling, or downregulation of cardiac receptor sensitivity.

STRATEGIES TO IMPROVE CARDIAC DIASTOLIC FUNCTION

Although not fully understood, the clinical significance of diastolic cardiac dysfunction is increasingly gaining recognition by clinicians who manage patients with HF. Only limited, randomized, double-blinded, placebo-controlled, multicenter trials have been conducted on patients with diastolic HF. The management strategies currently used are still based on empirical information, on clinical investigations in small groups of patients, and are based on traditionally believed pathophysiologic mechanisms.

Pathophysiology

Diastolic dysfunction is characterized by increased diastolic pressure in the left ventricle despite normal or subnormal diastolic volume. Histologic evidence supporting diastolic dysfunction shows hypertrophy of the cardiomyocytes, increased interstitial collagen deposition, and/or infiltration of the myocardium. These changes collectively lead to a deterioration in distensibility of the myocardium. The ventricle then behaves as a balloon made from abnormally thick rubber. Despite filling at high pressure, the volume cannot expand adequately. If the heart cannot fill with blood easily, either the cardiac output becomes diminished or compensation ensues to increase the ventricular diastolic pressure to higher than normal levels. When the LV diastolic pressure is increased, pressure rises in the atrium. This increase is transmitted back to the pulmonary venous system, thereby increasing its hydrostatic pressure and promoting pulmonary edema (defined as congestive HF) and dyspnea. Activation of neurohumoral systems, such as the renin-angiotensin system, is associated with cardiac hypertrophy, increases in central and systemic volumes, and fluid retentive states common to patients in HF. When a normal heart is overfilled with blood, it may show increased stiffness and decreased compliance characteristics, similar to a balloon overfilled with air. Blowing more air into the balloon becomes more difficult because the balloon is stiffer and less compliant at these high volumes. It is wrong to classify the volume-overloaded heart as having diastolic dysfunction just because it is stiffer and less compliant. The term diastolic dysfunction is often erroneously applied in this circumstance when increased fluid volume retention causes the heart to be overfilled.[12]

Management Strategies of Patients with Diastolic HF Include Symptom-targeted and Mechanism-targeted Approaches

Decrease diastolic pressure

It is important to decrease the LV diastolic pressure that is the root cause of a patient's symptoms. LV diastolic pressures can be decreased by decreasing central blood volume through decreasing venous return (nitrates), reducing total blood volume (through fluid and sodium restriction or use of diuretics), and blunting neurohumoral activation by using antagonist(s). Decreasing LV volume can be achieved by maintaining synchronous atrial contraction and increasing the duration of diastole by reducing heart rate. Treatment with diuretics and nitrates should be initiated at low doses to avoid symptomatic hypotension and fatigue. Hypotension can be a significant problem, because these patients have a steep diastolic pressure volume curve such that a small change in diastolic volume causes a large change in pressure and cardiac output. Because both basic and clinical studies suggest that hypertrophy is associated with activation of neurohumoral systems such as the renin-angiotensin-aldosterone system, the treatment of diastolic HF should include agents such as angiotensin-converting enzyme (ACE) inhibitors, type-1 angiotensin-II (AT1) receptor antagonists, and aldosterone antagonists. In addition to promoting fluid retention, neurohumoral activation can have direct effects on cellular and extracellular mechanisms that contribute to the development of diastolic HF. Modulation of neurohumoral activation may also affect fibroblast activity, interstitial fibrosis, intracellular calcium handling, and myocardial stiffness.[13]

Decrease heart rate

Tachycardia is poorly tolerated in patients with diastolic HF for several reasons. Shorter diastolic time compromises LV diastolic refilling. β-Blockers and some calcium channel blockers can therefore be used to prevent excessive tachycardia and produce a low-normal heart rate. Although the optimal heart rate must be individualized, an initial goal for therapy might be a resting heart rate of 60 to 70 beats/min with a blunted exercise-induced increase in heart rate.

Improve exercise tolerance

Poor exercise tolerance is common in patients with diastolic HF. Mechanisms responsible for this include (1) patients with HF have limited ability to use the Frank-Starling mechanism because of increased diastolic stiffness preventing the increase in LV end-diastolic volume that normally accompanies exercise; (2) the abnormal relaxation velocity versus heart rate relationship that exists in patients with diastolic HF prevents augmentation of relaxation velocity as heart rate increases during exercise. As a result, during exercise, diastolic pressure increases but the stroke volume fails to increase, and patients experience dyspnea and fatigue. In patients with diastolic HF, there is frequently an exaggerated increase in blood pressure in response to exercise that increases LV load and in turn further impairs myocardial relaxation and filling. β-Blockers, calcium channel blockers, and AT1 antagonists may have a salutary effect on symptoms and exercise capacity in many patients with diastolic HF. However, the beneficial effect of these agents on exercise tolerance is not always paralleled by improved LV diastolic function or increased relaxation rate. Nonetheless, several small clinical trials have shown that the use of these agents results in improvement in exercise capacity in patients with diastolic HF.[13]

Positive inotropes

Positive inotropic agents are generally not indicated in the treatment of patients with isolated diastolic HF because the ejection fraction is usually preserved. Current inotropic agents have been related to worse mid- and long-term prognosis, potentially because of worsened pathophysiologic processes, which adversely affect energetics, higher heart rate, induced ischemia, and dysrhythmia. However, short-term use of positive inotropic drugs may be beneficial in managing patients with pulmonary edema associated with diastolic HF because they enhance SR function, promote more rapid and complete relaxation, increase splanchnic blood flow, increase venous capacitance, and facilitate diuresis. During hemodynamic stress or ischemia, digitalis may promote or contribute to diastolic dysfunction. Therefore, the usefulness of digitalis in the treatment of diastolic HF remains unclear. Conceptually, an ideal therapeutic agent should target the underlying mechanisms that cause diastolic HF.

An ideal therapeutic agent should improve calcium homeostasis and energetics, blunt neurohumoral activation, and prevent or regress fibrosis. However, there is no drug in clinical use that meets these criteria. Some pharmaceutical agents that possess these characteristics are already in the development phase, but progress is slow. Current therapy has been well documented to benefit patients with diastolic HF. The clinical benefits of using ACE inhibitors were elucidated in the following studies: meta-analysis of 6 studies (2898 women and 11,674 men) in which treatment duration ranged from 6 to 42 months. The results indicate that women with symptomatic HF benefit when treated with ACE inhibitors, although the benefit may be somewhat less than that seen in men. Groups of patients with and without diabetes achieved reductions in mortality when treated with ACE inhibitors for HF. There was no significant difference in mortality reduction among black and white patients in theses studies. For β-blockers, meta-analysis of 5 studies (2134 women and 7885 men) indicated that both women and men with symptomatic diastolic HF have reduced mortality when treated with β-blockers. In patients with HF, with or without diabetes, β-blocker treatment is associated with reduced mortality. Bucindolol was associated with worse mortality outcomes in black patients compared with white patients.

There are similarities and differences in treating diastolic versus systolic cardiac dysfunction. Many drugs are used to treat both diastolic and systolic HF despite being based on different rationales, pathophysiology, and dosing regimens. For example, β-blockers are currently used for both diastolic and systolic HF. For systolic HF, β-blockers are used chronically to increase the inotropic state, change the adrenergic receptor gene expression, and modify LV remodeling. β-Blockers must be titrated slowly and carefully for an extended time period to avoid hypotension and fatigue. However, the rational for diastolic HF (to decrease heart rate and increase the duration of diastole) usually does not warrant slow titration. Diuretics are used in the treatment of both systolic and diastolic HF. However, the diuretic dose used to treat diastolic HF is generally less than the doses used in systolic HF. Some drugs are used only to treat either systolic or diastolic HF, but not both. For example, calcium channel blockers such as diltiazem, nifedipine, and verapamil have no place in the treatment of systolic HF. By contrast, each of these has been proposed for the treatment of diastolic HF.[13]

INTRAVENOUS ANTIHYPERTENSIVE DRUGS

Approximately 72 million people suffer from hypertension in the United States, which accounts for almost a third of the adult population. Hypertension is one of the most common chronic medical conditions among adult Americans. Hypertension affects more men than women, and almost twice as many African Americans as whites. The incidence of hypertension increases with age. Management of patients with chronic hypertension undergoing surgery is of major clinical importance because they experience an increased risk of morbidity and mortality after surgery. When managing patients with hypertensive crisis in the emergency room, it is ideal to have drugs that possess the following features: fast onset, short-acting, predictable dose responses, minimal titration time to desired blood pressure, minimal dose adjustments, minimal adverse effects, no effect on intracranial pressure, no cerebral or coronary steal, no negative effect on cardiac contractility and conduction, and no reliance on renal or hepatic function for their clearance. Although no such drug is available, several newer drugs, such as nicardipine and clevidipine, possess many desirable characteristics.

Nicardipine

Nicardipine hydrochloride (Cardene) is a calcium ion influx inhibitor (slow channel blocker or calcium channel blocker). Nicardipine hydrochloride is a dihydropyridine derivative with the International Union of Pure and Applied Chemistry (IUPAC) chemical name (±)-2-(benzyl-methyl amino) ethyl methyl 1,4-dihydro-2,6-dimethyl-4-(m-nitrophenyl)-3,5-pyridinedicarboxylate monohydrochloride. Its structure is shown in **Fig. 5**.

Nicardipine hydrochloride is a greenish-yellow, odorless, crystalline powder that melts at about 169°C. It is freely soluble in chloroform, methanol, and glacial acetic acid, sparingly soluble in anhydrous ethanol, slightly soluble in n-butanol, water, 0.01 M potassium dihydrogen phosphate, acetone, and dioxane, very soluble in ethyl acetate, and practically insoluble in benzene, ether, and hexane. It has a molecular weight of 515.99.

Pharmacology

Nicardipine is a dihydropyridine L-type calcium channel blocker. Its dose response is linear from 0.5 to 40 mg/h. Its rapid early distribution phase (α) half time is 2.7 minutes, intermediate phase (β) half time is 44.8 minutes, and its slow terminal phase (γ) half time is 14.4 hours. Intravenous nicardipine is more than 95% protein bound and its volume of distribution is about 8.3 L/kg. The total clearance of nicardipine is about 0.4 L/h/kg. Nicardipine is metabolized in the liver by P450 3A2. Nicardipine's onset time is 1 minute and peak time is 5 to 10 minutes after intravenous administration. Currently, nicardipine is available for both oral and intravenous formulations. Nicardipine for intravenous administration contains 25 mg of nicardipine hydrochloride per 250 mL (0.1 mg/mL) in either dextrose or sodium chloride. Premixed nicardipine injection is available as a ready-to-use, sterile, nonpyrogenic, clear, colorless to yellow, iso-osmotic solution for intravenous administration. Hydrochloric acid and/or sodium hydroxide may have been added to adjust pH to between 3.7 and 4.7. Solutions are in contact with the polyethylene layer of the container and can leach out certain chemical components of the plastic in small amounts within the expiration period. The suitability and safety of the plastic have been confirmed in tests in animals according to

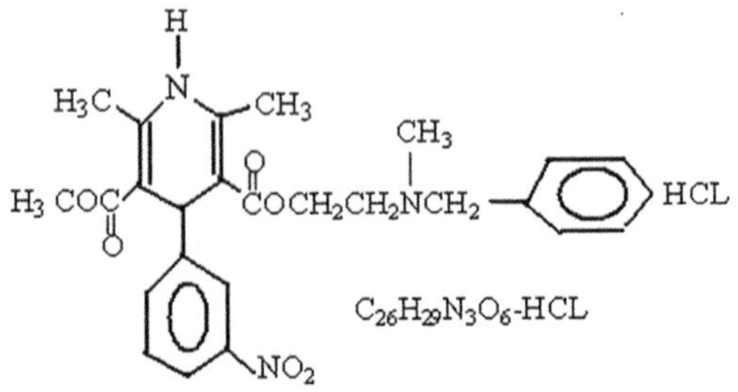

$C_{26}H_{29}N_3O_6 \cdot HCL$

Fig. 5. Nicardipine hydrochloride. (*Courtesy of* Henry Liu, New Orleans, LA.)

the United States Pharmacopeia biologic tests for plastic containers, as well as by tissue culture toxicity studies. If intravenous nicardipine is administered through a peripheral venous catheter, it may necessitate changing the venous site after a couple of days because of its potent venous irritant effect.

Clinical applications
Nicardipine intravenous administration has been compared with sodium nitroprusside (which is believed to be the gold standard of antihypertensive drugs) for hypertensive therapy after coronary artery bypass graft (CABG) surgery. Within 6 hours after surgery, 47 patients after CABG, with systolic blood pressure (SBP) of 150 mm Hg or greater, were randomized to receive either intravenous nicardipine or sodium nitroprusside. Both drugs were infused at 2 mg/kg/min for 10 minutes. The dosage was increased by 1 mg/kg/min every 10 minutes if the BP remained higher than the target BP and was decreased by 1 mg/kg/min when the target BP was achieved. No differences in SBP or heart rate were reported, but the duration of drug therapy and the total dose administered were lower for the nicardipine group compared with the sodium nitroprusside group. Cardiac index and stroke volume were higher and systemic vascular resistance (SVR) was lower in patients treated with nicardipine.[14] Nicardipine has also been used to treat cardiac diastolic dysfunction and it is used to prevent spasm of arterial graft for coronary artery bypass. The side effects of nicardipine include headache (14.6%), hypotension (5.6%), nausea and vomiting (4.9%), and tachycardia (3.5%).

Clevidipine

Clevidipine (Cleviprex) is a vasoselective, ultra–short-acting, third-generation dihydropyridine L-type calcium channel blocker. It was approved on August 4, 2008 by the US Food and Drug Administration (FDA) for the reduction of blood pressure when oral therapy is not feasible or desirable. Clevidipine is selective for arteriolar vasodilatation; thus, it lowers mean arterial pressure by decreasing SVR without reducing cardiac filling pressures. It produces little or no effect on myocardial contractility or cardiac conduction, a potentially favorable feature in patients after cardiac surgery. Clevidipine's selectivity for arterial vessels allows a direct reduction in peripheral vascular resistance without dilatation of the venous capacitance bed. Cleviprex is formulated as a lipid emulsion in 20% soybean oil (Intralipid) and contains approximately 0.2 g of fat per milliliter (2.0 kcal/mL). Clevidipine also contains glycerin (22.5 mg/mL), purified egg yolk phospholipids (12 mg/mL), and sodium hydroxide to adjust pH. Clevidipine has a pH of 6.0 to 8.0. Clevidipine is similar in structure to felodipine, an oral vasoselective dihydropyridine calcium channel antagonist, with the exception of an additional ester linkage that is responsible for its rapid metabolism. The molecular structure of nicardipine is shown in **Fig. 6**.

Pharmacology
Clevidipine butyrate is a racemic mixture of 2 enantiomers, S- and R-clevidipine. Like other dihydropyridine calcium channel antagonists, clevidipine exerts its effects by inhibiting transmembrane calcium influx through voltage-dependent L-type calcium channels with a high degree of vascular selectivity for arterial smooth muscle and no effect on venous capacitance vessels. Clevidipine is 3 to 6 times more potent at the lower resting membrane potentials that are seen in vascular smooth muscle, compared with cardiac myocytes that show a greater negative resting membrane potential. Because of this, the effect of clevidipine on myocardial contractility is limited.[15] A decrease in blood pressure is observed within 2 to 3 minutes after

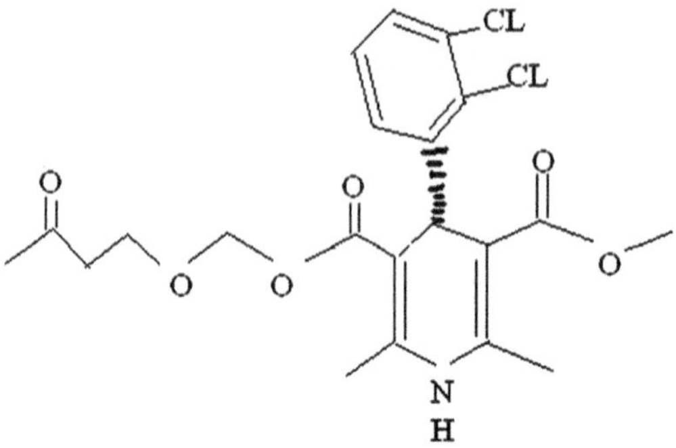

Fig. 6. Nicardipine. (*Courtesy of* Henry Liu, New Orleans, LA.)

intravenous administration of clevidipine. The blood pressure returns to pretreatment levels within 5 to 15 minutes of terminating the infusion, primarily as a result of the drug's high clearance rate (0.13 L/min/kg) and small volume of distribution at steady state (0.6 L/kg), resulting in an initial phase half-life of approximately 1 minute and terminal phase half-life of 10 to 15 minutes. At steady state, arterial blood concentration of clevidipine is twice that of venous blood, which results in an increased clearance rate (0.05 L/min/kg) and a smaller volume of distribution (0.17 L/kg); these arteriovenous concentration differences have also been observed in other short-acting compounds containing an ester linkage in their structure. More than 80% of the total area under the blood concentration-time curve is associated with the initial phase half-life owing to rapid elimination of drug rather than distribution, as is evident from postinfusion blood concentrations that decrease by 50% within 1 minute of stopping the infusion, regardless of the duration. Clevidipine is rapidly metabolized by esterases in the blood and extravascular tissues and, as such, it is unlikely to be affected by renal or hepatic insufficiency. Even in patients with pseudocholinesterase deficiency, it is rapidly metabolized. The major route of elimination is via the kidney, with 63% to 73% of radioactively labeled clevidipine recovered in the urine, and 10% to 20% recovered in the feces. Because of the lack of hepatic metabolism, clevidipine is not expected to be affected by changes in cytochrome P450 isoenzyme activity. The drug is highly protein bound (99.5%) in human plasma, in a non–concentration-dependent manner, and binding to specific plasma proteins, such as A-1-acid glycoprotein, has not been elucidated.

Clinical applications
Clevidipine is indicated for the reduction of hypertension when oral therapy is not feasible or desirable. In the perioperative patient population, clevidipine produces a 4% to 5% reduction in SBP within 2 to 4 minutes of starting a 1 to 2 mg/h infusion. In most patients, full recovery of blood pressure is achieved in 5 to 15 minutes after the infusion is stopped. In studies of up to 72 hours of continuous infusion, there was no evidence of tolerance. Varon and colleagues[16] conducted an open-label, single-group, multicenter study to evaluate the effect of clevidipine in 126 patients with acute hypertension (mean baseline SBP, 202 mm Hg) in the emergency department. The study included patients experiencing either hypertensive urgency or emergency. Long-term administration of clevidipine was evaluated for each patient (mean duration of infusion was 21.3 hours). Investigators determined a target SBP range (20–40 mm Hg from upper to lower limits) to be achieved within the first 30 minutes of clevidipine infusion initiation. The initial infusion rate was 2 mg/h (4 mL/h). Doses were then increased in

doubling increments every 3 minutes, not to exceed 32 mg/h, until the prespecified SBP was achieved. The mean infusion rate was 9.52 mg/h, with a mean maximum infusion rate of 17.5 mg/h. The median time to reach the target BP range was 10.9 minutes, and 88.9% of patients achieved the BP goal within 30 minutes of starting the infusion. By 18 hours (the minimum length of infusion defined by the study), SBP had been reduced by a mean of 26% from baseline. Most patients (90.5%) were treated with only clevidipine. Successful transition to oral therapy (defined as SBP remaining within the target range 6 hours after discontinuation of the clevidipine infusion) was accomplished in 91.3% of the patients. The most commonly reported adverse effects in this trial were headache (6.3%), nausea (4.8%), chest discomfort (3.2%), and vomiting (3.2%). Triglyceride levels were also evaluated 6 hours after infusion termination, and no differences were observed compared with baseline. Roughly 8.7% of patients who received clevidipine experienced 1 serious side effect (chest discomfort, dysrhythmia, and death). Clevidipine is contraindicated in patients with severe aortic stenosis, severe idiopathic hypertrophic subaortic stenosis, or allergies to soybeans, soy products, eggs, or egg products. Clevidipine has been found to have cardioprotective effects in animal studies. In pigs subjected to 45 minutes of myocardial ischemia followed by 4 hours of reperfusion, clevidipine infusions significantly reduced the final infarct size compared with placebo (mean percent of left ventricle at risk: 51% [8.2%] vs 80% [9.2%]), respectively; however, there are studies showing that clevidipine has no significant myocardial protective effects on reperfusion injury. There are also reports showing that clevidipine preserves renal reperfusion function in an experimental rat model in which acute ischemic renal failure was induced by occluding the left renal artery for 40 minutes. Either clevidipine or fenoldopam, a dopamine D1-receptor agonist, was infused for 60 minutes, beginning 10 minutes before reperfusion. Although there was no significant difference in glomerular filtration between clevidipine and fenoldopam, clevidipine was reported to reduce losses in both sodium and water after reperfusion (data not provided). This finding suggests that clevidipine may be more effective in protecting renal tubular function.[17]

REFERENCES

1. Lloyd-Jones D, Adams R, Carnethon M, et al. Heart disease and stroke statistics—2009 update: a report from the American Heart Association statistics committee and stroke statistics subcommittee. Circulation 2009;119(3):480–6.
2. Baggish AL, van Kimmenade RR, Pinto Y, et al. New York Heart Association class versus amino-terminal pro-B type natriuretic peptide for acute heart failure prognosis. Biomarkers 2010;15(4):307–14.
3. Kangawa K, Matsuo H. Purification and complete amino acid sequence of human atrial natriuretic polypeptide (alpha-hANP). Biochem Biophys Res Commun 1984; 118:131–9.
4. Bhardwaj A, Januzzi JL Jr. Natriuretic peptide-guided management of acutely destabilized heart failure: rationale and treatment algorithm. Crit Pathw Cardiol 2009;8(4):146–50.
5. Reichert S, Ignaszewski A. Molecular and physiological effects of nesiritide. Can J Cardiol 2008;24(Suppl B):15B–8B.
6. Elkayam U, Akhter MW, Singh H, et al. Comparison of effects on left ventricular filling pressure of intravenous nesiritide and high-dose nitroglycerin in patients with decompensated heart failure. Am J Cardiol 2004;93(2):237–40.
7. Available at: http://en.wikipedia.org/wiki/Cardiac_muscle. Accessed April 10, 2010.

8. Abraham WT, Adams KF, Fonarow GC, et al. In-hospital mortality in patients with acute decompensated heart failure requiring intravenous vasoactive medications: an analysis from the Acute Decompensated Heart Failure National Registry (ADHERE). J Am Coll Cardiol 2005;46:57–64.

9. Fellahi JL, Parienti JJ, Hanouz JL, et al. Perioperative use of dobutamine in cardiac surgery and adverse cardiac outcome: propensity-adjusted analyses. Anesthesiology 2008;108(6):979–87.

10. Teerlink JR. A novel approach to improve cardiac performance: cardiac myosin activators. Heart Fail Rev 2009;14(4):289–98.

11. Teerlink JR. Medscape. Available at: http://www.medscape.com/viewarticle/547591. Accessed April 10, 2010.

12. Available at: http://en.wikipedia.org/wiki/Diastolic_dysfunction#Pathophysiology. Accessed April 10, 2010.

13. Zile MR, Brutsaert DL. Causal mechanisms and treatment new concepts in diastolic dysfunction and diastolic heart failure: part II. Circulation 2002;105:1503–8.

14. Kwak YL, Oh YJ, Bang SO, et al. Comparison of the effects of nicardipine and sodium nitroprusside for control of increased blood pressure after coronary artery bypass graft surgery. J Int Med Res 2004;32:342–50.

15. Kenyon KW. Clevidipine: an ultra short-acting calcium channel antagonist for acute hypertension. Ann Pharmacother 2009;43(7):1258–65.

16. Varon J, Peacock W, Garrison N, et al. Prolonged infusion of clevidipine results in safe and predictable blood pressure control in patients with acute severe hypertension. Paper presented at the Annual Meeting of the American College of Chest Physicians. Chicago, October 20–25, 2007.

17. Nguyen HM, Ma K, Pham DQ. Clevidipine for the treatment of severe hypertension in adults. Clin Ther 2010;32:11–2.

Perioperative Statin Use: An Update

Phillip L. Kalarickal, MD, MPH[a], Charles J. Fox, MD[a],
Jeffrey Y. Tsai, MS[b], Henry Liu, MD[a],*, Alan D. Kaye, MD, PhD[c]

KEYWORDS

- Statins • Perioperative cardiac complications
- 3-hydroxyl 3-methylglutaryl coenzyme A reductase inhibitors
- Inflammation

Reducing the incidence of adverse perioperative outcomes has been pursued through various medical therapies. Pre-incision prophylactic antibiotics[1] and perioperative beta blockade[2] are just two examples of commonly used medical modalities directed toward reducing morbity and mortality in the perioperative period. 3-hydroxy 3-methylglutaryl coenzyme A (HMG CoA) reductase inhibitors (statins) have also demonstrated improvements in postoperative outcomes among patients taking them in the perioperative period. Many of the studies are in limited to select patient populations and/or select surgeries. This review will give an overview of the pharmacology of statins, summarize the mechanisms of the beneficial effects of statins, and provide an overview of evidence in the use of statins in the perioperative period.

PHARMACOLOGY OVERVIEW

Statins are competitive inhibitors of HMG-CoA reductase enzyme in cholesterol biosynthesis and prevent the conversion of HMG-CoA to mevalonate, the rate-limiting step in cholesterol biosynthesis. Initially, statins interfere with hepatic cholesterol synthesis, which enhances expression of the low-density lipoprotein (LDL) receptor gene in response to the reduced hepatic cholesterol level. Triggered transcription factors then signal the increasing synthesis of LDL receptors along with limited degradation of LDL receptors.[3,4] The increasing number of LDL receptors on the surface of hepatocytes amplifies the removal of LDL from the blood. Other theories have suggested that, similar to the effect of niacin, statins could reduce LDL levels in the triglyceride-lowering effect via removal of LDL precursors, very-low-density lipoprotein

The authors have nothing to disclose.
[a] Department of Anesthesiology, Tulane University Medical Center, 1430 Tulane Avenue, SL-4, New Orleans, LA 70112, USA
[b] LSUHSC-New Orleans, 1542 Tulane Avenue, New Orleans, LA 70112, USA
[c] Departments of Anesthesiology and Pharmacology, Louisiana State University School of Medicine, 1542 Tulane Avenue, Room 656, New Orleans, LA 70112, USA
* Corresponding author. 29 English Turn Drive, New Orleans, LA 70131.
E-mail address: henryliula@gmail.com

Anesthesiology Clin 28 (2010) 739–751
doi:10.1016/j.anclin.2010.08.007
1932-2275/10/$ – see front matter © 2010 Elsevier Inc. All rights reserved.

(VLDL) and intermediate density lipoprotein (IDL).[3,5] The increasing number of LDL receptors can eliminate apoB-100 of which VLDL and IDL consist.[3,6]

Statins were historically extracted from a genus of fungal class Ascomycetes, *Penicillium citrinum*, with the effect of interference of cholesterol synthesis. In vivo, mevastatin was the prototypical statin in humans studies. The first approved therapeutic statin was lovastatin, isolated from *Aspergillus terreus*.[3,7] The use of statins is major therapy in the treatment of coronary artery disease (CAD)[8–13] and atherothrombotic stroke.[7] Excellent clinical studies on the effects of statin therapy for medical patients is well documented.[14] There are six major clinical derivatives of statins: lovastatin, pravastatin, simvastatin, atorvastatin, fluvastatin, and rosuvastatin (**Fig. 1**). Due to their structural similarity to HMG-CoA, statins are reversible competitive inhibitors of HMG-CoA (**Fig. 2**).[3]

Statins have been demonstrated to provide reductions in coronary events in multiple patient populations, including men, women, African American, diabetics, smokers and hypertensive patients.[8–13] Reduction of LDL cholesterol concentration yields potential prevention of cardiovascular disease, such as myocardial infarction (MI). There is a 25%–30% reduction in mortality when statin derivatives are used for primary and secondary prevention of cardiovascular disease in patients between 60–80 years of age.[15]

MECHANISM OF LIPID-INDEPENDENT EFFECTS

Multiple studies suggest that statins provide additional cardiovascular benefits through cholesterol-independent or pleiotropic effects. These include, but are not limited to: anti-inflammatory response, anti-thrombosis, enhanced fibrinolysis and decreased platelet reactivity. These are described below and are outlined in **Fig. 3**.[16]

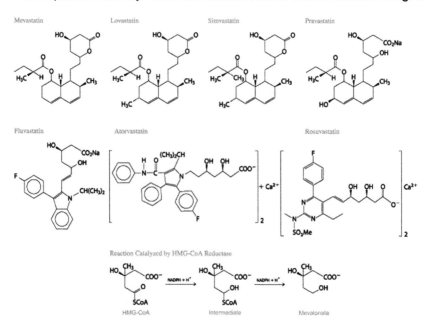

Fig. 1. Biochemical structure of the 7 HMG CoA reductase inhibitors. (*From* Brunton LL, Lazo JS, Parker KL. Goodman & Gillman's the pharmacologic basis of therapeutics. 11th edition. New York (NY): McGraw-Hill; 2006. Available at: http://www.accessmedicine.com. Copyright The McGraw-Hill Companies, Inc; with permission.)

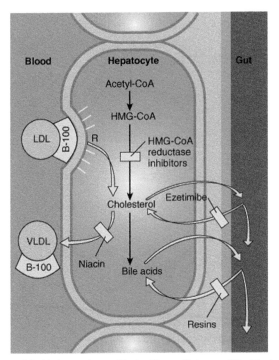

Fig. 2. Mechanism of lipid-dependent effects. (*From* Katzung BG, Masters SB, Trevor AJ. Basic and clinical pharmacology. 11th edition. New York: McGraw-Hill companies; 2009. Available at: http://www.accessmedicine.com/; with permission.)

Anti-Inflammatory Effects

Inhibition of HMG-CoA reductase by statins inhibit the generation of isoprenoids, which prevent downstream inflammatory signaling by obstructing Rho and Ras. These isoprenoids are also downstream products of the cholesterol synthesis pathway. Rho activates nuclear factor, NF-κB, which signals inflammatory responses and reduces endothelial nitric oxide synthetase. Statins inhibit Rho via reduction in C-reactive protein (CRP) and myeloperoxidase. Statins also inhibit cytokines IL-1, IL-6, and IL-8, which activate inflammatory cells and platelets. Also, they increase anti-inflammatory cytokines IL-10 and result in upregulation of endothelial nitric oxide synthetase. **Fig. 4** demonstrates these effects.[17] In total, statins stabilize and reduce imflammatory cells located in the fibrous cap, as well as, the lipid core and reduce the possibility of plaque rupture.[18,19] Fatal post-operative myocardial infarctions are secondary to plaque rupture as often as oxygen demand/supply mismatch.[19,20] This mechanism may account for reductions in perioperative adverse cardiac outcomes in medical patients.[8–13] Lastly, rebound increases in CRP and other inflammatory markers have been shown to occur within 2 days after discontinuation of statins and may be responsible for cardiovascular events after discontinuation of statins.[21]

Vasodilatory Effects

Statins are thought to prolong endothelial Nitric Oxide Synthetase.[22,23] The upregulation of endothelial nitric oxide synthetase by statin-induced inhibition of HMG-CoA

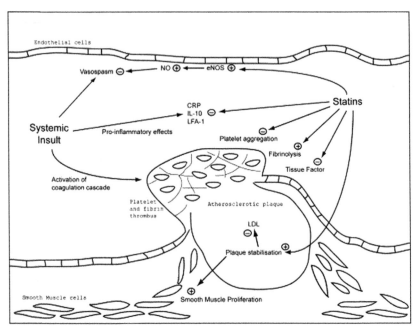

Fig. 3. Summary of relevant pleiotropic effects of statins. NO: nitric oxide; eNOS: endothelial nitric oxide synthase; CRP: C-reactive protein; IL-10: interleukin-10; LFA-1: leucocyte function antigen-1; LDL: low density lipoprotein. (*From* Gajendragadkar PR, Cooper DG, Walsh SR, et al. Novel uses for statins in surgical patients. Int J Surg 2009;7:285–90; with permission.)

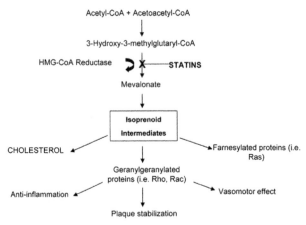

Fig. 4. Pharmacology of statins. The mevalonate pathway is demonstrated with the corresponding G-proteins affected by reduced flux through isoprenoid intermediates to formation of cholesterol. (*Modified from* Williams TM, Harken AH. Statins for surgical patients. Annals of Surgery 2008;247:30–7; with permission.)

reductase results in a rapid increase in nitric oxide bioavailability. Other vasodilatory effects by lipid independent effect of statins are mediated via:

1. Reduced expression of intercellular adhesion molecule, such as E-selectin,
2. Upregulation of heme-oxygenase 1 by monocytes,
3. Inhibition of angiotensin II–induced reactive oxygen species (ROS) production through down-regulation of angiotensin-1 receptors,
4. Inhibition of activation of Rac, a small G protein that contributes to nicotinamide adenine dinucleotide phosphate [NAD(P)H].

Anti-Thrombosis and Anti-Coagulation Effects

Antithrombotic effects of statins can be endothelium-dependent and endothelium-independent. Statins increase endothelial thrombotic expression and alter the balance between plasminogen activator inhibitor and tissue plasminogen activator favoring thrombolysis.[24] Moreover, statins can manipulate effects on coagulation factors V, VII, and XII, which mediate and anti-thrombosis actions derived from anti-inflammatory modulations. It is postulated that statins reduce the inflammatory atherosclerotic processes that lead to plaque instability.[18,20]

PHARMACOKINETICS

The primary mechanism of statins metabolism is through cytochrome P450 3A4 hydroxylation. After oral administration, intestinal absorption of the statins can reach up to 85%[3]. Atorvastatin, pravastatin, fluvastatin, and rosuvastatin, are administered in the β-hydroxy acid form, which is the form that inhibits HMG-CoA reductase. Simvastatin and lovastatin are administered as inactive lactones, which must be first transformed in the liver to their respective β-hydroxy acids, simvastatin acid and lovastatin acid. However, this form undergoes high intestinal clearance and first-pass metabolism, which results in low systemic availability, between 5% and 30% of administered doses. Food has been shown to reduce the rate of statin absorption as well. The maximum plasma concentration of statins absorption occurs in 2 to 4 hours. In the case of atorvastatin and rosuvastatin, which have half-lives of about 15 to 20 hours, the others have that of 1 to 4 hours.[7] The longer half-lives yield greater efficacy of cholesterol lowering.[25] The main drug elimination is via hepatic biliary excretion with less than 2% recovered in the urine.[26]

Adverse Effects

Hepatotoxicity

In addition to the beneficial aspect of statins in prevention of coronary heart disease, they have also demonstrated in clinical studies a low incidence of hepatic toxicity. The most common adverse effect is transaminitis, in which hepatic enzyme levels are elevated in the absence of proven hepatotoxicity. This side effect is usually asymptomatic, reversible, and dose-related.[27] However, there is increasing incidence of chronic liver diseases, including nonalcoholic fatty liver disease and hepatitis, when using statin in patients with high cardiovascular risk.[28] It is reasonable to measure alanine aminotransferase (ALT), which is elevated in hepatitis or other hepatotoxicity. The ALT has normal values of 10–40 U/L in male and 7–35 U/L in female.[3,28]

Myopathy

The most serious adverse effect of statins is rhabdomyolysis, which is an idiosyncratic destruction of muscle tissue, leading to renal failure. Although this may occur secondary to statin use only, this adverse effect is most commonly associated with drug-drug interactions especially in combinations with fibrates: gemfibrozil, 38%; cyclosporine, 4%; digoxin, 5%; warfarin, 4%; macrolide antibiotics, 3%, mibefradil, 2%; and azole antifungals, 1%.[27,28] The statin linked with the most complications, cerivastatin, is no longer commercially available. Cases of fatalities secondary to rhabdomyolysis after statin use are extremely rare. As of 2002, there have been 73 reported cases of fatal rhabdomyolysis. Thirty-one of these deaths are secondary to cerivastatin, which was removed from the market in 2001. The rate of deaths due to rhabdomyolysis is 0.15 deaths per 1 million prescriptions.[29] Despite this rare complication, statins are considered among the safest class of medications available today.[27,30]

Diabetes mellitus

In a relatively recent development, statins have been associated with a potential increased risk of developing diabetes.[31] In a meta-analysis of 13 large placebo controlled trials, Sattar and colleagues[32] found a 9% increase in risk of developing diabetes (OR 1.09, 95% CI 1.02-1.17). This is a small, but statistically significant risk. The risk appeared to be mostly in patients over 60 years of age. The authors calculated that the absolute risk of developing diabetes was one case per 1000 patient-years of statin treatment.

PERIOPERATIVE STATIN USE IN CARDIAC SURGERY

A number of studies have demonstrated patient who receive statins in the perioperative period for CABG or non-coronary cardiac surgery have had lower myocardial ischemia/infarction and lower all cause mortality. The following are the largest studies looking at the effects of perioperative statin use in cardiac surgical cases. Dotani and colleagues[33] in a retrospective chart review demonstrated decreased morbidity at 60 days and 1 year post CABG. Pan and colleagues[34] conducted a retrospective cohort study of 1663 patients undergoing primary coronary artery bypass graft surgery. 943 patients receiving prophylactic statins were compared with 720 patients not on antilipid therapy. After adjusting for demographic and clinical differences between the study and controls, there was an approximate 50% reduction in 30 day all-cause mortality after CABG. They found no association between statin therapy and perioperative atrial fibrillation, stroke, renal failure or MI. Clark and colleagues[35] performed a retrospective evaluation of effect of statin therapy in CABG or CABG/valve surgery. A total of 3892 patients (1044 statin, 2785 no statin) were examined and the authors demonstrated a 45% reduction in 30 day mortality (OR 0.55; 95% CI 0.32-0.93). Collard and colleagues[36] retrospectively studied 2666 patients undergoing primary coronary artery bypass grafting. Multivariate logistic regression analysis demonstrated a 75% reduction of mortality (0.3% vs 1.4%, $P<.03$) in patients taking statins. Discontinuation of statin therapy after CABG was associated with an increased rate of late cardiac and all-cause mortality compared with continuation of statin therapy postoperatively.

The literature is not uniform with regards to the beneficial effects of statins. Recent studies by Subramaniam and colleagues[37] and Ali and Buth[38] did not show a reduction in mortality or morbitity in patients undergoing cardiac surgery.

There are relatively few prospective randomized study of perioperative statin use in cardiac surgery patients. The most recent, by Mannacio and colleagues,[39] involved a randomized trial of 200 CABG patients that compared rosuvastatin 20 mg daily for 1 week before surgery compared with placebo. The rosuvastatin group had significantly lower proportion of patients with elevations of troponin I (35% vs 65%), myoglobin (39% vs 72%)and creatinine kinase (22% vs 40%) compared with the control group ($P<.001$).

Meta-analysis of these as well as other, smaller studies on perioperative effects of statins in cardiac surgery have been completed.[40,41] The Hindler analysis of 10 studies involving cardiac surgery demonstrated an overall 38% reduction in risk of mortality after cardiac surgery in patients receiving preoperative statin therapy (1.9% vs 3.1%, P = .0001).[40] Liakopoulos' meta-analysis included approximately 31,000 patients in 19 trials. Their analysis revealed a significant reduction in all-cause mortality (2.2% vs 3.7%, P<.0001), stroke (2.1% vs 2.9%, OR 0.74, 95%CI: 0.60–0.91), but not for MI (OR 1.11; 95%CI: 0.93–1.33) or renal failure (OR 0.78, 95%CI: 0.46–1.31).[41] Overall, the results demonstrate strongly that there is an association between perioperative statin therapy and reduced morbidity and mortality in cardiac surgery. The findings are limited, however, by the retrospective nature of the majority of the studies and the lack of a uniform protocol for medication, dosage, definition of "perioperative" period, and standardized outcome measures. Additionally, despite these encouraging findings, there is evidence that a significant number of patients that may potentially benefit significantly from statins are not being placed on them.[42]

The findings of the beneficial effects of statins in the periopertaive period are not limited to reductions in mortality and cardiac events. Katznelson and colleagues[43] analyzed 1059 patients undergoing cardiac surgery with CPB for an association between statin use and delirium postoperatively. They demonstrated a 46% reduction in the odds of delirium in the patient that took statins compared with those that did not. Statins have also been studied in the context of reducing post-CABG atrial fibrillation and have shown a reduced incidence of atrial fibrillation compared with controls in both retrospective[33,44–47] and prospective[48] studies. Liakopoulos' meta-analysis demonstrated a statistically significant reduction in atrial fibrillation (24.9% vs 29.3%; OR 0.67, 95% CI: 0.51–0.88).[41]

PERIOPERATIVE OUTCOMES OF STATIN USE IN VASCULAR SURGERY

The additional area in which significant literature exists with regards to the effects of perioperative statins is vascular surgery. The most recent and relevant findings are the results of the Dutch Echocardiographic Cardiac Risk Evaluation Appling Stress Echocardiography (DECREASE) III trial. Is a well-designed prospective, randomized trial of 497 patients that evaluated myocardial ischemia in vascular surgery patients. All enrolled patients had not previously been on statins but all patients were on beta blockers. The study group started fluvastatin XL 80 mg on average 37 days before surgery and continued them for at least 1 month after surgery. The statin group demonstrated a 47% reduction in myocardial ischemia (10.9% vs 19.0%, OR =0 .53; 95% CI: 0.32–0.88, P = .016). Additionally, the endpoint of cardiovascular mortality or non-fatal MI was also decreased from 10.1% to 4.8% (OR = 0.48; 95% CI 0.24-0.95, P = .039). Inflammatory markers (CRP and IL-6) and LDL-C were significantly decreased in the statin group.[49] The same group also prospectively evaluated perioperative statins in vascular surgery patients (DECREASE IV), but in patients that had not been on prior beta blockers or statins. The patients were randomized to receive beta blockade, statins, statins + beta blockade and control. Although the statin groups demonstrated a trend toward lower mortality, it did not reach the level of statistical significance.[50] Durazzo and colleagues[51] performed a prospective blinded randomized controlled trial of atorvastatin before vascular surgery. The statin group demonstrated a 68% reduction in the composite end point of death, acute nonfatal myocardial infarction, stroke or unstable angina (9.1% vs 28.3%, P = .03).

Multiple retrospective studies exist that demonstrate reductions in all-cause and cardiac morbidity and mortality in patients taking statins and undergoing vascular surgery.[52–55] Overall, there is quite strong prospective and retrospective data to support decreased mortality and morbidity in patients presenting for major vascular surgery if statin therapy is initiated perioperatively.

The effects of discontinuation of chronic statin therapy has been evaluated by 2 studies in the vascular surgery population. Schouten and colleagues evaluated the effect of withdrawal of statins in 298 patients after vascular surgery. Patients had an increased risk of postoperative troponin increase (Hazard Ratio = 4.6, CI: 2.2–9.6) and increased combination of post-op MI and cardiovascular death (HR = 7.5; 95% CI, 2.8–20.1).[56] Le Manach and colleagues[57] studied the effect on patients that had their statin discontinued postoperatively after infrarenal aortic surgery. They demonstrated that statin withdrawal greater than 4 days were associated with increased odds of myocardial ischemia (OR 2.9, CI 1.6-5.5). It is postulated that this may be due to the rebound increases in CRP and other inflammatory markers may be responsible for cardiovascular events after discontinuation of statins.[21]

RECOMMENDATIONS

Before 2002, there were no recommendations for the perioperative use of statins, but when Cerivastatin was voluntarily removed from the market in 2001 due to reports of fatal rhabdomyolysis that changed. In 2002, the American College of Cardiology/American Heart Association/National Heart Lung Blood Institute *Clinical Advisory on the Use and Safety of Statins* was organized to investigate the increased incidence of rhabdomyolysis noted with cervistatin and make recommendations for the use of statins. The risk factors linked with an increased incidence of rhabdomyolysis included advanced age, renal or hepatic dysfunction, diabetes, hypothyroidism, medications that interfere with statin metabolism(antifungals, calcium channel blockers, cyclosporins and amiodarone) and patients in the perioperative period. Because of this, the Advisory Committee suggested discontinuation of statins in the perioperative period.[58] Later, it was revealed that the few reported cases of rhabdomyolysis, in patients not on cerivastatin in the perioperative period, may have been related to medications other than statins. A study in 2005, by Schouten and colleagues[59] involving 981 patients found no increased risk of myopathy and no rhabdomyolysis in patients on statins in the perioperative period. It is now recognized that the rare incidence of rhabdomyolysis is heavily outweighed by the observed reduction in perioperative risk (postoperative death) in patients undergoing noncardiac surgery.

Also in 2002, the National Cholesterol Education Program Expert Panel on Detection Evaluation and Treatment of High Blood Cholesterol in Adults issued their recommendations for patients with known coronary artery disease, vascular disease, stroke or diabetes. They suggested that low-density lipoprotein cholesterol (LDL-C) levels be kept below 100 mg/dL.[60] By 2004, recommendations again suggested statin use to achieve a LDL-C levels below 100 mg/dL in patients with known coronary artery disease; however, suggested they should optimally be kept below 70 mg/dL in patients with known coronary artery disease who possess additional risk factors such as diabetes, hypertension, obesity, smoking and acute coronary syndromes.[61] Thus, by this profile, many operative patients would qualify for and receive statin therapy, but discontinue its use perioperatively.

In 2007, studies by LeManach and colleagues[57] and Schouten and colleagues looked at the effects of discontinuing statin therapy in the perioperative period for patients who were long term statin users and undergoing major vascular surgery. LeManach and colleagues explored the premise that statins were able to reduce mortality in the nonsurgical population undergoing an acute coronary syndrome.

They studied 669 patients who underwent major vascular surgery; 491 patients discontinued statin use in the perioperative period and 178 continued statin therapy throughout this period. The median delay in this study between discontinuation and continuation of statin therapy was 4 and 1 day respectively. The group which discontinued statin use was associated with an increased postoperative myonecrosis after major vascular surgery. Schouten and colleagues studied 298 statin users who underwent major vascular surgery. In a total of 70 patients, statin therapy was withdrawn in the perioperative period. The mean duration of statin therapy interruption was 3 days. When compared with the group who received statin therapy throughout the perioperative period, the patients with interrupted statin therapy experienced increased risk for troponin release, myocardial infarction and cardiovascular death. The lipid lowering effects from statins take days to weeks to reverse, so the effects from short term withdrawal could be linked to the lipid- independent or pleiotropic effects that are connected with their use. These pleiotropic effects (antioxidant, anti-inflammatory-decreases in C-reactive protein production, plaque- stabilizing actions, decreased endothelial-1 production, increases in nitric oxide synthetase production, and reduction in platelet aggregation) linked with statin use may be lost acutely and the main reason for the observed cardiovascular benefits found in patients who continue their use in the perioperative period.[56]

Patients presenting for coronary artery bypass grafting or vascular surgery should have statin therapy intiated before surgery. The American College of Cardiology/American Heart Association 2007 perioperative guidelines state "in patients undergoing vascular surgery with or without clinical risk factors, statin use is reasonable.[62]" The perioperative timing of statin initiation in these patients is not certain. A study involving patients with carotid artery disease found the patients who had received statin therapy 6 weeks before surgery were less likely to have symptoms four weeks before surgery. Durazzo and colleagues[51] studied vascular patients and found initiation at least 2 weeks before surgery and continued for 45 days post operatively produced statistically significant rate of cardiovascular complications at six months when compared with the placebo group. Patients with hypercholesterolemia may require more time for dose adjustment.

Most studies suggest that chronic statin users should be continued on therapy throughout the perioperative period. The ACC/AHA 2007 guidelines strongly recommend continuation of statin therapy in patients already on therapy undergoing noncardiac or cardiac surgery and deem it reasonable to consider statin therapy in patients with a risk factor undergoing intermediate-risk procedures.[62] Also, statins should be initiated immediately in patients who experience an acute coronary syndrome postoperatively[63] and logical to assume that patients, who qualify for chronic statin therapy, presenting for elective vascular surgery should be initiated on therapy before having surgery. One study found only 53% of patients presenting for elective abdominal aortic aneurysm surgery were on statins preoperatively,[64] while another study found only 48% of patients with peripheral vascular disease or critical ischemia were on statins preoperatively.[65] Clearly, the patients in these studies would qualify for chronic statin therapy and should be identified preoperatively by the anesthesiologist or surgeon.

Large scale prospective studies with standard outcome measures to provide pooled data do not exist at this time. Also, no standard definition for "perioperative period" is used with regards to beginning or ending statin therapy. Because of this, definitive information for the nonstatin user concerning dosage, timing of initiation and duration of therapy perioperatively for specific surgeries is not available at this time.[66] The physician must determine the lipid lowering effectiveness of the statin dose and have adequate time to rule out increases in hepatic transaminases, myopathies, or drug interactions before proceeding to surgery.

REFERENCES

1. Nichols RL. Surgical infections: prevention and treatment–1965 to 1995. Am J Surg 1996;172:68–74.
2. Bangalore S, Wetterslev J, Pranesh S, et al. Perioperative β blockers in patients having non-cardiac surgery: a meta-analysis. Lancet 2008;372(9654):1962–76.
3. Mahley RW, Bersot TP. Drug therapy for hypercholesterolemia and dyslipidemia. In: Brunton LL, Lazo JS, Parker KL, editors. Goodman & Gilman's the pharmacological basis of therapeutics. 11th edition. New York (NY): McGraw-Hill; 2006. Chapter 35.
4. Aguila-Salinas CA, Barrett H, Schonfeld G. Metabolic modes of action of the statins in the hyperlipoproteinemias. Atherosclerosis 1998;141:203–7.
5. Thompson GR, Nauumova RP, Watts GF. Role of cholesterol in regulating apolipoprotein D secretion by the liver. J Lipid Res 1996;37:439–47.
6. Katzung BG, Masters SB, Trevor AJ. Basic and clinical pharmacology. 11th edition. New York: McGraw-Hill companies; 2009.
7. Afilalo J, Duque G, Steele R, et al. Statinsfor secondary prevention in elderly patients: a hierarchical bayesian meta-analysis. J Am Coll Cardiol 2008;51: 37–45.
8. Randomized trial of cholesterol lowering in 4444 patients with coronary heart disease: the Scandinavian Simvastatin Survival Study (4S). Lancet 1994;344: 1383–9.
9. Shepherd J, Cobbe SM, Ford I, et al. Prevention of coronary heart disease with pravastatin in men with hypercholesterolemia. West of Scotland Coronary Prevention Study Group. N Engl J Med 1995;333:1301–7.
10. ALLHAT Officers and Coordinators for the ALLHAT Collaborative Research Group. The Antihypertensive and Lipid-Lowering Treatment to Prevent Heart Attack Trial. Major outcomes in moderately hypercholesterolemic, hypertensive patients randomized to pravastatin vs. usual care: the Antihypertensive and Lipid-Lowering Treatment of Prevent Heart Attack Trial (ALL HAT-LLT). JAMA 2002;288:2998–3007.
11. Heart Protection Study Collaborative Group. MRC/BHF Heart Protection study of cholesterol lowering with simvastatin in 20,536 high-risk individuals: a randomized placebo-controlled trial. Lancet 2002;306:7–22.
12. Sacks FM, Tonkin AM, Shepherd J, et al. Effect of pravastatin on coronary disease events in subgroups defined by coronary risk factors: the Prospective Pravastain Pooling Project. Circulation 2000;102:1893–900.
13. Downs JR, Clearfielf M, Weis S, et al. Primary prevention of acute coronoary events with lovastatin in men an dwomen with average cholesterol levels: results of AFCAPS/TexCAPS. Air Force/Texas Coronary Atherosclerosis Prrevention Study. JAMA 1998;279:1615–22.
14. Biccard BM. A peri-operative statin update for non-cardiac surgery. Part I: the effects of statin therapy on atherosclerotic disease and lessons learnt from statin therapy in medical (non-surgical) patients. Anaesthesia 2008;63:52–64.
15. Williams D, Feely J. Pharmacokinetic-pharmacodynamic drug interactions with HMG-CoA reductase inhibitors. Clin Pharm 2002;41(5):343–70.
16. Gajendragadkar PR, Cooper DG, Walsh SR, et al. Novel uses for statins in surgical patients. Int J Surg 2009;7:285–90.

17. Williams TM, Harken AH. Statins for surgical patients. Ann Surg 2008;247:30–7.
18. Rosenson RS, Tagney CC. Antiatherothrombotic properties of statins: implications for cardiovascular event reduction. JAMA 1998;279:1643–50.
19. Cohen MC, Artz TH. Histological analysis of coronary artery lesions in fatal postoperative myocardial infarction. Cardiovasc Pathol 1999;8:133–9.
20. Dawood MM, Gupta DK, Southern J, et al. Pathology of fatal perioperative myocardial infarction; implications regarding pathophysiology and prevention. Int J Cardiol 1996;57:37–44.
21. Li JJ, Li YS, Chen J, et al. Rebound phenomenon of inflammatory response may be a major mechanism responsible for increased cardiovascular events after abrupt cessation of statin therapy. Med Hypotheses 2006;66:1199–204.
22. Werner N, Nickenig G, Laufs U. Pleiotropic effects of HMG-CoA reductase inhibitors. Basic Res Cardiol 2002;97:105–16.
23. Wolfrum S, Jensen KS, Liao JK. Endothelium-dependent effects of statins. Arterioscler ThrombVasc Biol 2003;23:729–36.
24. Manach YL, Coriat P, Collard CD, et al. Statin therapy within the perioperative period. Anesthesiology 2008;108:1141–6.
25. Davidson MH. Rosuvastatin: a highly efficacious statin for the treatment of dyslipidaemia. Expert Opin Investig Drugs 2002;1:125–41.
26. Corsini A, Bellosta S, Baetta R, et al. New insights into the pharmacodynamic and pharmacokinetic properties of statins. Pharmacol Ther 1999;84:413–28.
27. Armitage J. The safety of statins in clinical practice. Lancet 2007;370:1781–90.
28. Calderon RM, Cubeddu LX, Goldberg RB, et al. Statins in the treatment of dyslipidemia in the presence of elevated liver aminotransferase levels: a therapeutic dilemma. Mayo Clin Proc 2010;85:349–56.
29. Ballantyne CM, Corsini A, Davidson MH, et al. Risk for myopathy with statin therapy in high-risk patients. Arch Intern Med 2003;163:553–64.
30. Black DM. A general assessment of the safety of HMG CoA reductase inhibitors (statins). Curr Artheroscler Rep 2002;4:34–41.
31. Ridker PM, Danielson E, Fonseca FA, et al. Rosuvastatin to prevent vascular events in men and women with elevated C-reactive protein. N Engl J Med 2008;359:2195–207.
32. Sattar N, Preiss D, Murray HM, et al. Statins and risk of incident diabetes: a collaborative meta-analysis of randomized statin trials. Lancet 2010;375:735–42.
33. Dotani MI, Elnicki DM, Jain AC, et al. Effect of preoperative statin therapy and cardiac outcomes after coronary artery bypass grafting. Am J Cardiol 2000;86:1128–30.
34. Pan W, Pintar T, Anton J, et al. Statins are associated with a reduced incidence of perioperative mortality after coronary artery bypass graft surgery. Circulation 2004;110(11 Suppl 1):1145–9.
35. Clark LL, Ikonomidis JS, Crawford FA Jr, et al. Preoperative statin treatment is associated with reduced postoperative mortality and morbidity in patients undergoing cardiac surgery: an 8 year retrospective cohort study. J Thorac Cardiovasc Surg 2006;131:679–85.
36. Collard CD, Body SC, Shernan SK, et al. Preoperative statin therapy is associated with reduced cardiac mortality after cornonary artery bypass graft surgery. J Thorac Cardiovasc Surg 2006;132:392–400.
37. Subramaniam K, Koch CG, Bashour A, et al. Preoperative statin intake and morbid events following isolated coronary artery bypass grafting. J Clin Anesth 2008;20:4–11.
38. Ali IS, Buth KJ. Preoperative statin use and outcomes following cardiac surgery. Int J Cardiol 2005;103:12–8.

39. Mannacio VA, Iorio D, De Amicis V, et al. Lipid-lowering effect of preoperative statin therapy on postoperative major adverse cardiac events after coronary artery bypass surgery. J Thorac Cardiovasc Surg 2007;134:1143–9.

40. Hindler K, Shaw AD, Samuels J, et al. Improved postoperative outcomes associated with preoperative statin therapy. Anesthesiology 2006;105:1079–80.

41. Liakopoulos OJ, Choi J, Haldenwang PL, et al. Impact of preoperative statin therapy on adverse postoperative outcomes in patients undergoing cardiac surgery: a meta-analysis of over 30,000 patients. Eur Heart J 2008;29:1548–59.

42. Khanderia U, Faulkner TV, Townsend KA, et al. Lipid-lowering herapy at hospital discharge after coronary artery bypass grafting. Am J Health Syst Pharm 2002; 59:548–51.

43. Kaznelson R, Djaiani GN, Borger MA, et al. Preoperative use of statins is associated with reduced early delirium rates after cardiac surgery. Anesthesiology 2009;110:67–73.

44. Marin F, Pascual DA, Roldan V, et al. Statins and postoperative risk of atrial fibrillation following coronary artery bypass grafting. Am J Cardiol 2006;97:55–60.

45. Ozaydin M, Dogan A, Varol E, et al. Statin use before by-pass surgery decreases the incidence and shortens the duration of postoperative atrial fibrillation. Cardiology 2007;107:117–21.

46. Mariscalco G, Lorusso R, Klersy C, et al. Observational study on the beneficial effect of preoperative statins in reducing atrial fibrillation after coronary surgery. Ann Thorac Surg 2007;84:1158–64.

47. Kourliouros A, De Souza A, Roberts N, et al. Dose-related effect of statins on atrial fibrillation after cardiac surgery. Ann Thorac Surg 2008;85:1515–20.

48. Patti G, Chello M, Candura D, et al. Randomized trial of atorvastatin for reduction of postoperative atrial fibrillation in patients undergoing cardiac surgery: results of the ARMYDA-3 (Atorvastatin for Reduction of Myocardial Dysrhythmia After cardiac surgery) study. Circulation 2006;114:1455–61.

49. Schouten O, Boersma E, Hoeks SE, et al. Fluvastatin and perioperative events in patients undergoing vascular surgery. N Engl J Med 2009;361:980–9.

50. Dunkelgrun M, Boersma E, Gemert AK, et al. Abstract 4536: bisopropol and fluvastatin for the reduction of reduction of perioperative cardiac mortality and myocardial infarction in intermediate risk patients undergoing non-cardiovascular surgery; a randomized controlled trial. Circulation 2008;118:S906–7.

51. Durazzo AE, Machado FS, Ikeoka DT, et al. Reduction in cardiovascular events after vascular surgery with atorvastatin: a randomized trial. J Vasc Surg 2004; 39:967–75.

52. Poldermans D, Bax JJ, Kertai MD, et al. Statins are associated with a reduced incidence of perioperative mortality in patients undergoing major noncardiac vascular surgery. Circulation 2003;107:1848–51.

53. O'Neil-Callhan K, Katsimaglis G, Tepper MR, et al. Statins decrease perioperative cardiac complications in patients undergoing non-cardiac vascular surgery: the Statins for Risk Reduction in Surgery (StaRRS) study. J Am Coll Cardiol 2005; 45:336–42.

54. Van Gestel YR, Hoeks SE, Sin DD, et al. Efect of statin therapy on mortality in patients with peripheral arterial disease and comparison of those with versus without associated chronic obstructive pulmonary disease. Am J Cardiol 2008; 102:192–6.

55. Kertai MD, Borsma E, Westerhout CM, et al. Association between long-term statin use and mortality after successful abdominal aortic aneurysm surgery. Am J Med 2004;116:96–103.

56. Schouten O, Hoeks SE, Welten G, et al. Effect of statin withdrawal on frequncy of cardiac events after vascular surgery. Am J Cardiol 2007;100:316–420.

57. Manach YL, Godet G, Coriat P, et al. The impact of postoperative discontinuation or continuation of chronic statin therapy on cardiac outcome after major vascular surgery. Anesth Analg 2007;104:1326–33.

58. American College of Cardiology/American Heart Association/National Heart Lung Blood Institute. Clinical advisory on the use and safety of Statins. J Am Coll Cardiol 2002;40:567–72.

59. Schouten O, Kertai MD, Bax JJ, et al. Safety of perioperative statin use in high-risk patients undergoing vascular surgery. Am J Cardiol 2005;95: 658–60.

60. National Cholesterol Education Program (NCEP) Expert Panel on Detection, Evaluation, and Treatment of High Blood Cholesterol in Adults (Adult Treatment Panel III). Third Report of the National Cholesterol Education Program (NCEP) Expert panel on detection evaluation and treatment of high blood cholesterol in adults (Adult Treatment Panel III) final report. Circulation 2002;106:3143–421.

61. Grundy SM, Cleeman JL, Merz CN, et al. Implications of recent trials for the national cholesterol education program adult treatment panel III guidelines. Circulation 2004;110:227–39.

62. Fleisher LA, Beckman JA, Brown KA, et al. ACC/AHA 2007 Guidelines on perioperative cardiovascular evaluation and care for noncardiac surgery. A report of the American College of Cardiology/American Heart Association Task Forceon practice guidelines. Circulation 2007;116:e418–99.

63. Fonarow GC, Wright RS, Spencer FA, et al. Effect of stain use within the first 24 hours of administration for acute myocardial infarction on early morbidity and mortality. Am J Cardiol 2005;96:611–6.

64. National Confidential Enquiry into Patient Outcome and Death. Report-abdominal aortic aneurysm: a service in need of surgery?. London: NCEPOD; 2005. Available at: http://www.ncepod.org.uk/2005report2/Downloads/AAA_report.doc2005. Accessed July 2, 2010.

65. Conte MS, Bandyk DF, Clowes AW, et al. Risk factors, medical therapies and perioperative events in limb salvage surgery: observations from the PREVENT III multicenter trial. J Vasc Surg 2005;42:829–36 [discussion: 836–7].

66. Bicard BM. A peri-operative statin update for non-cardiac surgery. Part II: Statin therapy for vascular surgery and peri-operative statin trial design. Anaesthesia 2008;63:162–71.

Levosimendan: Calcium Sensitizer and Inodilator

Daun Johnson Milligan, MD[a],*, Aaron M. Fields, MD[a,b]

KEYWORDS

- Levosimendan • Inodilators • Calcium sensitizer
- Decompensated heart failure

Levosimendan is a pyridazone-dinitrile derivative belonging to the novel class of heterogeneous inodilators. Levosimendan may improve mortality in patients with decompensated heart failure by 2 mechanisms. First, the drug enhances myocardial contractility in a unique manner by sensitizing the cardiac microfilament to calcium rather than by increasing calcium influx. The drug achieves this enhancement through functional stabilization of troponin C in a dose-dependent manner, which specifically improves the contractility, stroke volume, and thus cardiac output without inducing arrhythmias or increasing ATP levels or oxygen consumption. This effect is present only during the systole, thus not interfering with diastolic relaxation. Second, levosimendan decreases systemic vascular resistance and preload via venous pooling by initiating arteriolar and venous dilatations, respectively. This effect occurs throughout the body, including coronary and pulmonary vasculatures, by opening ATP-sensitive K^+ channels in smooth muscle. It is by this mechanism that levosimendan establishes a decrease in both preload and afterload. In addition, continuous infusions of levosimendan decrease the pulmonary capillary wedge pressure (PCWP), pulmonary vascular resistance, and pulmonary arterial pressure, which have not been demonstrated by dobutamine or catecholamine infusions.[1] These mechanisms make levosimendan a novel therapeutic option for decompensated congestive heart failure (CHF), which is defined as sustained deterioration of at least 1 New York Heart Association (NYHA) functional class with evidence of volume overload, without the adverse effects of traditional inotropic agents, which mainly rely on β-adrenergic stimulation.[2]

This work was not supported by a grant.
The authors have nothing to disclose.
[a] San Antonio Uniformed Services Health Education Consortium, Brooke Army Medical Center, Division of Anesthesiology and Critical Care, 3851 Roger Brooke Drive, Fort Sam Houston, TX 78234, USA
[b] Division of Anesthesiology and Critical Care, Wilford Hall Medical Center, 2200 Bergquist Drive, Lackland Air Force Base, TX 78236, USA
* Corresponding author.
E-mail address: daun.milligan@us.army.mil

Levosimendan may also be an alternative treatment of other conditions such as compensated CHF, postpartum cardiomyopathy (PPCM), pulmonary hypertension and right-sided heart failure, postmyocardial infarction (post-MI) or postcoronary artery bypass grafting (post-CABG), and severe chronic obstructive pulmonary disease (COPD).

Multiple human studies have shown the superiority of levosimendan over dobutamine in the treatment of acute decompensated heart failure (ADHF). The Levosimendan versus Dobutamine (LIDO) study was one of the earliest randomized control trials on humans to compare the efficacy of the 2 drugs and found that levosimendan statistically improved hemodynamic performance in adult patients with severe CHF.[3] LIDO was a multicenter, randomized, double-blind, double-dummy, parallel-group trial. Patients in the study group (103 patients) received an initial loading dose of levosimendan followed by an infusion, whereas patients in the control group (100 patients) received similar treatment with dobutamine. The primary end point was the proportion of patients demonstrating an increase of 30% or more in cardiac output and a decrease of 25% or more in PCWP at 24 hours. Analyses were by intention to treat. In this trial, 103 patients were assigned levosimendan and 100 dobutamine. The primary hemodynamic end point was achieved in a statistically significant more proportion of patients receiving levosimendan ($P = .022$).[3]

In 2004, the calcium sensitizer or inotrope or none in low-output heart failure (CASINO) study supported the findings of the LIDO trial.[4] The CASINO study was designed to evaluate the efficacy of intravenous levosimendan in patients who were hospitalized because of NYHA class IV decompensated heart failure with left ventricular (LV) dysfunction. The primary end point of mortality was evaluated at 1 month, 6 months, and 1 year in 600 patients. The patients were randomized to 24-hour infusion with levosimendan, dobutamine, or placebo. The results in favor of levosimendan were so compelling that the study was aborted by the safety monitoring board after interim analysis revealed the superiority of levosimendan over dobutamine or placebo treatments.[4]

The randomized multicenter evaluation of intravenous levosimendan efficacy versus placebo in the short-term treatment of decompensated heart failure (REVIVE-II) trial in 2004 was the first large, prospective, randomized, double-blind, controlled trial to compare the effects of levosimendan plus standard therapy with the effects of standard therapy alone during CHF. The standard therapy consisted of various combinations of inotropes and vasopressors. The primary end point was patients' self-rating of moderate to marked improvement at 6 hours, 24 hours, and 5 days. The grading system was as follows:

- Improved: moderately or markedly improved patient global assessment at 6 hours, 24 hours, and 5 days with no worsening.
- Unchanged: neither improved nor worse.
- Worse: death from any cause, persistent or worsening heart failure requiring intravenous medications (diuretics, vasodilators, or inotropes) at any time, or moderately or markedly worse patient global assessment at 6 hours, 24 hours, or 5 days.[5]

The study recruited 600 patients from 103 sites in the United States, Australia, and Israel. It was found that the group receiving levosimendan not only experienced a significant subjective improvement in CHF symptoms but also experienced more side effects of hypotension, ventricular tachycardia, and atrial fibrillation.[5] Although the data generated by the study were encouraging for the role of levosimendan in the treatment of acute heart failure, they merely sought to compare the efficacy of levosimendan with that of currently available drugs traditionally used to treat the condition. The data did not place emphasis on mortality as a primary end point.

A large, prospective, randomized trial monitoring long-term survival in patients with ADHF was held in 2007. The SURVIVal of patients with acutE heart failure in need of intravenous inotropic support (SURVIVE) trial was conducted in 8 European countries and Israel. SURVIVE was a double-blind controlled trial that randomized 1327 patients to either levosimendan or dobutamine. Inclusion criteria were left ventricular ejection fraction (LVEF) less than or equal to 30% and having failed a trial of vasodilators or diuretics. The 180-day all-cause mortality was not statistically different between the 2 groups. The levosimendan group did report dramatically low levels of brain natriuretic peptide (BNP), but the difference seemed to be unrelated to clinical response. Furthermore, the patients in the levosimendan group had significantly more reports of headache, hypokalemia, and arrhythmias than the patients in the dobutamine (control) group.[6] Despite these studies, there was still little human evidence that levosimendan lent any survival benefit to patients with CHF, and the data regarding risk to benefit ratio of the drug were lacking. The studies thus far had demonstrated poor recruiting and were only able to show trends that levosimendan might decrease the death rate in critically ill patients requiring inotropic support.

A recent meta-analysis of randomized controlled studies sought to show that levosimendan reduces the mortality in critically ill patients. Data from a total of 3350 patients from 27 trials supported the theory that levosimendan is associated with a reduction in mortality ($P = .001$) and reduction in the rate of MI ($P = .007$). As suggested by previous studies, it was also found that the levosimendan group again experienced significantly more episodes of hypotension ($P = .02$), most likely because of its prominent effect on systemic vascular resistance. Inclusion criteria for the meta-analysis included random allocation to treatment, no restriction in dose or timing of levosimendan, and mortality as the primary outcome. The secondary end points included hypotension, MI, and renal failure. No significant differences in the occurrence of renal failure between the levosimendan and control groups were found during the meta-analysis.[7]

In 2010, Bergh and colleagues[1] sought to establish the effect of using levosimendan in 60 patients with NYHA class III–IV heart failure who were concurrently on oral β-blockers in a multinational, randomized, double-blind, phase 4 study. At 1-month follow-up, it was found that a 24-hour infusion of levosimendan achieved an improvement in PCWP and/or cardiac index (CI) equal to that achieved by dobutamine at 24 hours and superior to that achieved by dobutamine at 48 hours. The effect was not thought to be caused by the tachyphylaxis of dobutamine because dobutamine had similar PCWP and CI at 24 hours and 48 hours. This finding is supportive of the post hoc analysis of the SURVIVE trial in 2009 by Mebazza and colleagues,[7] which showed that patients with ADHF receiving concomitant β-blocker therapy had a significantly lower mortality if given levosimendan as opposed to dobutamine. Again, levosimendan was associated with a significantly higher incidence of hypotension ($P = .007$). Overall, this study suggests that levosimendan may be a better therapeutic tool for patients with a history of CHF or on β-blocker therapy when they require support for acute exacerbations. This finding is also supported by the LIDO trial and the prospective but small efficacy and safety of short-term intravenous treatment with levosimendan versus dobutamine in decompensated HF patients treated with beta-blockers (BEAT-CHF) trial conducted in 2007.[3,8]

PPCM is a condition with a mortality rate as high as 60%. There is 1 human case report of a 42-year-old-woman surviving after treatment with levosimendan for 24 hours. Her pretreatment echocardiogram revealed an LVEF of 20%, and she required intubation, mechanical ventilation, and vasoactive drugs to counteract her hypotension. After only a few hours of levosimendan treatment, she was weaned from the ventilator, extubated, and taken off vasopressors. Echocardiography 3 months later revealed an LVEF of 50%.[9] The effect may be attributed to levosimendan's mechanism of increasing myocardial sensitivity to calcium without actually increasing the intracellular calcium concentration, which may augment apoptosis and induce arrhythmias.

The mechanisms that make levosimendan unique in the recovery of ADHF make it an attractive drug in the treatment of other diseases as well. In 2002, a study in cats revealed that levosimendan boasts significant vasodilating capacity in the pulmonary vasculature under conditions of high tone, such as pulmonary hypertension. Furthermore, the decreases in pulmonary vasculature tone were dose-dependent. It was this study by De Witt and colleagues[10] which suggested that levosimendan's vasodilatory properties were partially governed by the activation of ATP-sensitive K^+ channels because the effect of levosimendan was dramatically blocked by the concurrent administration of U-37883A, an ATP-sensitive K^+ channel inhibitor. It may be through this ATP-sensitive K^+ channel that levosimendan decreases the size and extent of MI. In addition, this study disproved the theory that levosimendan's vasodilating properties were modulated by cyclooxygenase or dependent on the synthesis of nitric oxide (NO). The study also demonstrated that levosimendan is a more potent vasodilator than siguazodan or rolipram, phosphodiesterase inhibitors 3 and 4, respectively, but could not rule out that levosimendan may in fact exert some of its vasodilatory properties via a phosphodiesterase-inhibiting mechanism.

In 2008, a study published in the *British Journal of Pharmacology* supported the idea that levosimendan does not induce or depend on the formation of NO. The investigators cited that levosimendan has been shown to have beneficial effects in human models of septic shock, both in adults and pediatric patients. They also cited that heart failure and septic shock have been associated with high levels of NO produced by the inducible NO synthase (iNOS) and proinflammatory cytokines. The investigators extrapolated a hypothesis that levosimendan reduces the production of NO during shock states. The study was an in vitro analysis of fibroblasts and macrophages exposed to inflammatory stimuli, mocking a shock state. Both levosimendan and its enantiomer dextrosimendan decreased murine NO production via the iNOS pathway in a dose-dependent manner; these drugs also reduced the production of interleukin 6 but not tumor necrosis factor α. This finding supports clinical evidence that levosimendan has antiinflammatory properties. The data suggest that NO production is inhibited by decreased iNOS promoter activity and nuclear factor κB–dependent transcription, which had previously not been demonstrated.[11]

A direct contrast to the discovery that levosimendan may decrease NO production came in 2009 with a study in porcine coronary endothelial cells (CECs) by Grossini and colleagues.[12] Building on recent published data that the addition of NO synthase (NOS) inhibitor abolishes the coronary vasodilation in anesthetized pigs, the study sought to prove that levosimendan exerted a direct effect on NO production and investigate the intracellular pathway involved. The investigators discovered that in porcine CECs, levosimendan created a concentration-dependent and potassium-dependent augmentation in the expression of NO through the endothelial NOS pathway, an effect amplified by an ATP-sensitive K^+ channel agonist found in mitochondria but not that found in the plasma membrane. Specifically, it was found that levosimendan accomplishes this feat through the production of cyclic adenosine monophosphate and the phosphorylation of certain protein kinases, including P13K/Akt, ERK/mitogen-activated protein kinases (MAPKs) and p38/MAPK. This finding lends evidence to the traditional but unproven notion that levosimendan elicits its positive inotropic effect not only by increasing myocardial sensitivity to calcium but also by inhibiting phosphodiesterase 3.

Levosimendan may have implications in the therapy for disease processes other than decompensated heart failure and pulmonary hypertension. For example, levosimendan has been found to cause a statistically significant enhancement in diaphragm muscle contractility in patients with severe COPD. It has been well established that levosimendan increases cardiac smooth muscle contractility by increasing calcium sensitivity of force contraction; this increase is accomplished through levosimendan binding cardiac troponin C in a calcium-dependent manner, thereby stabilizing the conformational changes in troponin C. However, it was not until the study by van Hees and colleagues[13] that the effect of levosimendan on skeletal muscle became clear. In this in vitro study, diaphragm muscle fibers from thoracotomized patients with and without COPD were exposed to a calcium solution with or without levosimendan. The results showed approximately 25% improved force generation in muscle fibers from 2 types of patients, those with and those without COPD; just as with myocardial fibers, the effect was achieved via increasing calcium sensitivity of force generation. Inspiratory muscle weakness heralds COPD and is often the cause of prolonged mechanical ventilation and death by respiratory failure. Diaphragm muscles from patients with COPD exhibit decreased calcium sensitivity, which is eliminated by the addition of levosimendan, at least in vitro. Implications of this discovery include the drug being a novel therapeutic tool in weaning from mechanical ventilation as well as a potential long-term therapeutic agent to decrease mortality in patients with COPD in general. The major limitations of this study include the fact it was in vitro, it did not consider the effect of levosimendan on other organ systems and vasculature, and it was small in size.

Another arena in which levosimendan may become useful is in overdose of medical agents, which causes dangerous levels of myocardial depression. The typical treatment of calcium antagonist overdose includes decreasing further absorption of the drug as well as the support of vital organ systems, particularly the myocardium. Typically, calcium antagonist intoxication produces hypotension, bradycardia, cardiac conduction abnormalities, and depression of myocardial muscle contractility. The normalization of sinus rhythm is established through the use of atropine, and the restoration of mean arterial pressure is achieved by infusions of catecholamines. There are instances, however, when a patient may be refractory to β-adrenergic stimulation and alternative support must be sought. Based on a case study in which levosimendan seemed to have saved a patient who had overdosed on verapamil, the effect of levosimendan on severe calcium antagonist overdose unresponsive to β-agonist therapy was studied in 2010 by Kurola and colleagues[14] The study included 12 pigs given escalating rates of infusion of intravenous verapamil and then, based on randomization into 2 separate groups, were given either intravenous saline (control) or intravenous levosimendan. The enhancement of myocardial performance was measured with respect to the change in the maximum of the positive slope of left ventricular pressure (LV dP/dt). Although the sample size was small and no statistically significant difference in hemodynamic performance or mortality was noted between the 2 groups, there was a noticeable association between the administration of levosimendan and improved survival. In contrast to data from previous studies, an intravenous bolus of levosimendan in these patients was well tolerated and failed to produce the deleterious side effect of profound hypotension. The investigators suggest this to be true, partly because the inotropic effects of levosimendan seem to be more prominent than the vasodilating properties.

Vasodilating drugs as well as inotropic agents are commonly used to wean patients from cardiopulmonary bypass (CPB) after CABG. Because levosimendan both increases contractility and causes vasodilation, it would be an ideal agent to use in this setting, without the side effects produced by the commonly used agents, such as dobutamine, epinephrine, and nitroglycerin. A small study in 2005 suggested that levosimendan may be useful in weaning patients from CPB after CABG.[15] A subsequent pilot study sought to investigate whether a short infusion of levosimendan (24 μg/kg/min for 10 minutes) before patients were being placed on CPB would provide myocardial protection and improve hemodynamics. Patients receiving the levosimendan infusion had lower troponin I concentrations for up to 48 hours postoperatively and higher cardiac indices than the controls. These data suggest that levosimendan may have a preconditioning effect on the myocardium.[16] Levosimendan may also serve as a more attractive alternative to intra-aortic balloon devices, which are invasive and have a high rate of complication. It has been shown that less than half of the patients requiring intra-aortic balloon devices as a bridge to recovery after severe postcardiotomy heart failure survive to hospital discharge. In 2006, Braun and colleagues[17] conducted a retrospective study on 41 patients who failed to wean from CPB and subsequently received an intra-aortic balloon device. Although the study was small, levosimendan provided statistically significant improvement in medium-term survival at both 14 and 180 days.

There have been much data generated on the positive inotropic effect of levosimendan on the LV; however, the effect of this calcium sensitizer on the left atrium (LA) was unknown until Duman and colleagues[18] compared the effect of levosimendan with that of dobutamine on LA function. In this study 74 patients with decompensated heart failure and an ejection fraction (EF) of 35% or less were enrolled to randomly receive levosimendan or dobutamine. Measurements of LA passive and active emptying fractions and the ratio of mitral inflow early diastolic velocity to annulus velocity were recorded using pulsed wave and tissue Doppler. Effect on BNP production was also analyzed, as had been done in previous studies on the effect of levosimendan on LV function. The results indicated that EF was significantly increased in both the levosimendan and dobutamine groups; however, the levosimendan group experienced a greater decrease in BNP and a greater increase in active emptying fraction at 24 hours. The ratio of mitral inflow early diastolic velocity to annulus velocity was significantly improved in the levosimendan group, and this improvement correlated with a decrease in BNP. This study was the first to demonstrate that levosimendan improves LA function and LV diastolic function in patients with heart failure.

The implications for levosimendan in the treatment of decompensated heart failure are vast. As the health care community faces an aging patient load populated by survivors of acute cardiac events, there will be a growing number of hospitalizations for acute episodes of decompensation in heart failure and accordingly a great demand for novel and appropriate treatment. And because most patients presenting as such will be on long-term β-blocker therapy, which may complicate traditional acute treatment, the possibility of using levosimendan and other calcium sensitizers will become more and more important.

Although levosimendan is available both in an oral and intravenous form, the bulk of clinical data have been generated on intravenous levosimendan. The drug's main pharmacokinetic parameters in the patient with CHF include linearity, 98% binding to plasma proteins, an elimination half-life of approximately 1 hour, and complete metabolism with some active metabolites. In fact, the highly active metabolite OR-1896 can cause an effect lasting between 70 and 80 hours in a patient with acute heart failure. Although some of the earlier human trials suggested multiple side effects, levosimendan seems to be fairly well tolerated. The main side effects, hypotension and headache, are most likely because of vasodilation and are a direct reflection of dosing. Other side effects include arrhythmias, particularly atrial fibrillation, extrasystoles, atrial or ventricular tachycardia, myocardial strain or ischemia, hypokalemia, or preexisting severe nausea.[19] The LIDO trial discovered that levosimendan was associated with fewer significant adverse events than the traditionally used drug dobutamine.[3] In addition, to date, levosimendan does not seem to cause drug interactions of any kind with drugs commonly used to treat heart failure, such as β-blockers, angiotensin-converting enzyme inhibitors, warfarin, digoxin, or nitrates. The typical dosage of intravenous levosimendan as used in most clinical trials is 12 μg/kg loading dose over 10 minutes followed by 0.05 μg/kg/min continuous infusion. Hemodynamic effects become visible several minutes into the loading dose, peak effect occurs at approximately 30 minutes, and duration of action is roughly 1 hour. Patients with mild to moderate renal failure or mild hepatic failure do not require reduction in dosing.[19] Contraindications to the usage of the drug include severe renal or hepatic impairment, severe ventricular filling or outflow obstruction, preexisting hypotension or tachycardia, or a history of torsades de pointes.[20]

Three main concerns for using levosimendan in the treatment of ADHF limit its usefulness. First, the drug is expensive. Second, there is not yet a specific time to start the therapy during an episode of decompensation and it is not clear whether levosimendan should be used solely or as an adjunct to traditional treatments.[20] Last, it is not yet available in the United States. Regardless, it is clear that more research and larger, prospective randomized clinical trials are warranted in the investigation of levosimendan and its role in certain chronic and common illnesses.

In summary, levosimendan is a unique therapeutic agent that decreases mortality in acute episodes of decompensated heart failure by increasing myocardial contractility without increasing oxygen consumption or ATP levels, decreasing preload, and decreasing afterload. The mechanism for each accomplishment is novel. The drug is a calcium sensitizer, which increases myocyte contractility by stabilizing troponin C rather than by increasing intracellular calcium. The vasodilatory properties are achieved by the opening of ATP-sensitive K^+ channels. The drug has been shown in a recent meta-analysis to be superior to the traditionally used dobutamine, and it may play a role in treating acute episodes of heart failure in patients on long-term β-blockers whose effect decreases the responsiveness to traditional treatment. The drug may have implications in numerous other common and chronic medical ailments, even in overdoses of drugs that stun and depress the myocardium.

REFERENCES

1. Bergh CH, Bert A, Dahlstrom U, et al. Intravenous levosimendan vs. dobutamine in acute decompensated heart failure patients in beta-blockers. Eur J Heart Fail 2010;12:404–10.
2. Mills RM, Hobbs RE. Drug treatment of patients with decompensated heart failure. Am J Cardiovasc Drugs 2001;1(2):119–25.
3. Follath F, Cleland JG, Just H, et al. Steering committee and investigators of the levosimendan infusion versus dobutamine (LIDO) study. Efficacy and safety of intravenous levosimendan compared with dobutamine in severe low-output heart failure (the LIDO study): a random double-blind trial. Lancet 2002;360:196–202.
4. Zairis MN, Apostolatos C, Anastasiadis P, et al. The effect of a calcium sensitizer or an inotrope or none in chronic low output decompensated heart failure: results from the Calcium Sensitizer or Inotrope or None in Low Output Heart Failure Study

(CASINO) [abstract 835–6]. Program and abstracts from the American College of Cardiology Annual Scientific Sessions 2004. New Orleans, LA, March 7–10, 2004.

5. Cleland JG, Freemantle N, Coletta A, et al. Clinical trials update from the American heart association: REPAIR-AMI, ASTAMI, JELIS, MEGA, REVIVE-II, SURVIVE, and PROACTIVE. Eur J Heart Fail 2006;8(1):105–10.

6. Landoni G, Mizzi A, Biondi-Zoccai G, et al. Levosimendan reduces mortality in critically ill patients. A meta-analysis of randomized controlled studies. Minerva Anestesiol 2010;76:276–86.

7. Mebazaa A, Nieminen MS, Filipattos G, et al. Levosimendan vs. dobutamine: outcomes for acute heart failure patients on beta-blockers in SURVIVE. Eur J Heart Fail 2009;11:304–11.

8. Bergh CH, Andersson B, Dahlstrom U, et al. Intravenous levosimendan versus dobutamine in acute decompensated heart failure patients treated with beta-blockers (BEAT-CHF study). Eur Heart J 2007;28:5388–9.

9. Uriate-Rodriguez A, Santa-Cabrera L, Sanchez-Palacios M, et al. Levosimendan use in the emergency management of decompensated peripartum cardiomyopathy. J Emerg Trauma Shock 2010;3(1):94.

10. De Witt BJ, Ibrahim IN, Bayer E, et al. An analysis of responses to levosimendan in the pulmonary vascular bed of the cat. Anesth Analg 2002;94:1427–33.

11. Sareila O, Korhonen R, Auvinen H, et al. Effects of levo- and dextrosimendan on NF-kappaB-mediated transcription, iNOS expression and NO production in response to inflammatory stimuli. Br J Pharmacol 2008;155:884–95.

12. Grossini C, Molinari C, Caimmi P, et al. Levosimendan induces NO production through p38 MAPK, ERK, and Akt in porcine coronary endothelial cells: role for mitochondrial K(ATP) channel. Br J Pharmacol 2009;156:250–61.

13. van Hees HW, Dekhuijzen PN, Heunks LM, et al. Levosimendan enhances force generation of diaphragm muscle from patients with chronic obstructive pulmonary disease. Am J Respir Crit Care Med 2009;179:41–7.

14. Kurola J, Leppikangas H, Magga J, et al. Effect of levosimendan in experimental verapamil-induced myocardial depression. Scand J Trauma Resusc Emerg Med 2010;18:12–9.

15. Siirila-Waris K, Suojaranta-Ylinen R, Harjola VP, et al. Levosimendan in cardiac surgery. J Cardiothorac Vasc Anesth 2005;19(3):345–9.

16. Tritapepe L, De Santis V, Vitale D, et al. Preconditioning effects of levosimendan in coronary artery bypass grafting–a pilot study. Br J Anaesth 2006;96(6):694–700.

17. Braun JP, Jasulaitis D, Moshirzadeh M, et al. Levosimendan may improve survival in patients requiring mechanical assist devices for post-cardiotomy heart failure. Crit Care 2006;10:R17.

18. Duman D, Palit F, Simsek E, et al. Effects of levosimendan versus dobutamine on left atrial function in decompensated heart failure. Can J Cardiol 2009;25(10): e353–6.

19. ISPUB. Dobutamine kills goods hearts! Levosimendan may not. Available at: http://www.ispub.com. Accessed April 3, 2010.

20. Levosimendan (INN)- drug information from Medic8.com. Available at: http://www.medic8.com/medicines/Levosimendan.html. Accessed April 10, 2010.

Molecular Approaches to Improving General Anesthetics

Stuart A. Forman, MD, PhD

KEYWORDS

- General anesthesia • Drug development • Drug discovery
- Mechanism • Trends • Etomidate • Xenon

Over the last several decades, the average age of patients has steadily increased, whereas the use of general anesthesia and deep sedation has grown largely outside the operating room environment. Currently available general anesthetics and delivery models represent limitations in addressing these trends. At the same time, research has tremendously expanded the knowledge of how general anesthetics produce their beneficial effects and also revealed evidence of previously unappreciated general anesthetic toxicities. The goal of this review is to highlight these important developments and describe translational research on new general anesthetics with the potential to improve and reshape clinical care.

DEMOGRAPHICS AND PRACTICE TRENDS AFFECTING ANESTHESIOLOGY

There are two large trends that affect the demands on anesthesia providers in the United States: (1) the demographic trend toward an aging population and (2) the increasing use of anesthesia for outpatient procedures, frequently outside the traditional operating room environment.

Between 1995 and 2010, the US population older than 65 years increased by approximately 20%, which is significantly faster than the total population.[1] In the next 15 years, the population aged 65 years or greater is expected to increase by more than 50% (**Table 1**). This group of patients has the highest incidence of chronic systemic diseases and also requires more procedures for management of such diseases. Older patients are also overrepresented among those undergoing inpatient

Funding: This work was supported in part by the Department of Anesthesia, Critical Care & Pain Medicine, MGH and by a grant from the National Institutes of Health (P01-GM58448).

Disclosure: The author is named as an inventor on patents for two derivatives of etomidate discussed in this article. At present, the author has no financial relationships deriving from these inventions.

Department of Anesthesia, Critical Care & Pain Medicine, Massachusetts General Hospital, Jackson 4, MGH, 55 Fruit Street, Boston, MA 02114, USA

E-mail address: saforman@partners.org

Table 1			
Growth in elderly US population			
Year	Estimated US Population	Percentage ≥65 y	Population ≥65 y
1995	265,066,000	12.8	33,928,000
2010	309,163,000	13.2	40,810,000
2025	337,361,000	18.5	62,412,000

Data from Campbell PR. Population projections for states by age, sex, race, and Hispanic origin: 1995 to 2025. Washington, DC: U.S. Government Printing Office; 1996 (U.S. Bureau of the Census, Population Division, PPL-47, 90 pages).

surgery.[2] Moreover, the high frequency of comorbidities among the elderly population increases their risk for surgical complications and toxicities associated with general anesthesia. Common toxicities of general anesthetics, such as hypotension, respiratory depression, and hypothermia, are exaggerated and dangerous in elderly patients. Advanced age is also an important risk factor for postoperative cognitive dysfunction (POCD). In summary, anesthetists are confronted with a rapidly increasing population of older patients having major procedures as inpatients and frequently burdened with systemic diseases.

The second trend influencing delivery of anesthesia care is the growth in the use of minimally invasive surgical and diagnostic approaches requiring general anesthesia but done on an outpatient basis. An assessment by the Agency for Healthcare Research and Quality reported that in 2003, more than 50% of surgeries in the United States were done on an outpatient basis.[2] As the number of ambulatory surgery centers continues to increase, the proportion of outpatient surgeries continues to grow. In these outpatient settings, the risk associated with general anesthesia is frequently greater than that posed by the concomitant procedure; thus, the burden to assure patient safety falls heavily on anesthesia personnel. In addition, recovery from general anesthesia is a particularly critical determinant of surgical productivity in the outpatient setting. For example, colonoscopic examinations typically require 20 minutes to complete, but recovery from sedatives frequently given during this procedure often takes an hour or more. Under these conditions, each gastroenterologist requires about 3 recovery beds and associated equipment and staffing to optimize the number of procedures performed. As a result, faster and more reliable recovery from general anesthesia has the potential to dramatically affect both efficiency and cost of care in these settings.

MECHANISMS OF GENERAL ANESTHESIA

Knowledge about how general anesthetics produce their beneficial and toxic effects is essential as a foundation on which researchers can design strategies for developing improved anesthetics. The last few decades have seen tremendous advances in the understanding of the mechanisms underlying general anesthesia.[3,4]

General anesthetic pharmacology is unique because so many types of molecules possess this activity, including simple gases, alcohols, alkanes, ethers, barbiturates, steroids, and other organic compounds. In the nineteenth century, Claude Bernard asserted that all general anesthetics produced their effects on animals via a common pathway (the Unitary Hypothesis), and Meyer and Overton both noted that general anesthetic potency was largely explained by a single biophysical property called hydrophobicity (or lipid solubility). These 2 seminal ideas led scientists to focus on lipid membranes as the primary site of general anesthetic action. A critical paradigm shift in research on mechanisms of general anesthesia was the change in focus from effects on membrane lipids to direct effects on membrane proteins and particularly on ion channels in neurons. Franks and Lieb[5] demonstrated that the nonspecific pharmacology of general anesthetics could be observed in a lipid-free protein enzyme. These experiments showed that lipids were no longer necessary to explain the association between anesthetic drug potency and hydrophobicity and instead suggested that anesthetics bind directly to sites on proteins. Using molecular biologic tools that enable the study of mutated proteins, research on neurotransmitter receptor channels has provided convincing evidence that general anesthetics do in fact act directly on channel proteins.[6,7]

Major research efforts to identify neuronal ion channels that are likely to mediate the actions of general anesthetics in the central nervous system identified several fast neurotransmitter receptor channels, including γ-aminobutyric acid type A (GABA$_A$) receptors, glycine receptors, nicotinic acetylcholine (nACh) receptors, and N-methyl-$_D$-aspartate (NMDA) sensitive glutamate channels.[3] Other major general anesthetic targets are the two-pore domain potassium (2PK) channels that produce background potassium leaks in neurons, stabilizing them in a nonexcitable state.[8] Some general anesthetics activate the 2PK channels, further increasing this stabilizing antiexcitatory current.

An important revelation emerged from studies on a variety of ion channel targets: groups of drugs with similar clinical properties often act at similar sets of ion channels (**Table 2**).[9,10] The important clinical actions produced by all general anesthetics include amnesia, hypnosis (unconsciousness), and immobilization during painful stimuli.[11] Other effects, such as analgesia and alterations in autonomic functions, vary widely among different anesthetics. Thus, propofol, etomidate, and alphaxalone are all potent intravenous amnestic or hypnotic drugs, but very high doses of these drugs are required to prevent movement in response to noxious stimulation. This group of drugs acts primarily by enhancing the activity of inhibitory GABA$_A$ receptors. A group of gaseous general anesthetics including nitrous oxide, xenon, and cyclopropane are weak immobilizers and hypnotics but they produce analgesia and autonomic stability. These gaseous agents, along with ketamine, act primarily by inhibiting excitatory ion channels such as glutamate and neuronal nACh receptors and act at 2PK channels as well. A third large group of general anesthetics includes the volatile agents and barbiturates. These drugs produce the classic effects of general anesthesia in a predictable manner as their concentration increases: amnesia, then hypnosis, and then immobility. Their molecular targets are widespread, including both inhibitory and excitatory neurotransmitter-gated channels, 2PK channels, proteins involved in presynaptic neurotransmitter release, and indirect modulators of neuronal excitability such as G protein–coupled receptors.

A small number of sites where general anesthetics interact with ion channels have been identified using photolabeling and mutational analysis. In nACh receptors, inhibition seems to be caused by the binding of the anesthetic to a discrete region within the transmembrane cation pore.[6] Photolabeling with long-chain alcohols also identified binding sites in the pore domains of nACh receptors.[12] In GABA$_A$ receptors, a photolabel analogue of etomidate was used to identify residues in transmembrane amino acids in which two subunits make contact within the membrane.[13] Mutations at the photolabeled sites affect interactions with etomidate, confirming that they are likely contact points between the protein and drug.[14]

In a growing number of cases, transgenic animal studies have strengthened inferences about the role of specific types of ion channels in the actions of general anesthetics. Mice containing GABA$_A$ receptor β2 or β3 subunit point mutations that dramatically reduce sensitivity to etomidate, propofol, and volatile anesthetics have

Table 2
Correlation between clinical profile and molecular targets of general anesthetics

	Group 1	Group 2	Group 3
Drugs	Etomidate, propofol, alphaxalone	Barbiturates, halogenated alkanes, and ethers	Nitrous oxide, xenon, ketamine, cyclopropane
Ratio of MAC-Immobility: MAC-Hypnosis	4+	2–3	1.5–2
Analgesia	None	None	Yes
Organ Protection	None	Ischemic preconditioning	Yes (xenon)
EEG effects	Reduced frequency	Reduced frequency	Minimal change or increased frequency
Molecular Targets	GABA$_A$ receptors, HCN1 (propofol)	GABA$_A$ receptors, glycine receptors, neuronal nACh receptors, 2PK channels, glutamate receptors, others	Glutamate receptors, neuronal nACh receptors, 2PK channels, others

Abbreviations: EEG, electroencephalogram; MAC, minimal alveolar concentration.

proved to be especially informative. Transgenic mice with a mutation in β3 subunits display markedly reduced sensitivity to the hypnotic and immobilizing actions of propofol and etomidate but only modestly reduced sensitivity to isoflurane.[15] In contrast, transgenic mice with mutated β2 subunits show reduced sensitivity to the sedative but not to the hypnotic and immobilizing actions of propofol and etomidate.[16] These data indicate that GABA$_A$ receptors containing β3 subunits play a particularly important role in neural pathways mediating major effects of intravenous anesthetics. Knockout mice lacking the gene for one anesthetic-sensitive 2PK channel (TASK3) display reduced sensitivity to the actions of specific volatile anesthetics.[17] Mutant mice lacking the ε1 subunit of NMDA receptors were shown to be resistant to the hypnotic effects of nitrous oxide.[18] However, these knockout mice were also shown to have globally enhanced monoaminergic tone and their resistance to immobilization by a variety of general anesthetics was sensitive to manipulation of excitatory amino acid levels.[19] Related experiments have been done in *Caenorhabditis elegans*, a flatworm with a simple nervous system. Knockout of the *C elegans* gene encoding a homologue of NMDA receptors made animals insensitive to nitrous oxide.[20] Knockout of another gene encoding a different glutamate receptor channel eliminated sensitivity to xenon.[21]

GENERAL ANESTHETIC TOXICITIES

The toxicities of general anesthetics vary, and the molecular targets underlying toxicities are known in only a few cases. The best understood example is a unique toxicity of etomidate, the only general anesthetic containing an imidazole group. Suppression of adrenal cortisol synthesis by etomidate was discovered a few years after its introduction into clinical practice.[22] The specific molecular target in the adrenal gland was identified as 11β-hydroxylase (CYP11B1), a mitochondrial cytochrome enzyme that converts 11-deoxycortisol to cortisol. Given the large number of imidazole derivatives that are known to inhibit various heme-containing enzymes, it is likely that the imidazole ring of etomidate forms a strong coordinate bond with the iron atom in the catalytic center of 11β-hyroxylase, blocking substrate access to this site.

Another unique and rare toxicity that is associated with prolonged sedation using propofol is the propofol infusion syndrome characterized by dysrhythmias, lipemia, fatty liver, metabolic acidosis, and rhabdomyolysis.[23] In this case, it is thought that the toxicity is not due to the anesthetic molecule but the lipid component of the drug vehicle, which is used to increase propofol solubility.

Other common toxicities of general anesthetics include respiratory depression, hypotension, hypothermia, and postoperative nausea and vomiting (PONV). There is a clear need for investigation of the molecular targets mediating these effects, which likely vary for each type of anesthetic. Some of these targets have been identified for some general anesthetics. For example, anesthetic-sensitive 2PK channels play critical roles in respiratory drive,[24] and drugs that selectively inhibit these channels are used as respiratory stimulants.[25] Thus, it is likely that anesthetic potentiation of 2PK channel activity contributes to respiratory depression and insensitivity to hypoxia/acidosis. Although etomidate and propofol both induce hypnosis and immobility through enhanced $GABA_A$ receptor activation, etomidate produces remarkable hemodynamic stability. It is likely that etomidate lacks activity at target molecules that mediate hypotension in the presence of other anesthetics, but molecular and transgenic animal studies also suggest that hemodynamic stability with etomidate is caused by its agonist activity at certain adrenergic receptors.[26] Similarly, propofol is widely favored as an induction agent for general anesthesia because it produces less PONV than other related drugs. Although the molecular targets triggering PONV by other anesthetics are not well defined, there is evidence that propofol possesses a unique antiemetic activity, apparently mediated indirectly through cannabinoid receptors.[27]

In addition to the short-term toxicities noted earlier, evidence of potential long-term neurotoxic effects of general anesthetics is a source of growing concern for patients and physicians.[28] POCD is a transient cognitive impairment characterized by problems with memory, concentration, language comprehension, and social integration.[29] It usually resolves within 1 year but is also associated with an increased risk of dementia developing years later.[30] Known risk factors for POCD include advanced age, low educational background, chronic diabetes and/or vascular disease, and coronary artery bypass graft surgery.[31,32] Notably, many of these symptoms and risk factors for POCD are similar to those for Alzheimer disease, a common form of dementia in the elderly. Preclinical models of POCD suggest that the type of anesthesia may be an important pathogenic factor as well,[33,34] although clinical studies have not consistently supported this hypothesis.[35] Nonetheless, evidence is accumulating that general anesthetics cause long-term changes to neuronal viability and function. In particular, volatile anesthetics have been shown to accelerate the oligomerization of amyloid-β (Aβ) peptide, which is thought to be an early step in the development of Alzheimer dementia.[36] Neurons exposed to both Aβ and volatile anesthetics undergo cell death at a significantly higher rate than those exposed to Aβ alone. Another hypothesized mechanism for POCD suggests that it is caused by an increased systemic inflammation associated with surgery and is perhaps enhanced by certain general anesthetics.[37] Surgery and anesthesia increase the release of several inflammatory mediators, including tumor necrosis factor (TNF) α, tissue growth factor β, and proinflammatory interleukins (IL-1β and IL-6). Again, clinical evidence does not strongly support this hypothesis,[38] but it is likely that POCD is multifactorial.

At the other extreme of age, concern is growing that general anesthetics may be harmful to the developing brain. There is convincing evidence that most known general anesthetics dramatically accelerate neuronal apoptosis (cell death) during critical phases of fetal brain development in both rodents and primates.[39,40] Rodent experiments also suggest that this damage can lead to abnormal learning and memory functions, although evidence of these manifestations in humans remains controversial while definitive studies are conducted. Mechanisms underlying this toxicity seem to be linked to the same ion channels that mediate the beneficial effects of general anesthesia. For example, a wide variety of general anesthetics that enhance GABA$_A$ receptor activity are hypothesized to produce excitotoxicity in developing neurons, which have different transmembrane chloride gradients than mature neurons. Although ketamine lacks GABA$_A$ receptor activity, it produces neuroapoptosis in developing animal brains.[41,42]

STRATEGIES FOR DEVELOPING NEW GENERAL ANESTHETICS

The issues reviewed in the previous sections represent a multidimensional framework for improving existing general anesthetics. The ideal general anesthetic would address all of these issues (**Box 1**), but in the real world, drug development efforts are often limited to a small number of goals. Broadly speaking, these efforts are aimed at (1) ameliorating the neurotoxic effects of current general anesthetics, (2) reducing or eliminating other clinically significant toxicities of specific agents through mechanism-based drug design, and (3) identifying novel general anesthetics.

Neuroprotection Strategies

Xenon is a monoatomic noble gas. It possesses anesthetic activity, and as an anesthetic, displays many desirable features.[43] It is odorless and nonpungent and produces no bronchial reactivity during inhalation. Xenon solubility in blood and tissue is lower than that of nitrous oxide, and therefore, xenon has even faster onset and offset kinetics. It is stable in storage, is nonflammable, undergoes zero metabolism, elicits no allergies, and produces minimal cardiovascular depression. Xenon itself is environmentally benign, although the amount of energy required to collect and purify it represents a considerable, albeit indirect, environmental effect. Toxicities of xenon include respiratory depression, hypothermia, and PONV. In addition, minimal alveolar concentration for xenon is 0.6 atm, and its use at high partial pressures is associated with expansion of trapped air spaces in the body. The major impediment to xenon as a clinical anesthetic is its cost (more than $10/L), which currently is prohibitive, but technologies to enable closed-circuit administration and reclamation of xenon in scavenged gas may reduce the overall cost of this anesthetic.

Box 1
Characteristics of an ideal general anesthetic

- Safety, high therapeutic index and no toxicities (perhaps even organ protective)
- Comfort, minimal pain on injection or minimal pungency if inhaled
- Rapid onset/offset
- Low metabolic burden and safe in renal/hepatic dysfunction (potent if intravenous, nonmetabolized if inhaled)
- Economical to make and store
- Environmentally benign

A research team at the Imperial College in London has renewed clinical interest in xenon as an anesthetic with unique neuroprotective properties. Their research in preclinical models has shown that xenon protects neurons and brain tissue from damage caused by anoxia,[44] cardiopulmonary bypass,[45] traumatic brain injury,[46] or volatile anesthetics in developing brain models.[47] Mechanistic studies demonstrate that xenon inhibits NMDA receptors, and molecular modeling suggests that unlike other drugs with similar activity, xenon may bind within the glycine coagonist sites of these proteins.[48]

Two clinical trials focusing on acute POCD have so far demonstrated no protective effect with xenon.[49,50] Two other clinical trials are investigating neuroprotection by xenon; one in the setting of brain ischemia in cardiac arrest and another in the setting of perinatal asphyxia.

Alternative neuroprotective strategies focus on compounds that lack anesthetic activity. Argon, like xenon, seems to have some neuroprotective activity in preclinical models.[51] In addition, inhibitors of inflammatory mediators, such as TNF-α, are also being investigated for their perioperative organ protective properties.

Mechanism-Based Drug Design

A detailed understanding of the mechanisms underlying both beneficial and toxic anesthetic actions enables researchers to identify ways that these actions can be independently manipulated. An excellent example is the development of the water-soluble propofol prodrug, fospropofol, thus both eliminating the need for lipid carrier and reducing the risk of propofol infusion syndrome.[52] Because of recently discovered problems with the assay used for fospropofol, the validity of clinical pharmacokinetic and pharmacodynamic studies, and their comparison with propofol, is questionable and a number of these studies have recently been retracted.[53] Nonetheless, this formulation may have clear advantages over propofol for long-term sedation.

A team at Harvard (of which S.A.F. is a member) has recently applied mechanism-based drug design in the development of 2 new etomidate analogues. Both new compounds have the potential to reduce adrenal toxicity. Methoxycarbonyl (MOC)-etomidate is a "soft" etomidate analogue.[54] Like esmolol and remifentanil, MOC-etomidate incorporates an accessible ester linkage, imparting rapid metabolism by nonspecific esterases in blood and tissues. Because it is metabolized at least 100 times faster than etomidate, MOC-etomidate is associated with a much shorter period of adrenal suppression. Assuming it can be used as an infusible general anesthetic for procedures of modest duration, MOC-etomidate may also provide for reliable rapid emergence. Carboetomidate is another etomidate analogue designed to retain the molecular shape of the parent drug while eliminating its adrenal toxicity.[55] This design was achieved by replacing the 5-membered imidazole ring of etomidate with a pyrrole ring and placing a carbon in the position of the nitrogen that was implicated in heme-binding interactions. Carboetomidate shows potent hypnotic activity in animals and seems to maintain other favorable clinical attributes of etomidate. In addition, its potency for the inhibition of 11β-hydroxylase is approximately 1000-fold lower than that of etomidate.

Screening for New General Anesthetics

Although the aforementioned strategies rely on exploitation of existing knowledge, the value of improving general anesthetics may have reached a tipping point where high-risk exploration strategies are justifiable. A research team at the University of Pennsylvania has combined two recent discoveries to launch such an effort. The first advance was the identification of a soluble protein that binds a wide variety of general anesthetics with high affinities. Apoferritin is a 24-subunit globular protein that binds and transports iron in all cells and tissues. Ferritin subunits each contain four helical domains, a structure similar to the four transmembrane helices of $GABA_A$ receptor subunits. The team at Penn discovered that apoferritin binds a variety of volatile anesthetics and propofol analogues with affinities that correlate nicely with the ability to potentiate GABA responses at $GABA_A$ receptors.[56,57] Furthermore, crystallographic studies showed that the anesthetic binding pocket in apoferritin is formed by helical domains at the interfaces between subunits, echoing the structure of anesthetic sites in $GABA_A$ receptors. The Penn team also discovered a fluorescent general anesthetic, 1-aminoanthracene, which binds selectively to neural tissues and also to apoferritin.[58] These two technologies were combined to create a high-throughput screening tool that uses fluorescence to detect novel compounds that compete with 1-aminoanthracene for occupation of the anesthetic site on apoferritin.[59] The initial screen identified 18 new compounds that are being further tested for general anesthetic activity.

SUMMARY

A variety of emerging factors are challenging anesthetists to improve safety, productivity, and the overall quality of patient experience. These factors include the (1) rapidly growing population of elderly patients, who have a high incidence of significant coexisting systemic diseases and who are likely to undergo a growing number of major surgical procedures as inpatients; (2) rapidly expanding use of outpatient diagnostic and therapeutic procedures requiring general anesthesia and rapid recovery; and (3) growing concern about long-term effect of general anesthesia on the brain and its functions, particularly POCD in the elderly and accelerated neuronal death in fetal development. Basic research during the last two decades has revealed a great deal about both mechanisms of general anesthesia and likely mechanisms of anesthetic toxicity. This knowledge is now being exploited in research projects aimed at meeting some of the clinical challenges ahead. Anesthetics such as xenon, which possess neuroprotective activity, are being reevaluated in clinical trials. It should be known soon whether benefit to patients at high risk for brain dysfunction after surgery and anesthesia will justify the high cost of xenon. Mechanism-based drug design has resulted in development of fospropofol, a water-soluble prodrug that eliminates the risk of devastating toxicity associated with long-term propofol infusion. Related strategies have been applied in development of two new etomidate derivatives. MOC-etomidate was developed based on a pharmacokinetic strategy, providing rapid metabolism by nonspecific esterases that promises to both reduce the duration of adrenal toxicity and provide more predictable/reliable recovery from general anesthesia. Carboetomidate uses a pharmacodynamic strategy to selectively eliminate etomidate toxicity while retaining etomidate's beneficial clinical features. Finally, the need for improved general anesthetics has fostered a search for new drugs. This high-risk approach may eventually lead to the discovery of entirely new classes of general anesthetics that may provide additional benefits to patients.

REFERENCES

1. Campbell PR. Population projections for states by age, sex, race, and Hispanic origin: 1995 to 2025. Washington, DC: U.S. Government Printing Office; 1996. (U.S. Bureau of the Census, Population Division, PPL-47, 90 pages).
2. Russo CA, Owens P, Steiner C, et al. Ambulatory surgery in U.S. hospitals, 2003. Rockville (MD): Agency for Healthcare Research and Quality; 2007. (HCUP Fact Book No. 9. AHRQ Publication No. 07-0007, 64 pages).
3. Alkire MT, Hudetz AG, Tononi G. Consciousness and anesthesia. Science 2008; 322:876.

4. Franks NP. General anaesthesia: from molecular targets to neuronal pathways of sleep and arousal. Nat Rev Neurosci 2008;9:370.
5. Franks NP, Lieb WR. Do general anaesthetics act by competitive binding to specific receptors? Nature 1984;310:599.
6. Forman SA, Miller KW, Yellen G. A discrete site for general anesthetics on a post-synaptic receptor. Mol Pharmacol 1995;48:574.
7. Mihic SJ, Ye Q, Wick MJ, et al. Sites of alcohol and volatile anaesthetic action on GABA(A) and glycine receptors. Nature 1997;389:385.
8. Franks NP, Honore E. The TREK K2P channels and their role in general anaesthesia and neuroprotection. Trends Pharmacol Sci 2004;25:601.
9. Solt K, Forman SA. Correlating the clinical actions and molecular mechanisms of general anesthetics. Curr Opin Anaesthesiol 2007;20:300.
10. Grasshoff C, Drexler B, Rudolph U, et al. Anaesthetic drugs: linking molecular actions to clinical effects. Curr Pharm Des 2006;12:3665.
11. Campagna JA, Miller KW, Forman SA. Mechanisms of actions of inhaled anesthetics. N Engl J Med 2003;348:2110.
12. Pratt MB, Husain SS, Miller KW, et al. Identification of sites of incorporation in the nicotinic acetylcholine receptor of a photoactivatible general anesthetic. J Biol Chem 2000;275:29441.
13. Li GD, Chiara DC, Sawyer GW, et al. Identification of a $GABA_A$ receptor anesthetic binding site at subunit interfaces by photolabeling with an etomidate analog. J Neurosci 2006;26:11599.
14. Stewart DS, Desai R, Cheng Q, et al. Tryptophan mutations at azi-etomidate photo-incorporation sites on α1 or β2 subunits enhance GABAA receptor gating and reduce etomidate modulation. Mol Pharmacol 2008;74:1687.
15. Jurd R, Arras M, Lambert S, et al. General anesthetic actions in vivo strongly attenuated by a point mutation in the GABA(A) receptor beta3 subunit. FASEB J 2003;17:250.
16. Reynolds DS, Rosahl TW, Cirone J, et al. Sedation and anesthesia mediated by distinct GABA(A) receptor isoforms. J Neurosci 2003;23:8608.
17. Linden AM, Sandu C, Aller MI, et al. TASK-3 knockout mice exhibit exaggerated nocturnal activity, impairments in cognitive functions, and reduced sensitivity to inhalation anesthetics. J Pharmacol Exp Ther 2007;323:924.
18. Sato Y, Kobayashi E, Murayama T, et al. Effect of N-methyl-D-aspartate receptor epsilon1 subunit gene disruption of the action of general anesthetic drugs in mice. Anesthesiology 2005;102:557.
19. Petrenko AB, Yamakura T, Kohno T, et al. Reduced immobilizing properties of isoflurane and nitrous oxide in mutant mice lacking the N-methyl-D-aspartate receptor GluR(epsilon)1 subunit are caused by the secondary effects of gene knockout. Anesth Analg 2010;110:461.
20. Nagele P, Metz LB, Crowder CM. Nitrous oxide (N(2)O) requires the N-methyl-D-aspartate receptor for its action in *Caenorhabditis elegans*. Proc Natl Acad Sci U S A 2004;101:8791.
21. Nagele P, Metz LB, Crowder CM. Xenon acts by inhibition of non-N-methyl-D-aspartate receptor-mediated glutamatergic neurotransmission in *Caenorhabditis elegans*. Anesthesiology 2005;103:508.
22. Wagner RL, White PF, Kan PB, et al. Inhibition of adrenal steroidogenesis by the anesthetic etomidate. N Engl J Med 1984;310:1415.
23. Corbett SM, Montoya ID, Moore FA. Propofol-related infusion syndrome in intensive care patients. Pharmacotherapy 2008;28:250.
24. Trapp S, Aller MI, Wisden W, et al. A role for TASK-1 (KCNK3) channels in the chemosensory control of breathing. J Neurosci 2008;28:8844.

25. Cotten JF, Keshavaprasad B, Laster MJ, et al. The ventilatory stimulant doxapram inhibits TASK tandem pore (K2P) potassium channel function but does not affect minimum alveolar anesthetic concentration. Anesth Analg 2006; 102:779.

26. Paris A, Philipp M, Tonner PH, et al. Activation of alpha 2B-adrenoceptors mediates the cardiovascular effects of etomidate. Anesthesiology 2003;99: 889.

27. Patel S, Wohlfeil ER, Rademacher DJ, et al. The general anesthetic propofol increases brain N-arachidonylethanolamine (anandamide) content and inhibits fatty acid amide hydrolase. Br J Pharmacol 2003;139:1005.

28. Perouansky M, Hemmings HC Jr. Neurotoxicity of general anesthetics: cause for concern? Anesthesiology 2009;111:1365.

29. Newman S, Stygall J, Hirani S, et al. Postoperative cognitive dysfunction after noncardiac surgery: a systematic review. Anesthesiology 2007;106:572.

30. Selnes OA, Grega MA, Bailey MM, et al. Cognition 6 years after surgical or medical therapy for coronary artery disease. Ann Neurol 2008;63:581.

31. Lee TA, Wolozin B, Weiss KB, et al. Assessment of the emergence of Alzheimer's disease following coronary artery bypass graft surgery or percutaneous transluminal coronary angioplasty. J Alzheimers Dis 2005;7:319.

32. Selnes OA, McKhann GM. Neurocognitive complications after coronary artery bypass surgery. Ann Neurol 2005;57:615.

33. Bianchi SL, Tran T, Liu C, et al. Brain and behavior changes in 12-month-old Tg2576 and nontransgenic mice exposed to anesthetics. Neurobiol Aging 2008;29:1002.

34. Culley DJ, Baxter MG, Yukhananov R, et al. Long-term impairment of acquisition of a spatial memory task following isoflurane-nitrous oxide anesthesia in rats. Anesthesiology 2004;100:309.

35. Rasmussen LS, Johnson T, Kuipers HM, et al. Does anaesthesia cause postoperative cognitive dysfunction? A randomised study of regional versus general anaesthesia in 438 elderly patients. Acta Anaesthesiol Scand 2003;47:260.

36. Eckenhoff RG, Johansson JS, Wei H, et al. Inhaled anesthetic enhancement of amyloid-beta oligomerization and cytotoxicity. Anesthesiology 2004;101:703.

37. Wan Y, Xu J, Ma D, et al. Postoperative impairment of cognitive function in rats: a possible role for cytokine-mediated inflammation in the hippocampus. Anesthesiology 2007;106:436.

38. McDonagh DL, Mathew JP, White WD, et al. Cognitive function after major noncardiac surgery, apolipoprotein E4 genotype, and biomarkers of brain injury. Anesthesiology 2010;112:852.

39. Istaphanous GK, Loepke AW. General anesthetics and the developing brain. Curr Opin Anaesthesiol 2009;22:368.

40. Loepke AW, Soriano SG. An assessment of the effects of general anesthetics on developing brain structure and neurocognitive function. Anesth Analg 2008;106: 1681.

41. Ikonomidou C, Bosch F, Miksa M, et al. Blockade of NMDA receptors and apoptotic neurodegeneration in the developing brain. Science 1999;283:70.

42. Ikonomidou C, Bittigau P, Ishimaru MJ, et al. Ethanol-induced apoptotic neurodegeneration and fetal alcohol syndrome. Science 2000;287:1056.

43. Lynch C 3rd, Baum J, Tenbrinck R. Xenon anesthesia. Anesthesiology 2000;92: 865.

44. Wilhelm S, Ma D, Maze M, et al. Effects of xenon on in vitro and in vivo models of neuronal injury. Anesthesiology 2002;96:1485.

45. Ma D, Yang H, Lynch J, et al. Xenon attenuates cardiopulmonary bypass-induced neurologic and neurocognitive dysfunction in the rat. Anesthesiology 2003;98:690.

46. Coburn M, Maze M, Franks NP. The neuroprotective effects of xenon and helium in an in vitro model of traumatic brain injury. Crit Care Med 2008;36:588.

47. Ma D, Williamson P, Januszewski A, et al. Xenon mitigates isoflurane-induced neuronal apoptosis in the developing rodent brain. Anesthesiology 2007;106:746.

48. Dickinson R, Peterson BK, Banks P, et al. Competitive inhibition at the glycine site of the N-methyl-D-aspartate receptor by the anesthetics xenon and isoflurane: evidence from molecular modeling and electrophysiology. Anesthesiology 2007;107:756.

49. Coburn M, Baumert JH, Roertgen D, et al. Emergence and early cognitive function in the elderly after xenon or desflurane anaesthesia: a double-blinded randomized controlled trial. Br J Anaesth 2007;98:756.

50. Hocker J, Stapelfeldt C, Leiendecker J, et al. Postoperative neurocognitive dysfunction in elderly patients after xenon versus propofol anesthesia for major noncardiac surgery: a double-blinded randomized controlled pilot study. Anesthesiology 2009;110:1068.

51. Loetscher PD, Rossaint J, Rossaint R, et al. Argon: neuroprotection in in vitro models of cerebral ischemia and traumatic brain injury. Crit Care 2009;13:R206.

52. Cooke A, Anderson A, Buchanan K, et al. Water-soluble propofol analogues with intravenous anaesthetic activity. Bioorg Med Chem Lett 2001;11:927.

53. Struys MM, Fechner J, Schuttler J, et al. Requested retraction of six studies on the PK/PD and tolerability of fospropofol. Anesth Analg 2010;110:1240.

54. Cotten JF, Husain SS, Forman SA, et al. Methoxycarbonyl-etomidate: a novel rapidly metabolized and ultra-short-acting etomidate analogue that does not produce prolonged adrenocortical suppression. Anesthesiology 2009;111:240.

55. Cotten JF, Forman SA, Laha JK, et al. Carboetomidate: a pyrrole analog of etomidate designed not to suppress adrenocortical function. Anesthesiology 2010; 112:637.

56. Liu R, Loll PJ, Eckenhoff RG. Structural basis for high-affinity volatile anesthetic binding in a natural 4-helix bundle protein. FASEB J 2005;19:567.

57. Vedula LS, Brannigan G, Economou NJ, et al. A unitary anesthetic binding site at high resolution. J Biol Chem 2009;284:24176.

58. Butts CA, Xi J, Brannigan G, et al. Identification of a fluorescent general anesthetic, 1-aminoanthracene. Proc Natl Acad Sci U S A 2009;106:6501.

59. Lea WA, Xi J, Jadhav A, et al. A high-throughput approach for identification of novel general anesthetics. PLoS One 2009;4:e7150.

Index

Note: Page numbers of article titles are in **boldface** type.

A

Abdominal laparoscopic surgery, efficacy of intravenous acetaminophen for acute pain after, 623–624

Acetaminophen, intravenous, **619–645**
  clinical efficacy in adults, 623–625, 626–634
    for fever, 624–625
    for postoperative pain, 623–624
    published randomized controlled trials, 626–634
  clinical efficacy in pediatric patients, 625, 635. 636–637
    published randomized controlled trials, 636–637
  clinical tolerability and safety, 635, 638
  pharmacokinetic and pharmacodynamic properties, 621–622

Acute pain, anesthesia in patients on buprenorphine maintenance, 615–616
  intravenous acetaminophen for, **619–645**
    clinical efficacy in adults, 623–625, 626–634
      after abdominal laparoscopic surgery, 623–624
      after total hip or knee arthroplasty, 623

Addiction, opioid, anesthesia for patients on buprenorphine for, **611–617**

ADP receptor antagonists, use in the perioperative period, 672

Adrenergic uptake inhibitors, in tramadol and tapentadol, **647–666**

Alpha-2 agonists, dexmedetomidine, **709–722**

Alternative medicine, herbal medications, use in the perioperative period, 673–675

Analgesia, buprenorphine for postoperative, **601–609**
  in patients on preoperative buprenorphine, 604–605
  intravenous acetaminophen, **619–645**
  patient-controlled, current and developing methods, **587–599**
    characteristics of specific opioids used for, 590–592
    intravenous, use for postoperative analgesia, 588–590
    systemic, advances in, 592–594
  tramadol and tapentadol, **647–666**

Anesthesia, for patients on buprenorphine, **611–617**
  general, molecular approaches to improving, **761–771**
  intravenous regional, dexmedetomidine as adjunct for, **709–722**

Anesthesiology, demographics and practice trends affecting, 761–762

Animal studies, dexmedetomidine, 711–712

Anti-inflammatory effects, of statins in the perioperative period, 741

Anticoagulants, new, use in the perioperative setting, **667–679**
  direct thrombin inhibitors, 670–671
  Factor Xa inhibitors, 668–670
  herbal medications and dietary supplements, 673–675
  monitoring, reversal and continuation through the perioperative period, 676–677
  new antiplatelet agents, 671–673

Anesthesiology Clin 28 (2010) 773–781
doi:10.1016/S1932-2275(10)00107-2
1932-2275/10/$ – see front matter © 2010 Elsevier Inc. All rights reserved.

United States Postal Service

Statement of Ownership, Management, and Circulation
(All Periodicals Publications Except Requestor Publications)

1. Publication Title	2. Publication Number	3. Filing Date
Anesthesiology Clinics	0 0 0 - 2 7 7	9/15/10

4. Issue Frequency	5. Number of Issues Published Annually	6. Annual Subscription Price
Mar, Jun, Sep, Dec	4	$268.00

7. Complete Mailing Address of Known Office of Publication (Not printer) (Street, city, county, state, and ZIP+4®)

Elsevier Inc.
360 Park Avenue South
New York, NY 10010-1710

Contact Person
Stephen Bushing

Telephone (Include area code)
215-239-3688

8. Complete Mailing Address of Headquarters or General Business Office of Publisher (Not printer)

Elsevier Inc., 360 Park Avenue South, New York, NY 10010-1710

9. Full Names and Complete Mailing Addresses of Publisher, Editor, and Managing Editor (Do not leave blank)

Publisher (Name and complete mailing address)

Kim Murphy, Elsevier, Inc., 1600 John F. Kennedy Blvd. Suite 1800, Philadelphia, PA 19103-2899

Editor (Name and complete mailing address)

Rachel Glover, Elsevier, Inc., 1600 John F. Kennedy Blvd. Suite 1800, Philadelphia, PA 19103-2899

Managing Editor (Name and complete mailing address)

Catherine Bewick, Elsevier, Inc., 1600 John F. Kennedy Blvd. Suite 1800, Philadelphia, PA 19103-2899

10. Owner (Do not leave blank. If the publication is owned by a corporation, give the name and address of the corporation immediately followed by the names and addresses of all stockholders owning or holding 1 percent or more of the total amount of stock. If not owned by a corporation, give the names and addresses of the individual owners. If owned by a partnership or other unincorporated firm, give its name and address as well as those of each individual owner. If the publication is published by a nonprofit organization, give its name and address.)

Full Name	Complete Mailing Address
Wholly owned subsidiary of	4520 East-West Highway
Reed/Elsevier, US holdings	Bethesda, MD 20814

11. Known Bondholders, Mortgagees, and Other Security Holders Owning or Holding 1 Percent or More of Total Amount of Bonds, Mortgages, or Other Securities. If none, check box ☐ None

Full Name	Complete Mailing Address
N/A	

12. Tax Status (For completion by nonprofit organizations authorized to mail at nonprofit rates) (Check one)
The purpose, function, and nonprofit status of this organization and the exempt status for federal income tax purposes:
☐ Has Not Changed During Preceding 12 Months
☐ Has Changed During Preceding 12 Months (Publisher must submit explanation of change with this statement)

PS Form 3526, September 2007 (Page 1 of 3 (Instructions Page 3)) PSN 7530-01-000-9931 PRIVACY NOTICE: See our Privacy policy in www.usps.com

---

13. Publication Title	14. Issue Date for Circulation Data Below
Anesthesiology Clinics	June 2010

15. Extent and Nature of Circulation			Average No. Copies Each Issue During Preceding 12 Months	No. Copies of Single Issue Published Nearest to Filing Date
a. Total Number of Copies (Net press run)			1711	1637
b. Paid Circulation (By Mail and Outside the Mail)	(1)	Mailed Outside-County Paid Subscriptions Stated on PS Form 3541. (Include paid distribution above nominal rate, advertiser's proof copies, and exchange copies)	585	515
	(2)	Mailed In-County Paid Subscriptions Stated on PS Form 3541 (Include paid distribution above nominal rate, advertiser's proof copies, and exchange copies)		
	(3)	Paid Distribution Outside the Mails Including Sales Through Dealers and Carriers, Street Vendors, Counter Sales, and Other Paid Distribution Outside USPS®	426	365
	(4)	Paid Distribution by Other Classes Mailed Through the USPS (e.g. First-Class Mail®)		
c. Total Paid Distribution (Sum of 15b (1), (2), (3), and (4))		▶	1011	880
d. Free or Nominal Rate Distribution (By Mail and Outside the Mail)	(1)	Free or Nominal Rate Outside-County Copies Included on PS Form 3541	123	106
	(2)	Free or Nominal Rate In-County Copies Included on PS Form 3541		
	(3)	Free or Nominal Rate Copies Mailed at Other Classes Through the USPS (e.g. First-Class Mail)		
	(4)	Free or Nominal Rate Distribution Outside the Mail (Carriers or other means)		
e. Total Free or Nominal Rate Distribution (Sum of 15d (1), (2), (3) and (4)		▶	123	106
f. Total Distribution (Sum of 15c and 15e)		▶	1134	986
g. Copies not Distributed (See instructions to publishers #4 (page #3))		▶	577	651
h. Total (Sum of 15f and g)		▶	1711	1637
i. Percent Paid (15c divided by 15f times 100)			89.15%	89.25%

16. Publication of Statement of Ownership

If the publication is a general publication, publication of this statement is required. Will be printed in the December 2010 issue of this publication.   ☐ Publication not required

17. Signature and Title of Editor, Publisher, Business Manager, or Owner	Date
Stephen R. Bushing – Fulfillment/Inventory Specialist	September 15, 2010

Stephen R. Bushing – Fulfillment/Inventory Specialist

I certify that all information furnished on this form is true and complete. I understand that anyone who furnishes false or misleading information on this form or who omits material or information requested on the form may be subject to criminal sanctions (including fines and imprisonment) and/or civil sanctions (including civil penalties).

PS Form 3526, September 2007 (Page 2 of 3)

Moving?

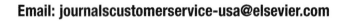

Make sure your subscription moves with you!

To notify us of your new address, find your **Clinics Account Number** (located on your mailing label above your name), and contact customer service at:

Email: journalscustomerservice-usa@elsevier.com

800-654-2452 (subscribers in the U.S. & Canada)
314-447-8871 (subscribers outside of the U.S. & Canada)

Fax number: 314-447-8029

Elsevier Health Sciences Division
Subscription Customer Service
3251 Riverport Lane
Maryland Heights, MO 63043

*To ensure uninterrupted delivery of your subscription, please notify us at least 4 weeks in advance of move.